T0139270

THROMBUS
AND STROKE

THROMBUS
AND STROKE

Edited by

Ajay K. Wakhloo
University of Massachusetts
Worcester, Massachusetts, USA

Matthew J. Gounis
University of Massachusetts
Worcester, Massachusetts, USA

Baruch B. Lieber
University of Miami
Coral Gables, Florida, USA

Robert A. Mericle
Vanderbilt University Medical Center
Nashville, Tennessee, USA

Italo Linfante
University of Massachusetts
Worcester, Massachusetts, USA

informa
healthcare

New York   London

Informa Healthcare U.S.A. Inc.
52 Vanderbilt Avenue
New York, NY 10017

© 2008 by Informa Healthcare U.S.A. Inc.
Informa Healthcare is an Informa business

No claim to original U.S. Government works
Printed in the United States of America on acid-free paper
10 9 8 7 6 5 4 3 2

International Standard Book Number-10: 0849341965(Hardcover)
International Standard Book Number-13: 9780849341960(Hardcover)

Library of Congress Cataloging-in-Publication Data

Thrombus and stroke/edited by Ajay K. Wakhloo ... [et al.].
   p.; cm.
   Includes bibliographical references and index.
   ISBN-13: 978-0-8493-4196-0 (hardcover : alk. paper)
   ISBN-10: 0-8493-4196-5 (hardcover : alk. paper)
   1. Thrombosis. 2. Cerebrovascular disesase--Treatment. I. Wakhloo, Ajay K.
   [DNLM: 1. Stroke--etiology. 2. Stroke--prevention & control. 3. Anticoagulants--
   therapeutic use. 4. Disease Models, Animal. 5. Thrombosis--physiopathology.
   6. Thrombosis--therapy. WL 355 T5318 2008]
RC694.3.T49 2008
616.1'35--dc22   2008015959

For Corporate Sales and Reprint Permissions call 212-520-2700 or write to:
Sales Department, 52 Vanderbilt Avenue, 16th floor, New York, NY 10017.

Visit the Informa Web site at
www.informa.com

and the Informa Healthcare Web site at

Preface

Stroke is no longer an untreatable or unpreventable condition. The management of stroke is changing rapidly as new developments appear for acute treatments, rehabilitation, and secondary prevention. In particular, it has been clearly demonstrated that patients with acute stroke need rapid assessment at the hospital following the onset of symptoms to be eventually treated with intravenous, intraarterial, or combination reperfusion therapy. Admission of stroke patients to specialized Stroke Units, with physicians specifically trained to treat stroke, improves their outcome. Hopefully in the near future, Stroke Units will be present not only in tertiary care centers but also in community hospitals.

With regard to primary and secondary stroke prevention, many potential candidates for anticoagulation still fail to receive appropriate treatment. To achieve effective prevention of stroke, more efforts should be spent on education to increase the number of treated subjects. Nevertheless, the widespread use of antiplatelet and cholesterol-lowering agents as well as the aggressive management of risk factors are shown to be effective in preventing stroke and improving outcomes. Epidemiological studies suggest that reducing the prevalence or shifting the distribution of risk factors across the entire population can be expected to reduce significantly the incidence of stroke, as is the case with coronary heart disease.

Further advances in stroke treatment will include combination therapies. The successful design of future drug therapies will result from a more complete understanding of not only the activity of these agents on platelet function and the coagulation cascade but also of their effects on the endothelium and within the brain parenchyma.

Why have we chosen to launch this publication when so many other publications on cerebrovascular disease and stroke are readily available?

The concept behind this volume is to integrate the basic science of clot formation and thrombolysis into the daily clinical practice of acute stroke treatment.

The first part of the volume provides an overview of how a clot forms, giving a brief review of the coagulation cascade at a cellular level and the interaction between clot formation/breakup and the flowing blood. Subsequently, research stroke models are evaluated for their use in basic and translational research. A chapter on assessment of thrombogenicity of vascular implants such as stents and grafts follows that we thought may be of use for the development of future implantable devices for stroke treatment.

The clinical implications and importance of the subject as it relates to stroke are then reviewed in the second part of the book. The latest methods of imaging stroke are surveyed. A chapter on immediate and chronic intervention in stroke follows. The most recent developments in endovascular treatments of ischemic stroke are summarized in the next chapter followed by a discourse on neuroprotection. Finally, the last chapter discusses the multimodality approach to acute stroke treatment.

We have on our panel a group of specialists who have through their dedicated efforts brought in the latest information about their subspecialty. We hope you will enjoy reading this inaugural issue. We also welcome your comments and suggestions to create an open forum for further discussion.

This book is being targeted at both basic scientists and clinicians who require a review of this subject, without the detailed descriptions found in other texts. This volume will allow the reader to formulate a basic understanding of what a clot is, how it forms, the clinical aspect of the problem, and the latest available treatment options in acute stroke.

We would like to thank all of the contributors involved in the production of this volume. Our special thanks go to the editors at Informa Healthcare, specifically to Dana Bigelow, the book development manager, Brian Kearns, the project editor, and Tintu Thomas, the typesetter. We also wish to thank Sandra Beberman, VP and managing director, US Books and Journals acquisitions, Chris DiBiase for the cover design, and Melissa King, our marketing manager. We would also like to express our thanks to Dagmar Schnau for editorial work in the early stages of the project.

I would like to thank Veronica, Albert, and Nathan for their love.

Ajay K. Wakhloo

Contents

Contributors

Danny Bluestein   State University of New York, Stony Brook, New York, U.S.A.

Marc Fisher   Department of Neurology, University of Massachusetts Medical School, Worcester, Massachusetts, U.S.A.

A.L. Frelinger   Center for Platelet Function Studies, University of Massachusetts Medical School, Worcester, Massachusetts, U.S.A.

Matthew J. Gounis   Department of Radiology, New England Center for Stroke Research, University of Massachusetts Medical School, Worcester, Massachusetts, U.S.A.

Jens O. Heidenreich   Case Western Reserve University and University Hospitals Health System, Cleveland, Ohio, U.S.A.

Michael A. Kurz   MA Consulting Services, Wayne, Pennsylvania, U.S.A.

Baruch Barry Lieber   University of Miami, Coral Gables, Florida, U.S.A.

Italo Linfante   Division of Neuroimaging and Intervention, Department of Radiology, University of Massachusetts Medical School, Worcester, Massachusetts, U.S.A.

Robert A. Mericle   Department of Neurosurgery, Vanderbilt University, Vanderbilt University Medical Center, Nashville, Tennessee, U.S.A.

Alan D. Michelson   Center for Platelet Function Studies, University of Massachusetts Medical School, Worcester, Massachusetts, U.S.A.

Chander Sadasivan   University of Miami, Coral Gables, Florida, U.S.A.

Kenneth M. Sicard   Department of Neurology, University of Massachusetts Medical School, Worcester, Massachusetts, U.S.A.

Sivaprasad Sukavaneshvar   Medical Device Evaluation Center, Salt Lake City, Utah, U.S.A.

Jeffrey L. Sunshine   Case Western Reserve University and University Hospitals Health System, Cleveland, Ohio, U.S.A.

Ajay K. Wakhloo   Department of Radiology, Neurology and Neurosurgery, University of Massachusetts Medical School, Worcester, Massachusetts, U.S.A.

Part 1

Basic Science

1 | Thrombus Formation

Alan D. Michelson and A.L. Frelinger, III

Center for Platelet Function Studies, University of Massachusetts Medical School, Worcester, Massachusetts, U.S.A.

INTRODUCTION

A blood clot that forms in response to injury, e.g., a cut, is a normal physiological process by which the body controls hemorrhage. Thrombosis is the formation of a blood clot in a pathological location, e.g., in response to the rupture of an atherosclerotic plaque in a cerebral artery. Thrombus formation can result in occlusion of blood flow with major clinical consequences, as discussed in detail elsewhere in this book. The purpose of this chapter is to discuss the basic science of thrombus formation. For simplicity, this chapter will be divided into two parts: (1) platelets and (2) the coagulation cascade. However, as discussed below, these two components of thrombus formation are an overlapping, intertwined continuum.

PLATELETS

Platelets are small cells (2.0–5.0 μm in diameter) of large importance in thrombus formation (1). In the venous system, low flow rates and stasis permit the accumulation of activated coagulation factors and the local generation of thrombin largely without the benefit of platelets (2). Although venous thrombi contain platelets, the dominant cellular components are trapped red cells. In the arterial circulation, higher flow rates limit fibrin formation by washing out soluble clotting factors (2). Hemostasis in the arterial circulation requires platelets to accelerate thrombin formation, to form a physical barrier, and to provide a base on which fibrin can accumulate. Hemostatic plugs and thrombi that form in the arterial circulation are therefore enriched in platelets and fibrin, giving them a different appearance from those formed in the venous circulation (2). This chapter will focus on the biological events underlying thrombus formation in the arterial circulation.

Platelet activation can be divided into three overlapping stages: initiation, extension, and perpetuation (Fig. 1). Initiation (Fig. 1A) can occur in more than one way (2). In the setting of trauma to the vessel wall, it may occur because circulating platelets are captured and then activated by exposed collagen and von Willebrand factor (vWF), forming a monolayer that supports thrombin generation and subsequent platelet aggregation (Fig. 2). Key to these events is the presence of receptors on the platelet surface that can bind to collagen (integrin $\alpha2\beta1$ and glycoprotein [GP] VI) and vWF (GPIbα and integrin αIIbβ3) and thereby initiate intracellular signaling (2). Platelet activation, particularly in thrombotic or inflammatory disorders, may also be initiated by thrombin, which activates platelets via G protein-coupled receptors (GPCRs) in the protease-activated receptor (PAR) family. Platelet activation may

A. Initiation (capture, adhesion, activation)

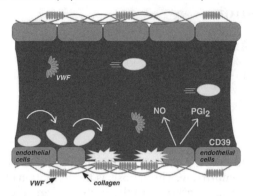

B. Extension (cohesion, secretion)

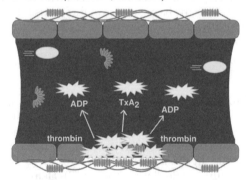

C. Perpetuation (stabilization)

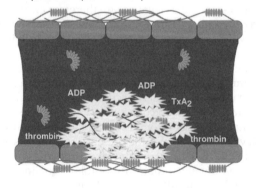

FIGURE 1 Steps in platelet plug formation. Prior to vascular injury, platelet activation is suppressed by endothelial cell-derived inhibitory factors. These include prostaglandin (PG) I_2 (prostacyclin), nitric oxide, and CD39, an ADPase on the surface of endothelial cells that can hydrolyze trace amounts of ADP that might otherwise cause inappropriate platelet activation. (*A*) Initiation. The development of the platelet plug is initiated by thrombin and by the collagen–vWF complex, which captures and activates moving platelets. Platelets adhere and spread, forming a monolayer. (*B*) Extension. The platelet plug is extended as additional platelets are activated via the release or secretion of thromboxane A_2 (TXA$_2$), ADP, and other platelet agonists, most of which are ligands for G protein-coupled receptors on the platelet surface. Activated platelets stick to each other via bridges formed by the binding of fibrinogen, fibrin, or vWF to activated αIIbβ3. (*C*) Perpetuation. Finally, close contacts between platelets in the growing hemostatic plug, along with a fibrin meshwork (shown in red), help to perpetuate and stabilize the platelet plug. *Source*: Reproduced with permission from Ref. (2). (See also color plate section.)

also occur because of the pathological activation of platelet FcγRIIA receptors, such as that occurs in some patients receiving heparin (3).

Extension (Fig. 1B) occurs when additional platelets are recruited and activated, resulting in platelet-to-platelet aggregation (Fig. 2) and accumulation on top of the initial monolayer (2). Thrombin can play an important role at this point,

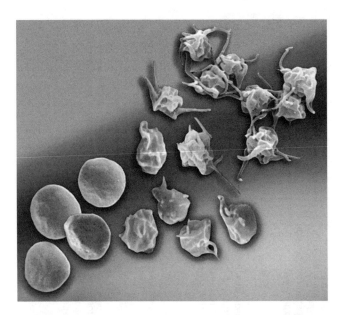

FIGURE 2 Platelet shape change and aggregation. Scanning electron micrographs of resting (*lower left*), partially activated (*lower middle*), and fully activated platelets (*upper right*), showing the accompanying shape changes, formation of filopodia and lamellipodia, and platelet aggregation. *Source*: Reproduced with permission from Ref. (2). (See also color plate section.)

as can secreted adenosine diphosphate (ADP) and released thromboxane A_2. Each of these agonists is able to activate phospholipase C in platelets, causing an increase in the cytosolic Ca^{2+} concentration (2). The receptors that mediate this response are members of the superfamily of GPCRs. The signals that they engender support the activation of integrin $\alpha IIb\beta 3$ (GPIIb-IIIa), making possible the cohesive interactions between platelets that are critical to the formation of the hemostatic plug (2).

Perpetuation (Fig. 1C) refers to the late events of platelet plug formation, when the intense, but often time-limited signals arising from GPCRs may have faded (2). These late events help to stabilize the platelet plug and prevent premature disaggregation. Such events typically occur after aggregation has begun and are facilitated by close contacts between platelets (2). Examples include outside-in signaling through integrins and signaling through receptor tyrosine kinases, including members of the Eph and Axl families that have membrane-bound ligands (Fig. 3).

Platelets localize, amplify, and sustain the coagulant response at the injury site (see below) and release procoagulant platelet-derived microparticles (4). Platelets also contain a variety of inflammatory modulators (e.g., CD40 ligand [CD40L] (5)) that are released on platelet activation (6).

Tests for the monitoring of antiplatelet therapy are shown in Table 1.

THE COAGULATION CASCADE

In 1964, two groups proposed a waterfall or cascade model of coagulation composed of a sequential series of steps in which activation of one clotting factor led to the activation of another, finally leading to a burst of thrombin generation (7, 8). Each clotting factor was believed to exist as a proenzyme that could be converted into an active

TABLE 1 An Alphabetical List of Currently Available Tests for the Monitoring of Antiplatelet Therapy

Name of Test	Principle	Advantages	Disadvantages	Frequency of Use
Aspirin Works®	Immunoassay of urinary 11-dehydrothromboxane B_2	Measures stable thromboxane metabolite	Indirect assay Not platelet-specific Renal function-dependent	Increasing use
Bleeding time	In vivo cessation of blood flow	Dependent upon COX-1 activity In vivo test Physiological POC	Insensitive Invasive Scarring High CV	Decreasing popularity
Flow Cytometry	Measurement of platelet glycoproteins and activation markers by fluorescence (e.g., VASP phosphorylation to monitor $P2Y_{12}$ inhibition)	Whole blood test Small blood volumes Wide variety of tests	Specialized operator Expensive	Widely used
HemoStatus® Device	Platelet procoagulant activity	Simple POC	Insensitive to aspirin and GPIb function	Used in surgery and cardiology
Ichor–Platelet-works®	Platelet counting pre- and post-activation	Rapid Simple POC Small blood volume	Indirect test measuring count after aggregation	Used in surgery and cardiology
Impact® cone-and-plate(let) analyzer	Quantification of high shear platelet adhesion/ aggregation onto surface	Small blood volume required High shear Rapid Simple Research (variable) and fixed versions available POC	Instrument not yet widely available.	Little widespread experience as only recently commercially available
Light Transmission Aggregometry (LTA)	Low shear platelet-to-platelet aggregation in response to classical agonists	Historical gold standard	Time consuming Sample preparation Expensive	Widely used in specialized labs

TABLE 1 (*Continued*)

Name of Test	Principle	Advantages	Disadvantages	Frequency of Use
PFA-100®	High shear platelet adhesion and aggregation during formation of a platelet plug	Whole blood test High shear Small blood volumes Simple Rapid POC	Inflexible vWF-dependent HCt-dependent Insensitive to clopidogrel	Widely used
Platelet Reactivity Index	Measurement of platelet aggregates in whole blood (modified Wu and Hoak method)	Simple Rapid Inexpensive	Requires blood counter Indirect test measuring count after aggregation	Little widespread experience
Serum Thromboxane B₂	Immunoassay	Dependent upon COX-1 activity	Prone to artefact Not platelet-specific	Widespread use
Thromboelastography (TEG® or ROTEM®)	Monitoring of rate and quality of clot formation	Global whole blood test POC	Measures clot properties only; largely platelet-independent unless platelet activators are used	Used in surgery and anesthesiology
VerifyNow®	Fully automated platelet aggregometer to measure antiplatelet therapy	Simple POC 3 test cartridges (aspirin, P2Y12 and GPIIb-IIIa)	Inflexible Cartridges can only be used for single purpose	Increasing use
Whole Blood Aggregometry	Monitors changes in impedance in response to classical agonists	Whole blood test	Older instruments require electrodes to be cleaned and recycled	Widely used in specialized labs although less than LTA

Abbreviations: COX-1, cyclooxygenase1; CV, coefficient of variation; GP, glycoprotein; HCt, hematocrit; LTA, light transmission aggregometry; PFA-100, platelet function analyzer 100; POC, point-of-care; VASP, vasodilator-stimulated phosphoprotein; vWF, von Willebrand factor.

Source: Reproduced with permission from Ref. (11).

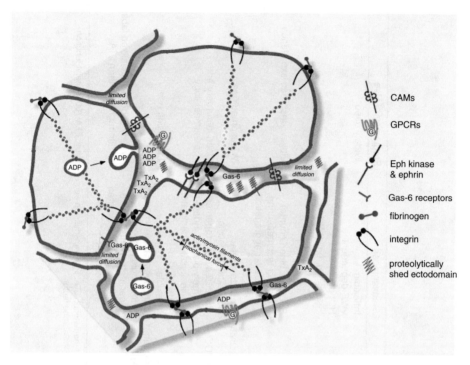

FIGURE 3 Contact-dependent and contact-facilitated events during thrombus formation. The onset of aggregation brings platelets into sufficiently close contact for integrins and other cell adhesion molecules to interact and for the activation of Eph receptor kinases by their cell surface ligands known as "ephrins." The space between platelets also provides a protected environment in which soluble agonists for G protein-coupled receptors (ADP, thrombin, and TXA$_2$) and receptor tyrosine kinases (Gas-6), and the proteolytically shed bioactive ectodomains of platelet surface proteins (CD40L) can accumulate. The mechanical forces generated by the contraction of actin/myosin filaments help to compress the space between platelets, improving contacts and possibly increasing the concentration of soluble agonists. *Abbreviations*: ADP, adenosine diphosphate; CAMs, cell adhesion molecules; Gas-6, growth-arrest specific gene 6; GPCRs, G protein-coupled receptors; TXA$_2$, thromboxane A$_2$. *Source*: Reproduced with permission from Ref. (2). (See also color plate section.)

enzyme (9). The original cascade models were subsequently modified to include the observation that some procoagulants were cofactors and did not possess enzymatic activity. The coagulation process is now often outlined in a Y-shaped scheme, with distinct intrinsic and extrinsic pathways initiated by factor XII (FXII) and FVIIa/tissue factor (TF), respectively, as outlined in Fig. 4. The pathways converge on a common pathway at the level of the FXa/FVa (prothrombinase) complex (9). The coagulation complexes require phospholipid and calcium for their activity.

As summarized by Hoffman and Monroe (9), subsequent findings have updated this view of the coagulation cascade. The demonstration that the FVIIa/TF complex activated not only FX but also FIX (10) suggested that the pathways were linked. Other important observations led to the conclusion that activity of the FVIIa/TF complex is the major initiating event in hemostasis in vivo (9). It was recognized from the earliest studies of coagulation that cells were important participants in the coagulation process. Normal hemostasis is not possible in the absence

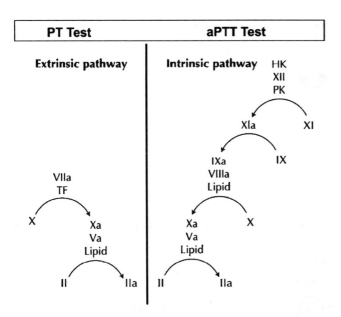

FIGURE 4 The extrinsic and intrinsic pathways in the cascade model of coagulation. These two pathways are conceived as each leading to the formation of the factor Xa/Va complex, which generates thrombin. Lipid indicates that the reaction requires a phospholipid surface. The extrinsic and intrinsic pathways are assayed clinically using the prothrombin time (PT) and activated partial thromboplastin time (aPTT), respectively. HK, high molecular weight kininogen; PK, prekallikrein. *Source*: Reproduced with permission from Ref. (9).

of platelets (9). In addition, TF is an integral membrane protein and thus its activity is normally associated with cells. Hoffman and Monroe (9) have therefore proposed a cell-based model of coagulation, as outlined below.

Step 1: Initiation of Coagulation on TF-Bearing Cells (9)
The goal of hemostasis is to produce a platelet and fibrin plug to seal a site of injury or rupture in the blood vessel wall. This process is initiated when TF-bearing cells are exposed to blood at a site of injury. TF is a transmembrane protein that acts as a receptor and cofactor for FVII.

Once bound to TF, zymogen FVII is rapidly converted into FVIIa. The resulting FVIIa/TF complex catalyzes activation of FX and activation of FIX. The factors Xa and IXa formed on the TF-bearing cells have distinct and separate functions in initiating blood coagulation. The FXa formed on the TF-bearing cell interacts with its cofactor Va to form prothrombinase complexes and generates a small amount of thrombin on the TF-bearing cells (Fig. 5A). By contrast, the FIXa activated by FVIIa/TF does not act on the TF-bearing cell and does not play a significant role in the initiation phase of coagulation. If an injury has occurred and platelets have adhered near the site of the TF-bearing cells, the FIXa can diffuse to the surface of nearby activated platelets. It can then bind to a specific platelet surface receptor, interact with its cofactor, FVIIIa, and activate FX directly on the platelet surface. Most of the coagulation factors can leave the vasculature and their activation peptides are found in the lymph. It is likely, therefore, that most (extravascular) TF is bound to FVIIa even in the absence of an

A

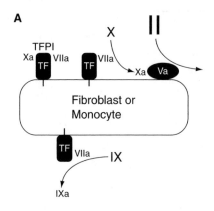

B

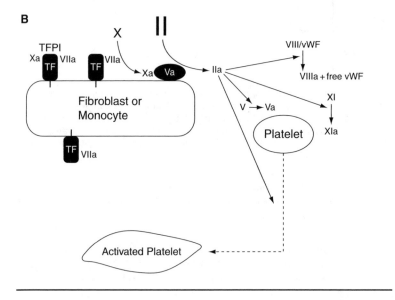

C

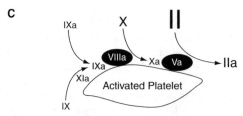

FIGURE 5 Steps in a cell-based model of coagulation. (*A*) Initiation occurs on the TF-bearing cell as activated FX combines with its cofactor, FVa, to activate small amounts of thrombin. (*B*) The small amount of thrombin generated on the TF-bearing cell amplifies the procoagulant response by activating cofactors, FXI, and platelets. (*C*) The large burst of thrombin required for effective hemostasis is formed on the platelet surface during the propagation phase. *Source*: Reproduced with permission from Ref. (9).

injury, and that low levels of FIXa, FXa, and thrombin are produced on TF-bearing cells at all times. This process is kept separated from key components of hemostasis by an intact vessel wall, however. The very large components of the coagulation process are platelets and FVIII bound to multimeric vWF. These components normally come into contact with the extravascular compartment only when an injury disrupts the vessel wall. Platelets and FVIII/vWF then leave the vascular space and adhere to collagen and other matrix components at the site of injury.

Step 2: Amplification of the Procoagulant Signal by Thrombin Generated on the TF-bearing Cell (9)

Binding of platelets to collagen or by way of vWF leads to partial platelet activation. The coagulation process is most effectively initiated, however, when enough thrombin is generated on or near the TF-bearing cells to trigger full activation of platelets and activation of coagulation cofactors on the platelet surface in the amplification step (Fig. 5B). Although this amount of thrombin may not be sufficient to clot fibrinogen, it is sufficient to initiate events that prime the clotting system for a subsequent burst of platelet surface thrombin generation. Experiments using a cell-based model have shown that minute amounts of thrombin are formed in the vicinity of TF-bearing cells exposed to plasma concentrations of procoagulants, even in the absence of platelets. The small amounts of FVa required for prothrombinase assembly on TF-bearing cells are activated by FXa or by noncoagulation proteases produced by the cells or are released from platelet that adhere nearby. The small amounts of thrombin generated on the TF-bearing cells are responsible for (a) activating platelets, (b) activating FV, (c) activating FVIII and dissociating FVIII from vWF, and (d) activating FXI. The activity of the FXa formed by the FVIIa/TF complex is restricted to the TF-bearing cell, because FXa that dissociates from the cell surface is rapidly inhibited by tissue factor pathway inhibitor or antithrombin in the fluid phase. In contrast to FXa, FIXa can diffuse to adjacent platelet surfaces because it is not inhibited by tissue factor pathway inhibitor and is inhibited much more slowly by antithrombin than is FXa.

Step 3: Propagation of Thrombin Generation on the Platelet Surface (9)

Platelets play a major role in localizing clotting reactions to the site of injury because they adhere and aggregate at the sites of injury where TF is also exposed. They provide the primary surface for generation of the burst of thrombin needed for effective hemostasis during the propagation phase of coagulation (Fig. 5C). Platelet localization and activation are mediated by vWF, thrombin, platelet receptors, and vessel wall components, such as collagen (see the section on Platelets). Once platelets are activated, the cofactors Va and VIIIa are rapidly localized on the platelet surface. As noted above, the FIXa formed by the FVIIa/TF complex can diffuse through the fluid phase and also bind to the surface of activated platelets. Likewise, FXI also binds to platelet surfaces and is activated by the priming amount of thrombin, bypassing the need for FXIIa. The platelet-bound FXIa can activate more FIX to IXa. Once the platelet tenase complex is assembled, FX from the plasma is activated to FXa on the platelet surface. FXa then associates with FVa to support a burst of thrombin generation of sufficient magnitude to produce a stable fibrin clot. The large amount of thrombin generated on the platelet surface is responsible for stabilizing the hemostatic clot in more ways than just promoting fibrin polymerization. In fact, most of the thrombin generated during the hemostatic process is produced after the initial fibrin

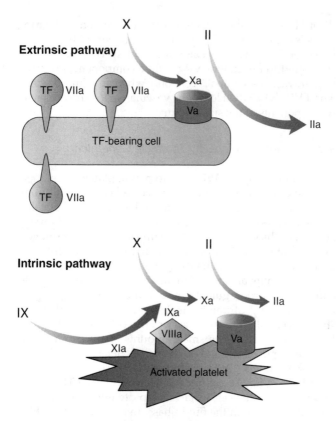

FIGURE 6 The extrinsic and intrinsic pathways in the cell-based model of coagulation. The role of the cell-based extrinsic pathway (*top*) is to act on the TF-bearing cell to generate the small amounts of thrombin (factor IIa) involved in initiating coagulation. The role of the cell-based intrinsic pathway (*bottom*) is to act on the platelet surface to generate the burst of thrombin needed to form a stable fibrin clot. TF, tissue factor. *Source*: Figure reproduced with permission from Ref. (9).

clot is formed. The platelet-produced thrombin also stabilizes the clot by (a) activating FXIII, (b) activating thrombin-activatable fibrinolysis inhibitor, (c) cleaving the platelet PAR-4 receptor, and (d) being incorporated into the structure of the clot.

The roles of the extrinsic and intrinsic pathways in the cell-based model of coagulation are summarized in Fig. 6.

REFERENCES

1. Michelson AD. Platelets. 2nd ed. San Diego: Elsevier/Academic Press, 2007.
2. Brass LF, Stalker TJ, Zhu L, Woulfe DS. Signal transduction during platelet plug formation. In: Michelson AD, ed. Platelets. San Diego: Elsevier/Academic Press, 2007:319–346.
3. Chong BH. Heparin-induced thrombocytopenia. In: Michelson AD, ed. Platelets. San Diego: Elsevier/Academic Press, 2007:861–886.
4. Nieuwland R, Sturk A. Platelet-derived microparticles. In: Michelson AD, ed. Platelets. San Diego: Elsevier/Academic Press, 2007:403–413.
5. Furman MI, Krueger LA, Linden MD, et al. Release of soluble CD40L from platelets is regulated by glycoprotein IIb/IIIa and actin polymerization. J Am Coll Cardiol 2004; 43:2319–2325.

6. Bergmeier W, Wagner DD. Inflammation. In: Michelson AD, ed. Platelets. San Diego: Elsevier/Academic Press, 2007.
7. Macfarlane RG. An enzyme cascade in the blood clotting mechanism, and its function as a biological amplifier. Nature 1964; 202:498–499.
8. Davie EW, Ratnoff OD. Waterfall sequence for intrinsic blood clotting. Science 1964; 145:1310–1312.
9. Hoffman M, Monroe DM. Coagulation 2006: a modern view of hemostasis. Hematol Oncol Clin North Am 2007; 21:1–11.
10. Østerud B, Rapaport SI. Activation of factor IX by the reaction product of tissue factor and factor VII: additional pathway for initiating blood coagulation. Proc Natl Acad Sci USA 1977; 74:5260–5264.
11. Harrison P, Frelinger AL 3rd, Furman MI, Michelson AD. Measuring antiplatelet drug effects in the laboratory. Thromb Res 2007; 120(3):323–336.

2 Blood Flow and Thrombus Formation

Danny Bluestein[1], Baruch B. Lieber[2], and Chander Sadasivan[2]

[1]State University of New York, Stony Brook, New York, U.S.A.
[2]University of Miami, Coral Gables, Florida, U.S.A.

BLOOD RHEOLOGY

To analyze blood flow and stresses that develop in it, and its interaction with the blood constituents, blood is traditionally considered a continuously deformable continuum in motion. Using this approach, blood can be characterized as a Newtonian fluid (in which the fluid deforms linearly as a function of the stress imposed) or a non-Newtonian fluid (in which the fluid deforms nonlinearly as a function of the stress). The Newtonian behavior of blood flow is relevant to most of the larger arteries in the vasculature. However, blood possesses a unique non-Newtonian viscosity behavior, which becomes apparent when it flows through the smaller vessels, such as arterioles and capillaries. This behavior is also observed when blood flow forms vortical structures, as may be found in flow through cardiovascular prostheses or in cardiovascular disease processes such as stenoses and aneurysms (1). In analyzing other aspects of hemodynamics such as the apparent reduction of viscosity and the migratory tendency of blood cells in the smaller scale vessels (i.e., the microcirculation), blood may be treated as a suspension of cells in plasma.

The non-Newtonian behavior exhibited by whole blood is due to fibrinogen molecules on the surface of red blood cells (RBC) that cause them to stack together in the rouleaux formation. This phenomenon is most pronounced during pregnancy, under pathological conditions, and when a large number of fibrinogen molecules are present on RBC surfaces. Such aggregation of cells in arterioles and small arteries is responsible for blood's deviation from Newtonian behavior (1). From a mechanics point of view, this behavior is a combination of Bingham and pseudoplastic fluid characteristics. That is, it has a yield stress; however even above this yield stress, the shear stress to shear rate relationship is nonlinear (Fig. 1).

A well-accepted, heuristic non-Newtonian model of blood is the Casson model. This behavior is most apparent in shear rates that are below 20 s^{-1}, with the region $20–100 \text{ s}^{-1}$ being the transition region. Above a shear rate of 100 s^{-1} blood behaves as a Newtonian fluid. However, in the non-Newtonian range, the shear stress does not exceed the yield stress in the central core flow region, and the core is merely carried along by the fluid in the annular region. Thus, the central core has a flat velocity profile (plug flow), which is carried by the annular region surrounding it, sustaining the bulk of the shear stress (1).

As blood consists of various kinds of cells such as erythrocytes (RBC), white blood cells (WBC or leukocytes), and platelets (thrombocytes) suspended in plasma, there is often a need to analyze its rheological properties in relation to its nature and to its cell-suspension properties. RBCs outnumber the other cells and assume major

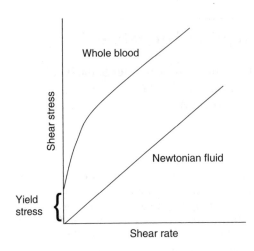

FIGURE 1   The non-Newtonian viscosity of blood.

rheological importance in addition to playing the vital role of carrying oxygen to all parts of the body because hemoglobin is contained within the RBC membrane. RBCs have a biconcave disk shape, approximately 7.2 μm in diameter and 2.2 μm thick. This shape represents an optimization between diffusion efficiency and mechanical strength, which enables RBCs to resist hemolysis (1). The percent volume concentration of RBCs in the whole blood is called the hematocrit, which normally ranges between 42% (for women) and 46% (for men). As expected for a suspension, the hematocrit value has an effect on the viscosity of blood.

There are two interrelated phenomena that occur when blood flows through narrow vessels such as arterioles. One is the tendency of RBCs to migrate toward the center of the flow channel, leaving a relatively cell-depleted layer of plasma (2). The other is the reduction of its apparent viscosity. Both phenomena were observed and reported first by Fahraeus and Lindqvist (2), subsequently supported and developed into the so-called marginal zone theory (3). The Fahraeus–Lindqvist effect predicts that the higher cell concentration in the central core, where the fluid flows faster, would make the concentration of cells appear to decrease while flowing through, creating an annular cell-depleted region around the core flow. When going down the scales of the vasculature, blood cell diameter is sufficiently close to the vessel diameter where blood may no longer be considered a continuum. Thus, thickness of the fluid layers is finite, which causes an apparent decrease in viscosity. This explains the amazing fluidity of blood when compared with true Newtonian fluids and enables it to overcome the inherent resistance offered by the microvasculature.

HEMODYNAMICS AND THEIR INTERACTION WITH BLOOD AND THE VESSEL WALL

One of the principal mechanisms leading to vessel narrowing (stenosis) is thrombus formation, which may be initiated by platelet activation. Shear rates and flow patterns (fluid dynamics factors), as well as a concentration of coagulation factors and platelet agonists (biological factors), modulate platelet function and may lead to platelet activation and aggregation (adhesion of platelets to each other in the presence of fibrinogen). Here we examine the flow-induced mechanisms leading to platelet activation in models of stenosed vessels.

Experimental and numerical methods were used to investigate and characterize the influence of the flow field on platelet activation. As it passes through pathological geometries, characteristic of arterial stenosis, a platelet is exposed to varying levels of shear stress. The cumulative effect of the shear stress level on the platelet and the duration of exposure determines whether it is brought beyond its activation threshold. Stress histories of individual platelets can be tracked within the flow field to locate the regions where activated platelets might be found and subsequently aggregate and/or adhere to the wall.

Numerous studies have shown that thrombi in narrowed arteries are rich in platelets. Although the role of platelets in hemostasis through their response to subendothelial damage by initiating the repair of vascular injuries is well documented, the mechanisms by which fluid flow stresses elicit similar responses in platelets, and the linkage between flow conditions and the potential level of shear activation, are still unclear. A quantitative depiction of the process by which fluid dynamics mechanisms lead to shear stress accumulation and, hence, platelet activation and aggregation would permit the formulation of an accountable model for platelet response under realistic flow conditions. Such models are essential for developing more potent therapeutic agents and effective preventive measures against platelet-mediated vessel occlusion.

CLINICAL PROBLEMS ASSOCIATED WITH ARTERIAL STENOSIS
Coronary Heart Disease
Arterial disease, characterized as stenosis by atherosclerotic plaque, is a leading cause of cardiovascular disease and a major healthcare problem in the Western world. Coronary heart disease (CHD) is the leading cause of death and accounts for almost one in four deaths in the United States, totaling about 500,000 deaths a year. It is the main cause of sudden and premature death and disability among American adults aged 35 years and older (4).

Mural thrombosis and embolization are frequently associated with arterial stenosis and play a central role in the development of unstable angina, myocardial infarction, and sudden ischemic death (5,6). Platelet aggregates were found to be larger and more frequent in coronary patients who died suddenly (7). Occlusions of more than 75% frequently induce occlusive thrombi (6). Further constriction occurs when platelet aggregates liberate the unopposed action of vasoconstrictors such as thromboxane A_2, serotonin, and thrombin. Eccentric coronary lesions are seen by angiography in 71% of patients with unstable angina (8). Platelet activation may occur (i) on exposure to abnormal flow patterns and high shear stresses during passage through a stenosis and (ii) in thrombus formation, which involves both platelet aggregation and fibrin formation. If the atherosclerotic plaque ruptures, coagulation is initiated and a thrombus rapidly forms, blocking the coronary artery, eventually leading to a heart attack and myocardial infarction (9). These observations correlate well with the clinical evidence that antiplatelet and fibrin-inhibiting medications are effective in preventing thrombosis (10).

Stroke
There are approximately 700,000 stroke cases annually in the United States with an estimated direct and indirect cost of $63 billion in 2007 (11). Stroke is the third largest

cause of death, ranking behind CHD and all forms of cancer combined. There are about 150,000 deaths attributed to stroke annually, and it is the leading cause of serious, long-term disability in the United States (11). Stroke can affect people of all ages, but the risk increases with age. Eighty-five percent of strokes are ischemic, with intracerebral and subarachnoid hemorrhages constituting the remainder of cases. The most common causes of ischemic stroke are cerebral artery thrombosis of a ruptured atherosclerotic plaque, cardioembolism, and small vessel occlusions (12,13). The classification of strokes into subtypes has largely followed the strategy set by the Trial of ORG 10172 in Acute Stroke Treatment (TOAST) investigators (12) although newer derivations (14,15) have been used to refine stroke etiology. Such classifications not only facilitate the proper management of patients or control over clinical trials but also serve to locate pathological flow mechanisms that may have originated any given stroke. Briefly, the TOAST classification categorizes strokes as due to large-artery atherosclerosis if brain imaging suggests >50% occlusion of a major brain artery or branch cortical artery with supporting clinical findings of cerebral cortical impairment or a history of transient ischemic attacks in the same vascular territory or carotid bruits (12,15). Strokes are classified as cardioembolic in origin if at least one cardiac source of an embolism such as bioprosthetic or mechanical heart valves (MHV), valvular disease, atrial fibrillation, endocarditis, left ventricular thrombus, myocardial infarction, or atrial septal aneurysms can be found. Lacunar strokes present with deep focal infarcts less than 1.5 cm in size with supporting clinical lacunar syndromes, whereas strokes due to unusual causes such as hypercoagulable states, hematologic disorders, or vasculopathies are classified as being of other determined etiology. Strokes that do not clearly fall into any of these classifications are categorized as being of undetermined etiology (12,15). Fig. 2 shows the distribution of ischemic stroke subtypes as per the TOAST criteria and based on data from the Stroke Data Bank of the National Institute of Neurological Disorders and Stroke (16,17) and a Rochester, Minnesota population-based study (18). It is to be noted that these percentages are based on US populations, and different populations may have varying degrees of atherothrombotic or cardioembolic

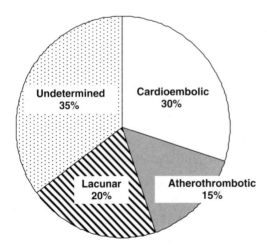

FIGURE 2 Approximate distributions of the subtypes of ischemic stroke. From the Stroke Data Bank (16,17) and a Minnesota population based study (18). Rare causes of stroke contribute another 2%–3%. The undetermined category is largely one of exclusion of the four other causes.

strokes (14). The TOAST criteria include emboli shed from atherosclerotic arteries as part of atherothrombotic strokes, and lacunar infarcts may be of embolic origin. The percentage of strokes purely due to emboli is thus difficult to ascertain. Studies involving patients with heart disease find that about 60% of strokes may be due to cardiac emboli, whereas co-existing atherosclerotic disease causes a large proportion of the remainder of strokes (15,19). Such studies note that atrial fibrillation causes 15% of ischemic strokes; presumably other abnormalities such as those mentioned above cause the remainder of embolisms. Studies on carotid artery stenoses show high rates of stroke in patients with asymptomatic stenosis of >75%, with increasing degrees of stenosis above this mark resulting in higher rates of stroke (19). High degrees of stenosis or plaque ruptures lead to atherothrombotic strokes by the same mechanisms mentioned above for CHD. The activation of platelets is involved in both embolus formation and thrombus formation (13).

PLATELETS' HEMOSTATIC RESPONSE

Platelets have long been regarded as the preeminent cell involved in physiologic hemostasis and pathologic thrombosis (10). In both hemostasis and thrombosis, von Willebrand factor (vWF) and platelets work together to affect the biologic response. Rheological factors mediate the binding of vWF to the platelet glycoprotein GPIb, with shear stress appearing to be equivalent to agonists such as ristocetin that evoke a similar response (20). Exposure to fluid shear stresses aggregates platelets irreversibly in the absence of any exogenous agonist, showing consistent "dose–" and time–response characteristics of equivalent chemical agonists (21).

On activation, platelets undergo dramatic morphological and biochemical changes, resulting in shape change (extrusion of pseudopods), aggregation, granule secretion, and clot retraction (22). When platelets are activated by flow (shear stress), increased binding of fibrinogen to platelets by way of the platelet glycoprotein GPIIb/IIIa occurs (23), leading to the secretion of procoagulant and self-stimulating substances from granules. Activated platelets then adhere to surfaces and aggregate. Aggregation is promoted by agonists secreted from the platelet α-granules (24,25) and by fibrinogen that binds to the platelet surface through GPIIb/IIIa (23).

Platelets also interact with other blood cells, enhancing the thrombotic state. Monocyte surface adhesive receptor Mac-1, bound to stimulated monocytes that express CD11b, binds coagulation factor X and activates the coagulation cascade (26). Thrombin is generated when factor Xa is assembled with cofactor Va on the surfaces of activated platelets expressing anionic phospholipids (27). The resulting prothrombinase complex cleaves the soluble fibrinogen into insoluble fibrin. The platelet α-granule-derived factor V (20% of its amount in blood) (28) dominates the prothrombinase complex and the rapid thrombin generation in the platelet-rich thrombus (29).

FLOW-INDUCED PLATELET ACTIVATION—"DOSE" AND TIME REVISITED

Under abnormal flow conditions, shear-induced platelet activation (SIPA) can cause both platelet aggregation and, through the provision of anionic phospholipid, thrombin generation. Platelet activation under tightly controlled flow shear stress has been investigated methodically in the past. Ramstack et al. (30) showed that platelet stimulation is a nonlinear phenomenon, where the extent of platelet trauma increases exponentially as a function of shear rate and time. The criteria for platelet activation under flow conditions have been established under constant bulk stress, for example in flow cytometers and cone-and-plate devices where the shear level was kept constant while measuring the time to reach activation. Constant stress experiments have established a threshold for platelet activation, forming the foundation for SIPA on a basic time-averaged blood flow model (31). Hellums et al. (32) compiled numerous experimental results in which the shear level was kept constant while measuring the time to reach activation, i.e., the exposure time, to depict a locus of incipient shear-related platelet activation on a shear stress-exposure time plane, which is commonly used as a standard for platelet activation threshold.

Yet, in arterial stenoses and in blood flow through prosthetic devices, the pathological blood flow patterns that arise are far more complicated. Rheologic variables related to pulsatility, eddy formation, and turbulence may predominate the platelets' response. Platelets exposed to pulsed and elongational stresses, as may be found in arterial occlusions and devices, are activated at lower shear rates and form larger aggregates (25,33,34). Applying Hellums' criterion, Boreda et al. (35) estimated maximal shear stress/exposure time combinations in moderate stenoses to reach approximately half the activation threshold. We measured platelet deposition in streamlined models of stenoses and conducted numerical simulations to establish a "level of activation" parameter based on a summation of the instantaneous product of the shear stress level and exposure time along turbulent trajectories (36). The cumulative effect of varying flow stresses and exposure times along individual platelet trajectories in stenosed arteries and past MHV indicates that platelet activation criteria should be established under more realistic flow conditions (36–42). The effect of the loading history of a blood corpuscle should also be taken into account (43).

FLUID MECHANICAL FACTORS IMPLICATED IN PLATELET ACTIVATION AND AGGREGATION

Fluid mechanical factors that have been implicated in platelet activation and aggregation include high rates of shear and deformation, turbulence, and areas of flow stagnation or recirculation that are characterized by low shear and longer retention time (44–46). Hemodynamic principles are fundamentally linked to thrombus formation, not only by inducing shear stresses that can cause platelet activation and aggregation but also by transporting cells and proteins to the thrombus (47). Folts et al. (48–50) described a canine model in which coronary artery constriction initiated a platelet-dependent thrombus formation. Using the same model, Strony et al. (51) demonstrated that the acceleration as platelets approach the converging stenotic region, and the deceleration downstream, can cause platelet deformation of 400%–800% and that the shear stress levels in stenosed human coronary arteries activated platelets within physiological transit times.

Vortex shedding, a complex flow phenomenon of interacting vortices in the wake of bluff bodies, has been observed experimentally in models of arterial stenosis and in various blood recirculating devices (36,52). These situations create the necessary conditions for the hemostatic reaction to proceed by providing optimal mixing for platelet aggregation, increasing the procoagulant surfaces needed for the coagulation reactions, and dispersing the clotting factors in the process. Prior activation and the extrusion of platelets' pseudopodia increase their effective hydrodynamic volume by several folds, resulting in an increased collision rate (53). The ensuing turbulent eddies enhance mixing and cascade energy to ever smaller spatial scales and dissipate it (Kolmogorov cascade). At cellular scales, eddies directly interact with the cells, damaging their membranes (54,55). The measured scale of turbulent eddies in stenosed arteries poses a direct threat to the platelets, resulting in much higher strain energy dissipated on their membranes, making them more prone to activation (56).

EXPERIMENTAL AND NUMERICAL FLOW STUDIES

Previous experimental studies using methods such as Laser Doppler Anemometry, photo-chromic tracer, and Digital Particle Image Velocimetry have further elucidated poststenotic flow patterns (36,57–59). Several investigators observed transition of the flow to turbulence, accompanied by a breakdown of waves and stream-wise vortices that were shed in the high shear layer, in axisymmetric stenoses with area reduction of 65%, 75% (59), 84% (36), and 90% (60–62). The poststenotic flow became unstable during this vortex generation phase of the cycle, resulting in intense fluctuations in wall shear stress. Steady flow through an axisymmetric stenosis has been investigated extensively, with some studies using an analytical approach (63). In situations of severe stenosis and/or high Reynolds number, a flow separation and recirculation region develops distal to the stenosis, and as a result, the poststenotic region may become turbulent. Using a finite difference, Deshpande et al. (64) computed flow patterns that corroborated the experimental results of Young and Tsai (65). We observed that turbulence produced by stenotic jets increased the wall shear stress by more than one order of magnitude (37). They also computed the platelets' activation potential along pertinent turbulent trajectories and found that it underwent a step jump during the passage of a platelet through the stenosis. Tu et al. (66) and Tu and Deville (67) simulated both steady and pulsatile flows through axisymmetric stenoses. Rosenfeld and Einav (68) studied pulsatile flow in a stenotic channel with varying degrees of obstruction. Vortices were generated during systole and were washed out during diastole. More recently, Rappitsch and Perktold (69), Buchanan and Kleinstreuer (70), and Deplano and Siouffi (71) reported their numerical studies on pulsatile flows in axisymmetric stenosis with 75% area reduction. Although these studies have served to identify regions of flow separation and vortex motion and have provided numerical estimates of wall shear stress, in many cases certain simplifying assumptions were applied, e.g., sinusoidal instead of arterial flow waveforms, flow symmetry instead of fully 3D simulations, and Newtonian instead of non-Newtonian fluid properties. Furthermore, in most cases, laminar flow models and, in very few cases, simplified turbulence models that cannot handle turbulent flow in the transition range characterizing stenotic jet flows were used.

FLOW AND THROMBOLYSIS

Fibrinolysis of thrombi formed on arterial surfaces is also strongly mediated by the local flow regimes. It has been shown, for example, that cultured human endothelial cells produce three times as much tissue plasminogen activator (t-PA) when subjected to a shear stress of 25 dyn/cm^2 as compared with cells under stationary flow, whereas varying degrees of shear stress do not effect the secretion rate of plas-minogen activator inhibitor-1 (72). All blood-surface interactions are governed by the transport of fluid elements to the surface, protein–cell reactions at the surface, and the removal of reaction products from the surface (46). The transport of fluid elements to the surface is in turn governed by the mechanism of convection along the flow direction in regions farther from the surface and by diffusion transverse to the flow direction in regions close to the surface. Fibrinolysis is dependent on these transport mechanics. The rates of dissolution of thrombi are dependent on factors such as the levels of plasminogen activators and plasminogen being transported to the thrombus surface, rates of binding of t-PA to the fibrin clot or degradation of the fibrin mesh by plasmin, and removal of degraded fibrin products from the fluid–solid interface. The primary motivation of investigations into the effects of flow on the fibrinolytic cascade has been to develop effective thrombolytic therapies for ischemic stroke, myocardial infarction, or peripheral artery disease (73).

The dynamics of flow-mediated thrombolysis differ depending on whether the thrombus is occlusive (thrombus plug occluding entire arterial cross-section) or nonocclusive (partially occluding thrombus formed on arterial surface or recana-lized thrombus). In occlusive plugs, the transport of plasmin or plasminogen acti-vators through the clot is due to permeation (convection) driven by the pressure difference between the proximal and distal ends of the clot. This notion is supported by the observation that initial recanalization can be achieved in occlusive thrombi within minutes to hours, whereas if the process were driven solely by diffusion, recanalization would take on the order of hours to days. The process of permeation hastens the rate of clot lysis by 10- to 100-fold as compared with lysis by diffu-sion alone, and lysis rates increase with increasing pressure gradients across the clots (74). This also affects the mode of delivery of a thrombolytic agent as systemic infusions may be suitable only for short clots with a high pressure gradient across them. Longer clots with smaller pressure gradient across the occlusion may be bet-ter treated by local delivery of the lytic to optimize its concentration at the thrombus surface. There may also be regions of flow stasis proximal to occlusive thrombi, which could retard systemically infused thrombolysis agents from reaching the thrombus. Additionally, when the thrombus is eventually recanalized by a channel or channels, the permeation-driving pressure gradient drops considerably and the residual thrombus tends to undergo lysis by the much slower process of radial dif-fusion of the thrombolytic agent (74).

Numerical simulations of flow-mediated thrombolysis usually solve differ-ential equations characterizing the convective-diffusive transport of species to the thrombus surface, flow through a porous medium for occlusive thrombi, and the reaction kinetics at the surface to investigate different features. Species interactions such as free plasminogen activation, free plasmin inhibition by $\alpha2$-antiplasmin, free t-PA binding to the clot, and fibrin degradation based on plasmin concentration can be simulated (75). Control over the simulations is achieved by making simplifying assumptions such as single reactive species (76), single lumped reaction constant (77), or single reaction time (78) to enhance complexity in other areas such as the use of higher dimensional models or analytical expressions. Numerical simula-tions of occlusive thrombi show the propagation of finger-like channels through the thrombus in correlation with experimental observations (78). Varying the structure of the fibrin mesh shows these "dissolution fingers" to propagate faster through high permeability (low resistance) regions of the clot potentially leaving recanalized thrombus on the wall, or the fingers propagating around regions of high fibrin density and potentially dissolving the clot, but initiating emboli of these high-density clumps (76). Simulations of nonocclusive thrombi can also quantify the role of viscous shear forces in mechanically degrading the clot with one such study suggesting a 250-fold slower dissolution of clot in a low-velocity regime as compared with a high-velocity regime (Reynolds number ratio ~20) (77).

THROMBOEMBOLISM IN BLOOD RECIRCULATING DEVICES

The advent of implantable blood recirculating devices has provided life-saving solutions to patients with severe cardiovascular diseases. The REMATCH (Randomized Evaluation of Mechanical Assistance for the Treatment of Congestive Heart Failure) study demonstrated a 48% decrease in mortality with left ventricular assist devices (LVAD) compared with drug therapy, paving the way for their ultimate use as a long-term therapy for patients not eligible for heart transplants (79,80). In North America, there are over 45,000 patients in end-stage heart disease awaiting transplant annually, with only 2000 transplants available (data from the American Heart Association (11) and the Organ Procurement and Transplantation Network). The implantable total artificial heart may eventually offer a solution to this chronic shortage.

The LVAD, if approved for destination therapy, has only a 30% 2-year survival and a still unacceptable complication rate of thrombosis/stroke. Currently, prosthetic heart valves (PHV) are routinely used for replacing diseased heart valves. However, all these devices share a common problem: significant complications such as hemolysis, platelet destruction, and thromboembolism often arise after their implantation. This, combined with the attendant risk for cardioembolic stroke, remains an impediment to these devices. Compounding the problem, even the mandatory life-long anticoagulant drug regimen they require, which induces vulnerability to hemorrhage and is not a viable therapy for some patients, does not eliminate the thromboembolic risk.

Patients with a PHV, for example, develop thromboembolic complications at a linearized rate of between 0.7% and 6.4% per patient-year (81–84). In those patients, it has been shown that platelets are chronically activated (85–85). An example of flow-induced PHV thromboembolism is the Medtronic Parallel valve, which was withdrawn voluntarily during clinical trials due to an unacceptable incidence of thrombus formation in valve recipients (89). Thromboembolism is also one of the major complications with vascular assist devices (VAD), occurring in 3%–35% of bridge-to-transplant patients and resulting in strokes in 16% of destination therapy VAD patients of the REMATCH study (90–92).

Transcranial Doppler ultrasound (TCD) has been used to detect microembolic events in patients with MHV (93). The amount of events varies significantly according to the prosthesis implicating local flow conditions in their genesis (94–96). The measurement of hemostatic indexes in conjunction with TCD in patients with VAD (97) supports the hypothesis that microembolic signals (MES) are related to increased hemostatic activity, even in the presence of aggressive anticoagulant therapy. Neurobiochemical markers indicating cerebral embolic events were elevated in valve replacement patients compared with patients who have undergone coronary artery bypass grafting (98).

One of the major culprits in blood recirculating devices is the emergence of nonphysiologic (pathologic) flow patterns that enhance the hemostatic response.

Elevated flow stresses that are present in the nonphysiologic geometries of these devices enhance their propensity to initiate thromboembolism. In recent years it has been demonstrated that flow-induced thrombogenicity, caused by chronic platelet activation and the initiation of thrombus formation, is the salient aspect of this blood trauma. This lends itself to the premise that thromboembolism in prosthetic blood recirculating devices is initiated and maintained primarily by the nonphysiological flow patterns and stresses that activate and enhance the aggregation of blood platelets, thus increasing the risk of thromboembolism and cardioembolic stroke.

DEVICE THROMBOEMBOLISM AND ITS CONSISTENCY

The mechanisms underlying flow-induced thromboembolic complications are poorly understood. One of the culprits in PHVs and similar blood recirculating devices is nonphysiologic flow patterns characterized by elevated shear stresses, with portions of the flow cycle becoming turbulent (42,56,99–102). Linear discriminant analysis measurements revealed that elevated turbulent stresses within the valve's hinges were linked to the thrombus formation (56,103). Current standards of the Food and Drug Administration and the International Standards Organization are under re-examination in lieu of these findings. Further, thromboembolism and the attendant risk for stroke (2%–47%) (104–105) remain hurdles to chronic VAD application (106). VADs induce changes to the coagulation system by activating platelets despite aggressive anticoagulant therapy (97,107–109). The flow patterns within VADs have been implicated as the underlying risk for thromboembolism (110). Fewer thrombi were recorded in the high shear regions, and platelet-like features were common in lower shear stress regions, likely due to varied fluid dynamics within the VAD blood sac (111). After removal of the annular tissue during PHV implantation surgery, the larger annulus is a tempting target for an oversized prosthesis, sometimes implanted by "wedging" the valve. Inadequate orientation of the valve may distort its presentation to the axis of blood flow, exceeding the normal restraints of the prosthesis design (112). An oblique tilt of 5 or more degrees, which is difficult to visualize at operation, can result in one of the leaflets opening past the axis of flow with a delayed, asynchronous, closure, and resultant regurgitation (113), as well as higher maximal transprosthetic velocity, pressure gradients, and marked turbulence (114). Blood clots may also form because of poor contractile function of the ventricles, atrial fibrillation, septic complications, and insufficient anticoagulation. Simultaneously, bleeding complications can occur as a consequence of anticoagulant treatment and/or platelet defects (115). However, flow-induced thromboembolic complications in devices, mostly overlooked in the past, appear to be a central mechanism, which is directly related to the device hemodynamics.

Platelet aggregates or gaseous microemboli were suggested as the source of high-intensity transient signals (HITS) measured with TCD in patients (93,116). HITS associated with solid emboli were measured in rabbit aorta (117,118) and in the distal carotid artery of sheep (119). Thrombi were excluded as an underlying embolic material because of a lack of correlation with thrombin markers (120). However, as platelet markers were not used in that study, microemboli rich in platelets were inherently excluded. Platelet microthrombi and microemboli from cardiopulmonary bypass were quantified in organs using radioactive-labeled platelets (37). Recently, a method was developed to monitor platelet microemboli formation

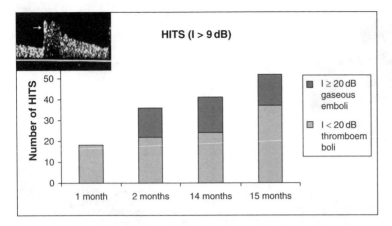

FIGURE 3 High-intensity transient signals (HITS) measurements following mechanical heart valve implantation in sheep. The number of microembolic signals, specifically thromboemboli, increased over time. *Source*: Reproduced with permission from Ref. (122).

in vivo (121). In a more recent study on sheep (122), in which HITS were measured and correlated to platelet activity measurements, the number of HITS (MES), specifically thromboemboli, increased over time following the MHV implantation (Fig. 3). This was correlated to the sheep platelet activity measurements using the PAS assay that indicated a significant increase in platelet activity in the sheep with implanted MHV 15 months post implantation (Fig. 4).

A significant effect of valve rotation and orientation on downstream turbulence and HITS frequency was found for two valve designs (bileaflet vs. monoleaflet)

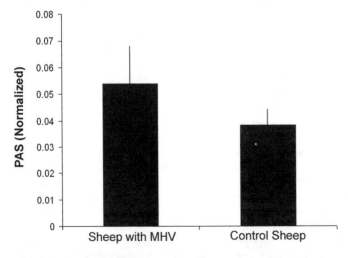

FIGURE 4 Increased platelet activation in sheep with mechanical heart valves (15 months post-implantation) as measured with the Platelet Activity State (PAS) assay. *Source*: Adapted from Ref. (41) with permission of Future Drugs Ltd.

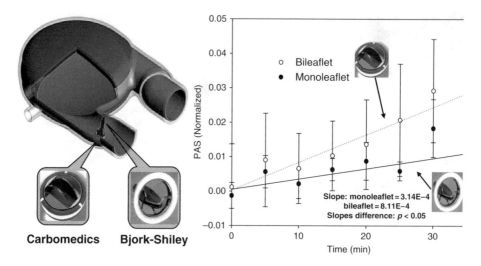

FIGURE 5 In vitro platelet activity measurements in left ventricular assist devices: the bileaflet mechanical heart valve (MHV) generated higher platelet activity than the monoleaflet MHV ($p < 0.05$). *Abbreviation*: PAS, platelet activity state. *Source*: Adapted from Ref. (41) with permission of Future Drugs Ltd. (See also color plate section.)

implanted in patients (123,124) and in pigs (94). The higher number of HITS for bileaflet versus monoleaflet MHV in patients (124) correlated well to in vitro measurements of platelet activity in an LVAD with the same type of valves (125). The results from this comparative study, performed with the MHV mounted in a LVAD system, are presented in Fig. 5 showing more than twofold increase in the slope of the platelet activity state (PAS) for the bileaflet MHV as compared with the monoleaflet MHV.

THE SIGNIFICANCE OF STUDYING PLATELET ACTIVATION OVER HEMOLYSIS IN DEVICES

In the past, mechanically induced blood trauma in blood recirculating devices was almost exclusively studied with respect to RBC damage (hemolysis) (126–128). However, in recent years it has been shown that platelet activation and the initiation of thrombus formation is the salient aspect of mechanically induced blood trauma (129). RBCs are much more resistant to mechanical damage because of their "tank-treading" motion and membrane flexibility. RBCs experience fewer shear forces than platelets (130,131) as they predominantly flow in core regions (Fahraeus–Lindqvist effect). The relative rigidity of the platelet membrane as compared with RBC is a major mechanism for a higher strain to dissipate across the platelet membrane (56). Hemolysis occurs with shear stress levels of 1500–2500 dyn/cm² and exposure time of 10^2 s (132–135), whereas platelet activation occurs at stress levels almost one order of magnitude lower at 100–300 dyn/cm² and 10^2 s (30,136). The smaller size of platelets causes them to respond more exclusively to viscous shearing because they are smaller than the typical Kolmogorov length scales characterizing the turbulent energy cascade in MHV flows (54,137). Recent studies (56) contrasted hemolysis by leakage flow through MHV (138) with platelet activation measurements and demonstrated that while hemoglobin levels (hemolysis indicator) barely increased, platelet activation markers such as annexin V were greatly increased. This is further supported by an in vitro study in a Couette-type device that found that hemolysis started at critical shear rates of about 80,000 s^{-1}, whereas significant impact on platelets occurred at lower shear rates (starting at 55,000 s^{-1}) (137). These new findings are followed closely by the FDA, which is likely to set more stringent limits to the design layout of devices based on platelet activation rather than hemolysis.

MEASURING THE THROMBOGENIC POTENTIAL OF DEVICES

The growing recognition that thrombosis, rather than hemolytic anemia, is the primary clinical problem associated with blood recirculating devices suggests that markers of thrombogenic potential should be studied, rather than markers of hemolysis. This is further accentuated by the pioneering AbioCor Implantable Replacement Heart System that was implanted in several patients in recent years and eventually not supported for continued development by the FDA. Morbidity and mortality associated with these devices were often stroke-related, whereas no evidence of significant hemolysis was observed in either animals (139) or humans (140–142). Regrettably, few data on flow-induced thrombogenic aspects are currently available because of the complexity of the blood coagulation system (143). Several approaches for studying device-induced thrombogenicity are in progress by only a few groups (56,126,144–146). A subsequent chapter in this volume (Part 1, Chapter 4) reviews platelet assays that enable near real-time measurements of the thrombogenic potential induced by flow through devices. Other techniques have been applied to in vitro measurements of flow-induced platelet activation in MHV mounted in a LVAD (40,125), and this methodology is now utilized to measure the thrombogenicity of bioprosthetic and new generation polymer valves (147)

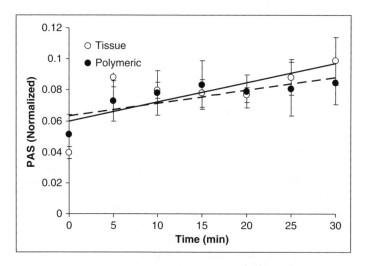

FIGURE 6 Platelet activity comparison in left ventricular assist devices between a St. Jude tissue and a trileaflet polymeric prosthetic heart valve—no significant difference was observed. *Abbreviation*: PAS, platelet activity state. *Source*: Reproduced with permission from Ref. (147).

that are targeted for minimally invasive percutaneous valve delivery (148–150)—the breakthrough technique with a huge promise for patients who cannot tolerate cardiothoracic surgery. The goal of the polymer valves, which are better suited for stented delivery than bioprosthetic valves, is to have a thrombogenic potential comparable to the latter so as not to require mandatory anticoagulation therapy. Recent measurements of the thrombogenic potential of an innovative polymer valve design (Innovia LLC Trileaflet composite polymeric valve) as compared with that of a St. Jude Toronto SPV™ stentless porcine bioprosthetic tissue valve indicated that there was no significant difference between the two valves (Fig. 6) (147).

STENT/COIL THROMBOSIS

Currently, the treatment of cerebral aneurysms is largely accomplished by the deposition of microcoils into the aneurysmal sac. One of the primary sources of morbidity related with this procedure is the occurrence of thromboembolic events, which are estimated to range from 2% to 11%, with permanent deficits occurring in 2%–5% of cases (151–153). To prevent aneurysmal recanalization over the long term after coil embolization, dense packing of coils at the aneurysmal neck is advocated. This must, however, be balanced with the possibility of the coil mass extending out of the sac and potentially creating a surface for acute thrombus formation on the coils at the aneurysm–parent artery interface (153). Another source of acute thrombus formation is the protrusion of individual coil loops into the parent artery during the deposition of additional coils, particularly in wide-necked aneurysms. Thrombotic material can potentially shear off the treatment site and be carried distally as emboli that eventually occlude smaller vessels. A study conducted to evaluate arterial occlusion with detachable coils provides some insight into the production of flow-related emboli (154). Coils were deposited in canine common femoral arteries, with flow arrest by a proximal balloon in some cases and without flow arrest in others. A Doppler probe was situated distal to the coil occlusion site to record embolic events. In arteries in which coils were deposited without flow arrest, there were at least 15 times as many embolic events as compared with those arteries occluded with coils under flow arrest.

To alleviate these shortcomings of aneurysm coiling, stents have been developed for use in the neurovasculature, where they are deployed across the aneurysmal neck to confine coils to the aneurysmal sac or to press protruded coil loops against the artery wall. Stents provide the additional benefit of redirecting the flow away from the aneurysm, thus inducing aneurysmal flow stasis and subsequent intraaneurysmal thrombosis. Stents, however, have themselves been known to occlude with thrombus, thereby obstructing parent artery flow (155). As neurovascular stents have a high porosity by design to provide them with flexibility, they may be unsuccessful in completely eliminating coil prolapse into the artery, possibly worsening the situation (156). As neurovascular stenting is a relatively new procedure, only a few reports are available on acute and delayed thrombosis (155). The phenomenon of stent thrombosis has, however, been studied extensively in the coronary circulation, where stents are deployed to maintain arterial patency.

Predisposing factors to stent thrombosis include inherent thrombogenicity of stents, due to their metallic nature, and arterial injury during stent deployment, which exposes the underlying thrombogenic surfaces such as collagen and tissue factor. In the coronary circulation, stents are deployed in diseased arteries that may contain ruptured plaque and thrombus. Studies with intravascular ultrasound previously revealed that major contributors to stent thrombosis were the under-expansion of stents and poor stent apposition to the arterial wall. Although initially there was a high incidence (~20%) of stent thrombosis with bare metal stents, it was subsequently reduced to approximately 2% or less due to high-pressure balloon stent expansions and appropriate pharmaceutical management (141,142). These recent improvements have been critical because mortality rates associated with stent thrombosis are reported to be as high as 15%–20% (157,158).

Various other factors, such as small-diameter arteries, longer stents, complex lesions, treatment of multiple vessels requiring multiple stents, and stenting of bifurcation lesions, have been found to also promote stent thrombosis. Although the advent of drug-eluting stents has significantly reduced restenosis rates, incidence rates and correlated factors of stent thrombosis are similar to those for bare metal stents (159). Recent reports on complications with drug-eluting stents describe the phenomenon of late stent thrombosis (>30 days after treatment) in approximately 0.4% of cases, resulting in myocardial infarctions (160). Interestingly, these reports suggest a correlation between the discontinuation of clopidogrel therapy and late stent thrombosis. The drug coatings possibly delay endothelialization of stent struts, which does not present as a problem as long as dual antiplatelet therapy is continued. Other possible causes of this phenomenon include the formation of a dysfunctional endothelial surface due to drug therapy or an inflammatory reaction to the polymer coating once the drugs have dissolved (160). These findings provide additional support to the notion that it is difficult to artificially regulate flow-related thrombosis as its mechanisms are not yet completely understood.

It must be recognized that the phenomenon of acute thrombosis under arterial blood flow is mediated by different biochemical interactions than thrombosis related to hemostasis. Acute thrombi are rich in platelets (white clots) as opposed to clots associated with flow stasis, such as venous thrombi or pulmonary emboli, which are rich in erythrocytes (red clots). The reduction or cessation of flow increases the residence time of soluble coagulation factors, increasing their local concentration and thereby promoting clotting. This is supported by the observation that antico-agulants such as heparin and warfarin are effective treatments against this disease. Under arterial flow conditions with concomitant high shear rates, however, circulat-ing factors are washed away rapidly and weak bindings are not tolerated. Thrombi formed under such conditions have been suggested to be vWF-mediated platelet aggregations, where vWF in flowing blood binds to exposed thrombogenic surfaces on the arterial wall, activates platelets by interacting with GPIb receptors, and firmly binds platelets through GPIb and GPIIb-IIIa receptors (161). This concept explains the effectiveness of antiplatelet therapies, such as aspirin or clopidogrel, in prevent-ing and reducing acute thrombosis. Patients undergoing interventional procedures such as stenting or coiling are thus managed with long-term antiplatelet medica-tion. Recently, GPIIb-IIIa receptor inhibitors such as abciximab have been used dur-ing interventional procedures to reduce the incidence of complications due to acute thrombosis (150,151). Treatment regimens with these pharmaceuticals, however, have yet to be defined precisely; lessons are still being learned empirically, such as with late stent thrombosis of drug-eluting stents, hemorrhage with the use of GPIIb-IIIa receptor inhibitors, or thrombolytics during coiling of ruptured cerebral aneurysms. Experiments that elucidate the effects of these pharmaceutical regimens are invaluable. An ex vivo flow chamber system used to test platelet aggregation in

samples of human blood with different coronary stent designs and different pharmaceutical regimens found evidence that supports the use of dual antiplatelet therapy (aspirin and clopidogrel) over aspirin alone (146). GPIIb-IIIa receptor inhibitors
were also found to be more potent inhibitors of platelet thrombus formation than an
anti-GPIb antibody (162). Another in vitro study with similar aims but much better
simulation of the hemodynamic conditions in coronary arteries used closed loops of
plastic tubing containing thawed fresh frozen plasma and fresh platelet concentrations rotating in a pulsatile manner about the same central axis (163). Flow cessation
within any tube, as monitored by an ultrasonic flow probe, was used to evaluate the
relative thrombogencities of the stents deployed within the tubes. Computational
models of flow-related thrombosis in the presence of artificial materials have also
been developed over the years (164). One such numerical analysis that resolved species convection-diffusion and reaction equations under low shear conditions to predict thrombus initiation and growth matched results obtained for thrombus location
and growth rate in a corresponding in vitro experiment (165).

SUMMARY
Blood is a complex fluid containing suspended cells that exhibits varying rheological and biochemical properties depending on the region through which it is flowing.
Although this behavior serves to optimize and maintain the supply of nutrients to
the various organs, pathological or artificial alterations to the flow domains offset
the balance in ways that are as yet incompletely understood. One of the most severe
consequences of the disruption of homeostatic flow states is the formation of thrombus leading to ischemic stroke, which causes as much as 1.5 million deaths in the
world every year. Platelets are crucial to thrombus formation, and their activation
and aggregation are modulated by fluid mechanical factors such as high rates of
shear and deformation or low shear areas of flow stagnation or recirculation that
facilitate longer residence time of platelet agonists and coagulation factors. The two
primary sources of abnormal flow patterns that generate platelet-rich thrombi and
lead to ischemic stroke are atherosclerotic disease associated with high degrees of
arterial stenosis or unstable plaques and cardiac disease associated with atrial fibrillation or devices such as PHV. The magnitudes and exposure times leading to SIPA
under complex flow patterns such as pulsatility, acceleration–deceleration regions,
eddy formation, or turbulence are only recently being investigated in detail. The
extent to which thrombi can be lysed is also mediated by fluid dynamics factors
such as the convective and diffusive transport of lysis agonists and antagonists to
and through the thrombus or clot permeation of these agents through pressure gradients. Fluid mechanics thus plays a critical role in triggering atherothrombotic and
cardioembolic events. The therapeutic benefit of medical devices such as artificial
heart valves, ventricular assist devices, stents, or coils could be greatly enhanced by
a more thorough appreciation of how they alter blood flow patterns.

REFERENCES
1. Lih MM-S. Transport phenomena in medicine and biology. New York: Wiley-Interscience,
   1975.
2. Fahraeus R, Lindqvist T. The viscocity of the blood in narrow capillary tubes. Am
   J Physiol 1931; 96:562–568.
3. Maude AD, Whitmore RL. Theory of the flow of blood in narrow tubes. J Appl Physiol
   1958; 12(1):105–113.

4. National Institutes of Health. National Heart, Lung, and Blood Institute report of the task force on research in epidemiology and prevention of cardiovascular diseases. Bethesda, MD: Public Health Service. 1994.

5. Stein B, Fuster V. Antithrombotic therapy in acute myocardial infarction: prevention of venous, left ventricular and coronary artery thromboembolism. Am J Cardiol 1989; 64(4):33B–40B.

6. Sakariassen KS, Barstad RM. Mechanisms of thromboembolism at arterial plaques. Blood Coagul Fibrinolysis 1993; 4(4):615–625.

7. Haerem JW. Sudden coronary death: the occurrence of platelet aggregates in the epicardial arteries of man. Atherosclerosis 1971; 14(3):417–432.

8. Ambrose JA, Hjemdahl-Monsen CE, Borrico S, et al. Angiographic demonstration of a common link between unstable angina pectoris and non-Q-wave acute myocardial infarction. Am J Cardiol 1988; 61(4):244–247.

9. Kristensen SD, Andersen HR, Falk E. What an interventional cardiologist should know about the pathophysiology of acute myocardial infarction. Semin Interv Cardiol 1999; 4(1):11–16.

10. Antiplatelet Trialists' Collaboration. Secondary prevention of vascular disease by prolonged antiplatelet treatment. Br Med J (Clin Res Ed) 1988; 296(6618):320–331.

11. American Heart Association Statistics Committee and Stroke Statistics Subcommittee. Heart disease and stroke statistics—2007 update: a report from the American Heart Association Statistics Committee and Stroke Statistics Subcommittee. Circulation 2007; 115(5):e69–e171.

12. Adams HP Jr, Bendixen BH, Kappelle LJ, Biller J, Love BB, Gordon DL, Marsh EE 3rd. Classification of subtype of acute ischemic stroke. Definitions for use in a multicenter clinical trial. TOAST. Trial of Org 10172 in Acute Stroke Treatment. Stroke 1993; 24(1):35–41.

13. Hennerici MG. The unstable plaque. Cerebrovascular Dis 2004; 17(suppl 3):17–22.

14. Han SW, Kim SH, Lee JY, Chu CK, Yang JH, Shin HY, Nam HS, Lee BI, Heo JH. A new subtype classification of ischemic stroke based on treatment and etiologic mechanism. Eur Neurol 2007; 57(2):96–102.

15. Benbir G, Uluduz D, Ince B, Bozluolcay M. Atherothrombotic ischemic stroke in patients with atrial fibrillation. Clin Neurol Neurosurg 2007; 109(6):485–490.

16. Foulkes MA, Wolf PA, Price TR, Mohr JP, Hier DB. The Stroke Data Bank: design, methods, and baseline characteristics. Stroke 1988; 19(5):547–554.

17. Sacco RL, Ellenberg JH, Mohr JP, Tatemichi TK, Hier DB, Price TR, Wolf PA. Infarcts of undetermined cause: the NINCDS Stroke Data Bank. Ann Neurol 1989; 25(4):382–390.

18. Petty GW, Brown RD Jr, Whisnant JP, Sicks JD, O'Fallon WM, Wiebers DO. Ischemic stroke subtypes: a population-based study of incidence and risk factors. Stroke 1999; 30(12): 2513–2516.

19. Kistler JP, Furie KL. Carotid endarterectomy revisited. N Engl J Med 2000; 342(23): 1743–1745.

20. O'Brien JR. Platelet activation at high and low shear is followed by inactivation:the clinical relevance. Platelets 1995; 6(4): 242–243.

21. O'Brien JR. Shear-induced platelet aggregation. Lancet 1990; 335(8691):711–713.

22. Gerrard JM, White JG. The structure and function of platelets, with emphasis on their contractile nature. Pathobiol Annu 1976; 6:31–59.

23. Janes SL, Wilson DJ, Chronos N, et al. Evaluation of whole blood flow cytometric detection of platelet bound fibrinogen on normal subjects and patients with activated platelets. Thromb Haemost 1993; 70(4):659–666.

24. Tuszynski GP, Rothman VL, Murphy A, et al. Thrombospondin promotes platelet aggregation. Blood 1988; 72(1):109–115.

25. Merten M, Chow T, Hellums JD, et al. A new role for P-selectin in shear-induced platelet aggregation. Circulation 2000; 102(17):2045–2050.

26. Altieri DC, Edgington TS. The saturable high affinity association of factor X to ADP-stimulated monocytes defines a novel function of the Mac-1 receptor. J Biol Chem 1988; 263(15):7007–7015.

27. Bevers EM, Comfurius P, Zwaal RF. Changes in membrane phospholipid distribution during platelet activation. Biochim Biophys Acta 1983; 736(1):57–66.

28. Tracy PB, Eide LL, Mann KG. Human prothrombinase complex assembly and function on isolated peripheral blood cell populations. J Biol Chem 1985; 260(4):2119–2124.

29. Nesheim M, Blackburn MN, Lawler CM, et al. Dependence of antithrombin III and thrombin binding stoichiometries and catalytic activity on the molecular weight of affinity-purified heparin. J Biol Chem 1986; 261(7):3214–3221.

30. Ramstack JM, Zuckerman L, Mockros LF. Shear-induced activation of platelets. J Biomech 1979; 12(2):113–125.

31. Kroll MH, Hellums JD, McIntire LV, et al. Platelets and shear stress. Blood 1996; 88(5):1525–1541.

32. Hellums JD, Peterson DM, Stathopoulos NA, et al. Studies on the mechanisms of shear-induced platelet activation. In: Hartman A, Kuschinsky W, eds. Cerebral Ischemia and Hemorheology. Berlin, New York: Springer-Verlag, 1987:80–89.

33. Sutera SP, Nowak MD, Joist JH, et al. A programmable, computer-controlled cone-plate viscometer for the application of pulsatile shear stress to platelet suspensions. Biorheology 1988; 25(3):449–459.

34. Purvis NB Jr, Giorgio TD. The effects of elongational stress exposure on the activation and aggregation of blood platelets. Biorheology 1991; 28(5):355–367.

35. Boreda R, Fatemi R, Rittgers S. Potential for platelet stimulation in critically stenosed carotid and coronary arteries. J Vasc Invest 1995; 1:26–37.

36. Bluestein D, Gutierrez C, Londono M, et al. Vortex shedding in steady flow through a model of an arterial stenosis and its relevance to mural platelet deposition. Ann Biomed Eng 1999; 27(6):763–773.

37. Bluestein D, Niu L, Schoephoerster RT, et al. Fluid mechanics of arterial stenosis: relationship to the development of mural thrombus. Ann Biomed Eng 1997; 25(2):344–356.

38. Cao J, Rittgers SE. Particle motion within in vitro models of stenosed internal carotid and left anterior descending coronary arteries. Ann Biomed Eng 1998; 26(2):190–199.

39. Bluestein D, Li YM, Krukenkamp IB. Free emboli formation in the wake of bi-leaflet mechanical heart valves and the effects of implantation techniques. J Biomech 2002; 35(12):1533–1540.

40. Bluestein D, Yin W, Affeld K, et al. Flow-induced platelet activation in mechanical heart valves. J Heart Valve Dis 2004; 13(3):501–508.

41. Bluestein D. Research approaches for studying flow induced thromboembolic complications in blood recirculating devices. Expert Rev Med Devices 2004; 1(1):65–80.

42. Bluestein D, Rambod E, Gharib M. Vortex shedding as a mechanism for free emboli formation in mechanical heart valves. J Biomech Eng 2000; 122(2):125–134.

43. Grigioni M, Daniele C, Morbiducci U, et al. The power-law mathematical model for blood damage prediction: analytical developments and physical inconsistencies. Artif Organs 2004; 28(5):467–475.

44. Alevriadou BR, Moake JL, Turner NA, et al. Real-time analysis of shear-dependent thrombus formation and its blockade by inhibitors of von Willebrand factor binding to platelets. Blood 1993; 81(5):1263–1276.

45. Folie BJ, McIntire LV. Mathematical analysis of mural thrombogenesis. Concentration profiles of platelet-activating agents and effects of viscous shear flow. Biophys J 1989; 56(6):1121–1141.

46. Slack SM, Turitto VT. Fluid dynamic and hemorheologic considerations. Cardiovasc Pathol 1993; 2(3 suppl):11S–21S.

47. Wootton DM, Ku DN. Fluid mechanics of vascular systems, diseases, and thrombosis. Annu Rev Biomed Eng 1999; 1:299–329.

48. Folts JD, Crowell EB Jr, Rowe GG. Platelet aggregation in partially obstructed vessels and its elimination with aspirin. Circulation 1976; 54(3):365–370.

49. Folts JD, Gallagher K, Rowe GG. Hemodynamic effects of controlled degrees of coronary artery stenosis in short-term and long-term studies in dogs. J Thorac Cardiovasc Surg 1977; 73(5):722–727.

50. Folts JD, Gallagher K, Rowe GG. Blood flow reductions in stenosed canine coronary arteries: vasospasm or platelet aggregation? Circulation 1982; 65(2):248–255.
51. Strony J, Beaudoin A, Brands D, et al. Analysis of shear stress and hemodynamic factors in a model of coronary artery stenosis and thrombosis. Am J Physiol 1993; 265 (5 Pt 2):H1787–H1796.
52. Hoerner SF. Fluid Dynamic Drag. Midland Park, NJ: Author, 1958.
53. Wurzinger LJ, Opitz R, Blasberg P, et al. Platelet and coagulation parameters following millisecond exposure to laminar shear stress. Thromb Haemost 1985; 54(2):381–386.
54. Jones SA. A relationship between Reynolds stresses and viscous dissipation: implications to red cell damage. Ann Biomed Eng 1995; 23(1):21–28.
55. Liu JS, Lu PC, Chu SH. Turbulence characteristics downstream of bileaflet aortic valve prostheses. J Biomech Eng 2000; 122(2):118–124.
56. Travis BR, Marzec UM, Ellis JT, et al. The sensitivity of indicators of thrombosis initiation to a bileaflet prosthesis leakage stimulus. J Heart Valve Dis 2001; 10(2):228–238.
57. Ahmed SA, Giddens DP. Pulsatile poststenotic flow studies with laser Doppler anemometry. J Biomech 1984; 17(9):695–705.
58. Gijsen FJ, Palmen DE, van der Beek MH, et al. Analysis of the axial flow field in stenosed carotid artery bifurcation models—LDA experiments. J Biomech 1996; 29(11):1483–1489.
59. Ojha M, Cobbold RSC, Johnston KW, et al. Pulsatile flow through constricted tubes: an experimental investigation using photochromic tracer methods. J Fluid Mech 1989; 203:173–197.
60. Lieber BB, Giddens DP. Apparent stresses in disturbed pulsatile flows. J Biomech 1988; 21(4):287–298.
61. Lieber BB, Giddens DP. Post-stenotic core flow behavior in pulsatile flow and its effects on wall shear stress. J Biomech 1990; 23(6):597–605.
62. Lieber BB, Giddens DP, Kitney RI, et al. On the discrimination between band-limited coherent and random apparent stresses in transitional pulsatile flow. J Biomech Eng 1989; 111(1):42–46.
63. Smith FT. Separating flow through a severely constricted symmetric tube. J Fluid Mech 1979; 90:725–754.
64. Deshpande MD, Giddens DP, Mabon RF. Steady laminar flow through modelled vascular stenoses. J Biomech 1976; 9(4):165–174.
65. Young DF, Tsai FY. Flow characteristics in models of arterial stenoses. II. Unsteady flow. J Biomech 1973; 6(5):547–559.
66. Tu C, Deville M, Dheur L, et al. Finite element simulation of pulsatile flow through arterial stenosis. J Biomech 1992; 25(10):1141–1152.
67. Tu C, Deville M. Pulsatile flow of non-Newtonian fluids through arterial stenoses. J Biomech 1996; 29(7):899–908.
68. Rosenfeld M, Einav S. The effect of constriction size on the pulsatile flow in a channel. J Fluids Eng 1995; 117:571–576.
69. Rappitsch G, Perktold K. Pulsatile albumin transport in large arteries: a numerical simulation study. J Biomech Eng 1996; 118(4):511–519.
70. Buchanan JR Jr, Kleinstreuer C. Simulation of particle-hemodynamics in a partially occluded artery segment with implications to the initiation of microemboli and secondary stenoses. J Biomech Eng 1998; 120(4):446–454.
71. Deplano V, Siouffi M. Experimental and numerical study of pulsatile flows through stenosis: wall shear stress analysis. J Biomech 1999; 32(10):1081–1090.
72. Diamond SL, Eskin SG, McIntire LV. Fluid flow stimulates tissue plasminogen activator secretion by cultured human endothelial cells. Science 1989; 243(4897):1483–1485.
73. Kolev K, Longstaff C, Machovich R. Fibrinolysis at the fluid-solid interface of thrombi. Curr Med Chem Cardiovasc Hematol Agents 2005; 3(4):341–355.
74. Blinc A, Francis CW. Transport processes in fibrinolysis and fibrinolytic therapy. Thromb Haemost 1996; 76(4):481–491.
75. Pleydell CP, David T, Smye SW, Berridge DC. A mathematical model of post-canalization thrombolysis. Phys Med Biol 2002; 47(2):209–224.

76. Anand S, Kudallur V, Pitman EB, Diamond SL. Mechanisms by which thrombolytic ther-
     apy results in nonuniform lysis and residual thrombus after reperfusion. Ann Biomed
     Eng 1997; 25(6):964–974.
77. Sersa I, Vidmar J, Grobelnik B, Mikac U, Tratar G, Blinc A. Modelling the effect of laminar
     axially directed blood flow on the dissolution of non-occlusive blood clots. Phys Med
     Biol 2007; 52(11):2969–2985.
78. Zidansek A, Blinc A, Lahajnar G, Keber D, Blinc R. Finger-like lysing patterns of blood
     clots. Biophys J 1995; 69(3):803–809.
79. Rose EA, Moskowitz AJ, Packer M, et al. The REMATCH trial: rationale, design, and end
     points. Randomized Evaluation of Mechanical Assistance for the Treatment of Conges-
     tive Heart Failure. Ann Thorac Surg 1999; 67(3):723–730.
80. Stevenson LW, Miller LW, Desvigne-Nickens P, et al. Left ventricular assist device as des-
     tination for patients undergoing intravenous inotropic therapy: a subset analysis from
     REMATCH (Randomized Evaluation of Mechanical Assistance in Treatment of Chronic
     Heart Failure). Circulation 2004; 110(8):975–981.
81. Butchart EG, Ionescu A, Payne N, et al. A new scoring system to determine thromboem-
     bolic risk after heart valve replacement. Circulation 2003; 108(suppl 1):II68–II74.
82. Butchart EG, Lewis PA, Grunkemeier GL, et al. Low risk of thrombosis and serious
     embolic events despite low-intensity anticoagulatio. Experience with 1,004 Medtronic
     Hall valves. Circulation 1988; 78(3 Pt 2):I66–I177.
83. Butchart EG, Lewsi PA, Kulatilake EN, et al. Anticoagulation variability between centres:
     implications for comparative prosthetic valve assessment. Eur J Cardiothorac Surg 1988;
     2(2):72–81.
84. Butchart EG, Li HH, Payne N, et al. Twenty years' experience with the Medtronic Hall
     valve. J Thorac Cardiovasc Surg 2001; 121(6):1090–1100.
85. Edmunds LH Jr. Is prosthetic valve thrombogenicity related to design or material? Tex
     Heart Inst J 1996; 23(1):24–27.
86. Pumphrey CW, Dawes J. Platelet alpha granule depletion: findings in patients with pros-
     thetic heart valves and following cardiopulmonary bypass surgery. Thromb Res 1983;
     30(3):257–264.
87. Edmunds LH Jr. Thrombotic and bleeding complications of prosthetic heart valves. Ann
     Thorac Surg 1987; 44(4):430–445.
88. Edmunds LH Jr, Mckinlay S, Anderson JM, et al. Directions for improvement of substi-
     tute heart valves: National Heart, Lung, and Blood Institute's Working Group report on
     heart valves. J Biomed Mater Res 1997; 38(3):263–266.
89. Bodnar E. The Medtronic Parallel valve and the lessons learned. J Heart Valve Dis 1996;
     5(6):572–573.
90. Piccione W Jr. Left ventricular assist device implantation: short and long-term surgical
     complications. J Heart Lung Transplant 2000; 19(8 suppl):S89–S94.
91. Portner PM, Jansen PG, Oyer PE, et al. Improved outcomes with an implantable left
     ventricular assist system: a multicenter study. Ann Thorac Surg 2001; 71(1):205–209.
92. Lazar RM, Shapiro PA, Jaski BE, et al. Neurological events during long-term mechanical
     circulatory support for heart failure: the Randomized Evaluation of Mechanical Assis-
     tance for the Treatment of Congestive Heart Failure (REMATCH) experience. Circulation
     2004; 109(20):2423–2427.
93. Grosset DG, Georgiadis D, Kelman AW, et al. Detection of microemboli by transcranial
     Doppler ultrasound. Tex Heart Inst J 1996; 23(4):289–292.
94. Kleine P, Perthel M, Hasenkam JM, et al. Downstream turbulence and high intensity
     transient signals (HITS) following aortic valve replacement with Medtronic Hall or
     St. Jude Medical valve substitutes. Eur J Cardiothorac Surg 2000; 17(1):20–24.
95. Georgiadis D, Kaps M, Berg J, et al. Transcranial Doppler detection of microemboli in
     prosthetic heart valve patients: dependency upon valve type. Eur J Cardiothorac Surg
     1996; 10(4):253–257; discussion 257–258.
96. Nötzold A, Droste DW, Hagedorn G, et al. Circulating microemboli in patients after
     aortic valve replacement with pulmonary autografts and mechanical valve prostheses.
     Circulation 1997; 96(6):1843–1846.

97. Wilhelm CR, Ristich J, Knepper LE, et al. Measurement of hemostatic indexes in conjunction with transcranial Doppler sonography in patients with ventricular assist devices. Stroke 1999; 30(12):2554–2561.
98. Herrmann M, Ebert AD, Galazky I, et al. Neurobehavioral outcome prediction after cardiac surgery: role of neurobiochemical markers of damage to neuronal and glial brain tissue. Stroke 2000; 31(3):645–650.
99. Sabbah HN, Stein PD. Fluid dynamic stresses in the region of a porcine bioprosthetic valve. Henry Ford Hosp Med J 1982; 30(3):134–138.
100. Stein PD, Sabbah HN, Lakier JB, et al. Frequency content of heart sounds and systolic murmurs in patients with porcine bioprosthetic valves: diagnostic value for the early detection of valvular degeneration. Henry Ford Hosp Med J 1982; 30(3):119–123.
101. Stein PD, Walburn FJ, Sabbah HN. Turbulent stresses in the region of aortic and pulmonary valves. J Biomech Eng 1982; 104(3):238–244.
102. Bluestein D, Einav S, Hwang NH. A squeeze flow phenomenon at the closing of a bileaflet mechanical heart valve prosthesis. J Biomech 1994; 27(11):1369–1378.
103. Healy TM, Ellis JT, Fontaine AA, et al. An automated method for analysis and visualization of laser Doppler velocimetry data. Ann Biomed Eng 1997; 25(2):335–343.
104. McCarthy PM, Nakatani S, Vargo R, et al. Structural and left ventricular histologic changes after implantable LVAD insertion. Ann Thorac Surg 1995; 59(3):609–613.
105. Vetter HO, Kaulbach HG, Schmitz C, et al. Experience with the Novacor left ventricular assist system as a bridge to cardiac transplantation, including the new wearable system. J Thorac Cardiovasc Surg 1995; 109(1):74–80.
106. Kasirajan V, McCarthy PM, Hoercher KJ, et al. Clinical experience with long-term use of implantable left ventricular assist devices: indications, implantation, and outcomes. Semin Thorac Cardiovasc Surg 2000; 12(3):229–237.
107. Rothenburger M, Wilhelm MJ, Hammel D, et al. Treatment of thrombus formation associated with the MicroMed DeBakey VAD using recombinant tissue plasminogen activator. Circulation 2002; 106(12 suppl 1):I-189–I-192.
108. Korn RL, Fisher CA, Livingston ER, et al. The effects of Carmeda Bioactive Surface on human blood components during simulated extracorporeal circulation. J Thorac Cardiovasc Surg 1996; 111(5):1073–1084.
109. Wilhelm MJ, Hammel D, Schmid C, et al. Clinical experience with nine patients supported by the continuous flow Debakey VAD. J Heart Lung Transplant 2001; 20(2):201.
110. Jin W, Clark C. Experimental investigation of unsteady flow behaviour within a sac-type ventricular assist device (VAD). J Biomech 1993; 26(6): 697–707.
111. Yamanaka H, Rosenberg G, Weiss WJ, et al. Multiscale analysis of surface thrombosis in vivo in a left ventricular assist system. ASAIO J 2005; 51(5):567–577.
112. DeWall RA, Ellis RL. Implantation techniques: a primary consideration in valve surgery. Ann Thorac Surg 1989; 48(3 suppl):S59–S60.
113. Antunes MJ, Colsen PR, Kinsley RH. Intermittent aortic regurgitation following aortic valve replacement with the Hall-Kaster prosthesis. J Thorac Cardiovasc Surg 1982; 84(5):751–754.
114. Omoto R, Matsumura M, Asano H, et al. Doppler ultrasound examination of prosthetic function and ventricular blood flow after mitral valve replacement. Herz 1986; 11(6):346–350.
115. Gruber EM, Seitelberger R, Mares P, et al. Ventricular thrombus and subarachnoid bleeding during support with ventricular assist devices. Ann Thorac Surg 1999; 67(6):1778–1780.
116. Mackay TG, Georgiadis D, Grosset DG, et al. On the origin of cerebrovascular microemboli associated with prosthetic heart valves. Neurol Res 1995; 17(5):349–352.
117. Braekken SK, Reinvang I, Russell D, et al. Association between intraoperative cerebral microembolic signals and postoperative neuropsychological deficit: comparison between patients with cardiac valve replacement and patients with coronary artery bypass grafting. J Neurol Neurosurg Psychiatry 1998; 65(4):573–576.
118. Russell D, Madden KP, Clark WM, et al. Detection of arterial emboli using Doppler ultrasound in rabbits. Stroke 1991; 22(2):253–258.

119. Markus H, Loh A, Brown MM. Detection of circulating cerebral emboli using Doppler ultrasound in a sheep model. J Neurol Sci 1994; 122(1):117–124.
120. Georgiadis D, MacKay TG, Kelman AW, et al. Differentiation between gaseous and formed embolic materials in vivo. Application in prosthetic heart valve patients. Stroke 1994; 25(8):1559–1563.
121. van Gestel MA, Heemskerk JW, Slaaf DW, et al. Real-time detection of activation patterns in individual platelets during thromboembolism in vivo: differences between thrombus growth and embolus formation. J Vasc Res 2002; 39(6):534–543.
122. Yin W, Krukenkamp IB, Saltman AE, Gaudette G, Suresh K, Bernal O, Jesty J, Bluestein D. Thrombogenic performance of a St. Jude bileaflet mechanical heart valve in a sheep model. ASAIO J 2006; 52(1):28–33.
123. Laas J, Kleine P, Hasenkam MJ, et al. Orientation of tilting disc and bileaflet aortic valve substitutes for optimal hemodynamics. Ann Thorac Surg 1999; 68(3):1096–1099.
124. Laas J, Kseibi S, Perthel M, et al. Impact of high intensity transient signals on the choice of mechanical aortic valve substitutes. Eur J Cardiothorac Surg 2003; 23(1):93–96.
125. Yin W, Alemu Y, Affeld K, et al. Flow-induced platelet activation in bileaflet and monoleaflet mechanical heart valves. Ann Biomed Eng 2004; 32(8):1058–1066.
126. Paul R, Marseille O, Hintze E, et al. In vitro thrombogenicity testing of artificial organs. Int J Artif Organs 1998; 21(9):548–552.
127. Schima H, Müller MR, Papantonis D, et al. Minimization of hemolysis in centrifugal blood pumps: influence of different geometries. Int J Artif Organs 1993; 16(7):521–529.
128. Schima H, Siegl H, Mohammad SF, et al. In vitro investigation of thrombogenesis in rotary blood pumps. Artif Organs 1993; 17(7):605–608.
129. Schima H, Wieselthaler G. Machanically induced blood trauma: are the relevant questions already solved, or is it still an important field to be investigated? Artif Organs 1995; 19(7):563–564.
130. Yeh C, Calvez AC, Eckstein EC. An estimated shape function for drift in a platelet-transport model. Biophys J 1994; 67(3):1252–1259.
131. Yeh C, Eckstein EC. Transient lateral transport of platelet-sized particles in flowing blood suspensions. Biophys J 1994; 66(5):1706–1716.
132. Brown CH 3rd, Lemuth RF, Hellums JD, et al. Response of human platelets to sheer stress. Trans Am Soc Artif Intern Organs 1975; 21:35–39.
133. Sutera SP, Croce PA, Mehrjardi M. Hemolysis and subhemolytic alterations of human RBC induced by turbulent shear flow. Trans Am Soc Artif Intern Organs 1972; 18(0):335–341, 347.
134. Sutera SP, Mehrjardi M. Deformation and fragmentation of human red blood cells in turbulent shear flow. Biophys J 1975; 15(1):1–10.
135. Brown CH 3rd, Leverett LB, Lewis CW, et al. Morphological, biochemical, and functional changes in human platelets subjected to shear stress. J Lab Clin Med 1975; 86(3):462–471.
136. Hung TC, Hochmuth RM, Joist JH, et al. Shear-induced aggregation and lysis of platelets. Trans Am Soc Artif Intern Organs 1976; 22:285–291.
137. Klaus S, Körfer S, Mottaghy K, et al. In vitro blood damage by high shear flow: human versus porcine blood. Int J Artif Organs 2002; 25(4):306–312.
138. Lamson TC, Rosenberg G, Geselowitz DB, et al. Relative blood damage in the three phases of a prosthetic heart valve flow cycle. ASAIO J 1993; 39(3):M626–M633.
139. Dowling RD, Etoch SW, Stevens KA, et al. Current status of the AbioCor implantable replacement heart. Ann Thorac Surg 2001; 71(3 suppl):S147–S149; discussion S183–S184.
140. Dowling RD, Gray LA Jr, Etoch SW, et al. Initial experience with the AbioCor implantable replacement heart system. J Thorac Cardiovasc Surg 2004; 127(1):131–141.
141. Dowling RD, Gray LA Jr, Etoch SW, et al. The AbioCor implantable replacement heart. Ann Thorac Surg 2003; 75(6 suppl):S93–S99.
142. Samuels LE, Holmes EC, Entwistle JC 3rd. Swan-Ganz monitoring of the AbioCor artificial heart. Ann Thorac Surg 2005; 80(3):1133.

143. Charron M, Follansbee W, Ziady GM, et al. Assessment of biventricular cardiac function in patients with a Novacor left ventricular assist device. J Heart Lung Transplant 1994; 13(2):263–267.

144. Jesty J, Bluestein D. Acetylated prothrombin as a substrate in the measurement of the procoagulant activity of platelets: elimination of the feedback activation of platelets by thrombin. Anal Biochem 1999; 272(1):64–70.

145. Jesty J, Yin W, Perrota P, et al. Platelet activation in a circulating flow loop: combined effects of shear stress and exposure time. Platelets 2003; 14(3):143–149.

146. Kawahito K, Adachi H, Ino T. Platelet activation in the gyro C1E3 centrifugal pump: comparison with the terumo capiox and the Nikkiso HPM-15. Artif Organs 2000; 24(11):889–892.

147. Yin W, Gallocher S, Pinchuk L, et al. Flow-induced platelet activation in a St. Jude mechanical heart valve, a trileaflet polymeric heart valve, and a St. Jude tissue valve. Artif Organs 2005; 29(10):826–831.

148. Shemin RJ. Percutaneous valve intervention: a surgeon's perspective. Circulation 2006; 113(6):774–775.

149. Feldman T. Percutaneous valve repair and replacement: challenges encountered, challenges met, challenges ahead. Circulation 2006; 113(6):771–773.

150. Mesana T. Percutaneous valve technology: an historical opportunity for cardiac surgeons. Curr Opin Cardiol 2006; 21(2):94.

151. Song JK, Niimi Y, Fernandez PM, et al. Thrombus formation during intracranial aneurysm coil placement: treatment with intra-arterial abciximab. AJNR Am J Neuroradiol 2004; 25(7):1147–1153.

152. Pelz DM, Lownie SP, Fox AJ. Thromboembolic events associated with the treatment of cerebral aneurysms with Guglielmi detachable coils. AJNR Am J Neuroradiol 1998; 19(8):1541–1547.

153. Workman MJ, Cloft HJ, Tong FC, et al. Thrombus formation at the neck of cerebral aneurysms during treatment with Guglielmi detachable coils. AJNR Am J Neuroradiol 2002; 23(9):1568–1576.

154. Hughes SR, Graves VB, Kesava PP, et al. The effect of flow arrest on distal embolic events during arterial occlusion with detachable coils: a canine study. AJNR Am J Neuroradiol 1996; 17(4):685–691.

155. Fiorella D, Albuquerque FC, Han P, et al. Preliminary experience using the Neuroform stent for the treatment of cerebral aneurysms. Neurosurgery 2004; 54(1):6–16; discussion 16–17.

156. Lee YJ, Kim DJ, Suh SH, et al. Stent-assisted coil embolization of intracranial wide-necked aneurysms. Neuroradiology 2005; 47(9):680–689.

157. Cutlip DE, Baim DS, Ho KK, et al. Stent thrombosis in the modern era: a pooled analysis of multicenter coronary stent clinical trials. Circulation 2001; 103(15):1967–1971.

158. Uren NG, Schwarzacher SP, Metz JA, et al. Predictors and outcomes of stent thrombosis: an intravascular ultrasound registry. Eur Heart J 2002; 23(2):124–132.

159. Kuchulakanti PK, Chu WW, Torguson R, et al. Correlates and long-term outcomes of angiographically proven stent thrombosis with sirolimus- and paclitaxel-eluting stents. Circulation 2006; 113(8):1108–1113.

160. Ong AT, McFadden EP, Regar E, et al. Late angiographic stent thrombosis (LAST) events with drug-eluting stents. J Am Coll Cardiol 2005; 45(12):2088–2092.

161. Goto S, Handa S. Coronary thrombosis. Effects of blood flow on the mechanism of thrombus formation. Jpn Heart J 1998; 39(5):579–596.

162. Sakakibara M, Goto S, Eto K, et al. Application of ex vivo flow chamber system for assessment of stent thrombosis. Arterioscler Thromb Vasc Biol 2002; 22(8):1360–1364.

163. Kolandaivelu K, Edelman ER. Low background, pulsatile, in vitro flow circuit for modeling coronary implant thrombosis. J Biomech Eng 2002; 124(6):662–668.

164. Basmadjian D, Sefton MV, Baldwin SA. Coagulation on biomaterials in flowing blood: some theoretical considerations. Biomaterials 1997; 18(23):1511–1522.

165. Goodman PD, Barlow ET, Crapo PM, et al. Computational model of device-induced thrombosis and thromboembolism. Ann Biomed Eng 2005; 33(6):780–797.

3 In Vivo Experimental Models of Focal Ischemic Stroke

Matthew J. Gounis[1], Kenneth M. Sicard[2], Ajay K. Wakhloo[3], and Marc Fisher[2]

[1]*Department of Radiology, New England Center for Stroke Research, University of Massachusetts Medical School, Worcester, Massachusetts, U.S.A.*

[2]*Department of Neurology, University of Massachusetts Medical School, Worcester, Massachusetts, U.S.A.*

[3]*Department of Radiology, Neurology and Neurosurgery, University of Massachusetts Medical School, Worcester, Massachusetts, U.S.A.*

INTRODUCTION

More than 80% of strokes in humans are ischemic (1), generally resulting either from an embolus of material originating elsewhere in the vasculature that blocks flow to the brain or from thrombosis of a diseased cerebral vessel. Animal models of focal cerebral ischemia are used to understand the evolution of brain tissue damage secondary to an ischemic event and to develop strategies to protect the brain from infarct. These models further serve to study the effects of reperfusion after restoring blood flow through the occluded vessel and mechanisms of hemorrhagic transformation of the ischemic tissue. Modeling cerebral ischemia in animals has been researched for more than a century, and thus a myriad of publications exists on the subject. As most human ischemic strokes are caused by occlusion of the middle cerebral artery (MCA) (2), we will review nonprimate animal models of focal ischemic stroke with a special emphasis on MCA embolic models used to evaluate physical or pharmacologic flow restoration. These models aim to satisfy the following criteria (3): (i) to mimic the pathophysiological changes found in human stroke, (ii) to create reproducible lesions, (iii) to employ procedures that are relatively simple and noninvasive, (iv) to enable monitoring of physiologic parameters and analysis of brain tissue for outcome measures, and (v) to be of practical financial cost.

As with all animal models of any disease state, it is essential to employ the model most appropriate to the question being addressed. In many instances, the hypothesis is too complex for any one model system to adequately provide definitive confirmation. Therefore, it is becoming more common to formulate a research plan that employs multiple models designed to study potential therapies. In models of cerebral ischemia, the selection of the animal model depends on three fundamental decisions: (i) the species in which to create the stroke, (ii) the method employed to produce ischemia, and (iii) the vascular territory that will be affected. This chapter is organized by using the above decision tree.

ANIMAL MODELS OF FOCAL ISCHEMIC STROKE
Rodent Models
Many higher animal species fulfill the aforementioned stroke-modeling criteria; however, rats are the most commonly used animals for several reasons, including (4–6): (i) the ability to induce reproducible infarcts, (ii) their small size that enables easy analysis of physiology and brain tissue, (iii) their low cost, (iv) the remarkable genetic homogeneity within strains, and (v) greater public and institutional ethical acceptability of use relative to larger animals. The disadvantages of using rodent models are (i) the small size that limits the ability to test new devices for the treatment of stroke and (ii) lissencephalic brains that are anatomically and functionally different from humans.

Although there are numerous animal models of focal cerebral ischemia, here, special focus is paid to the intraluminal MCA occlusion, thromboembolic, and microsphere embolus models because of their widespread use in the development of treatments for stroke. Importantly, these methods can also be performed on mice, allowing for the use of transgenic models to study the pathophysiology of stroke. However, it should be noted that in mice the long-term survivability following surgical procedures is lower than that in rats (7).

Intraluminal Middle Cerebral Artery Occlusion Model
This model was originally described by Koizumi et al. (8) and has since been modified by others. It is the most commonly used rat model for stroke because of its relative simplicity and noninvasive character. After surgical exposure of the neck, the MCA is occluded by inserting a monofilament suture into the internal carotid artery (ICA). The blood flow to the MCA is blocked either permanently or transiently by keeping the filament in place or withdrawing it, respectively. Several manuscripts describe in detail the technical and procedural features of this model (8–13).

This model typically induces infarcts in the lateral caudate-putamen complex and fronto-parietal cortex (14) (Fig. 1A). The infarct is reproducible, and there is a significant ischemic penumbra early after MCA occlusion, making this model suitable for testing neuroprotective agents (15). However, several technical factors may influence infarct size, such as (i) physical differences in the employed monofilament suture (16), (ii) insertion distance of the suture (17), (iii) the strain and vendor of the animals (18), and (iv) accidental premature reperfusion (19). It is therefore essential that standardized surgical and technical procedures be used by adequately trained personnel to generate reproducible lesions. There are also some complications with the intraluminal MCA occlusion model such as subarachnoid hemorrhage secondary to suture-induced arterial rupture (9), spontaneous hyperthermia when the duration of ischemia is longer than 2 h (20), and mechanical damage of endothelium that can complicate reperfusion (20,21). The complication rates may be reduced by using silicone-coated sutures (9).

The suture MCA occlusion model has recently been modified to induce ischemia in a magnetic resonance imaging (MRI) unit by remotely advancing the suture occluder (14). This in-bore (within the magnet) occlusion method has achieved a high reproducibility rate and enables investigators to monitor in vivo ischemic changes at preocclusion, acute, subacute, and chronic postocclusion time points (14). Combined with multiparametric MR techniques, the MCA occlusion model enables anatomic, diffusion, perfusion, and functional data to be obtained longitudinally and noninvasively in the same animal (22,23), making it a powerful tool for studying the pathophysiology of brain ischemia.

A

B

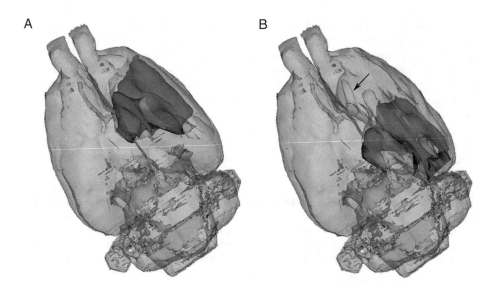

FIGURE 1 Comparison of the suture (*A*) and the thromboembolic (*B*) middle cerebral artery (MCA) occlusion models acquired 30 min after the onset of ischemia. 3D renderings of the evolving stroke with superimposed apparent diffusion coefficient (red) and cerebral blood flow (green) lesion volumes are shown. Note the increased perfusion–diffusion mismatch and the presence of a smaller perfusion lesion in the anterior component of the MCA territory (*arrow*). The authors hypothesize that this second lesion could be the result of clot fragmentation and migration. Finally, the lesion volume of the thromboembolic model extends further into the posterior aspect of the cerebrum. *Source*: Reproduced with permission from Macmillan Publishers Ltd: Ref. (27) (Sprague-Dawley rats, 300 g). (See also color plate section.)

Thromboembolic Model
Although thromboembolic ischemia can be induced by a photochemical method (24), the most commonly used thromboembolic model is blood clot injection, first applied in dogs by Hill et al. (25) and later applied to the rat (26,27) (Fig. 1B). This model is of great interest to researchers because of its close resemblance to human thromboembolic ischemic stroke and its utility in evaluating thrombolytic therapies (28). Thrombolytic therapy with recombinant tissue plasminogen activator (t-PA) administered intravenously within 3 h of onset of ischemic stroke in select patients is the only FDA-approved treatment for human stroke and has been shown to improve neurological outcome (29). Recently, there has been heightened interest in studying the efficacy of combining thrombolytic and neuroprotective agents in the treatment of stroke (30), giving thromboembolic animal models an increasingly important role in this respect.

Several disadvantages were common to the early thromboembolic models, such as diffuse and inhomogenous infarction in the MCA territory from microemboliza-tion to peripheral branches (26). Additionally, spontaneous recanalization frequently occurred, making it difficult to study thrombolytic therapies (14). Infarct sizes were variable, contralateral strokes were common, and ischemia caused by multiple small clots did not mimic typical clinical ischemic stroke (14). Later, it was determined that size (length and diameter) and the biological characteristics of the blood clot (fibrin-rich) are crucial to the relevance and reproducibility of this model (14).

Busch et al. (31) developed a rat clot model that surmounted the above issues in which a single fibrin-rich autologous clot was injected to produce reliable occlusion of the proximal MCA segment with consistent reduction of cerebral blood flow (CBF). No spontaneous thrombolysis was observed, and reproducible histological damage of the MCA perfusion territory was seen. In separate experiments a successful recanalization of the occluded MCA with thrombolytic therapy using t-PA (31) or prourokinase (32) was achieved. Recently, Henninger et al. (33) used the embolic model in conjunction with multimodal MRI to investigate the pathophysiological mechanisms underlying the relatively rare clinical phenomenon of "spectacular shrinking deficit" in stroke patients, which refers to an acute hemispheric ischemic stroke that rapidly resolves leaving only mild clinical symptoms (Fig. 2).

In conclusion, the single fibrin-rich clot model induces reproducible infarcts in the MCA territory similar to those produced by the intraluminal MCA occlusion model. The clot model has the added advantages of bearing closer similarity to the mechanism underlying human ischemic stroke and better utility for studying thrombolytic therapy. Combined with modern imaging techniques, thromboembolic models have the potential to take the experimental study of stroke to new frontiers.

Microsphere Embolus Model

Many materials such as carbon, plastic microspheres, silicone cylinders, and air can be injected into the common or internal carotid arteries to induce ischemia (34–36). The magnitude and severity of the ischemic damage depends on the number and size of the injected emboli (37). These models were previously characterized by diffuse distribution and inhomogenous infarction, making their experimental utility questionable. However, recent refinements have led to reproducible infarcts, with injection of 0.3–0.4-mm ceramic spheres into the common carotid artery, and results are promising (38). The disadvantage of all these models is that they do not allow a reperfusion of the ischemic tissue or the evaluation of thrombolytic treatment. Recent advancements in the design of thromboembolic models, as discussed above, may render the microsphere models obsolete.

Photothrombosis-Induced Focal Ischemia

Watson et al. first described the photothrombotic stroke model (39,40) in the rat. The model is created using a photosensitive dye, rose bengal, that is administered systemically. When the dye is irradiated with an excitation beam of green light that passes through the intact skull, singlet oxygen production in the irradiated area leads to focal endothelial damage and platelet activation producing microvascular occlusion (39,40). The model has the advantage that by controlling physical parameters, such as the intensity and wavelength of the light and the duration of irradiation, the resulting ischemia may be reliably altered. With a low level of invasiveness, small infarcts may be placed within distinct functional subdivisions of the cortex. The lack of subcortical involvement allows not only acute studies but also long-term survival for chronic studies. Moreover, this technique may be modified for use in mice (41). However, the disadvantages of this model include the damage of the endothelium that results in vasogenic edema (42). The simultaneous insult to the blood–brain barrier along with the evolving infarction produces both vasogenic and cytotoxic edema that is not consistent with stroke in humans (43). Moreover, the lack of collateral circulation to the ischemic area brings into question the accuracy of

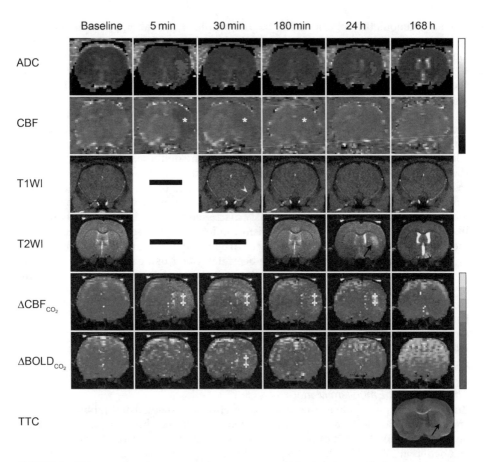

FIGURE 2 This montage shows magnetic resonance and histology images before and at various points after the onset of ischemic stroke using the rat thromboembolic model. In the case shown here, the middle cerebral artery (MCA) spontaneously recanalized within 15 min after injection of the clot. Shown are the results of apparent diffusion coefficient (ADC), cerebral blood flow (CBF), T1-weighted, T2-weighted, and changes to CBF and blood oxygenation level-dependent (BOLD) signal in response to hypercapnia (ΔCBF_{CO_2} and $\Delta BOLD_{CO_2}$, respectively) imaging. The gray scale bar provides the range of ADC values from 0 to 0.001 mm^2/s and CBF from 0 to 3 ml/g per min; and the color scale gives the ΔCBF_{CO_2} range from 0% to 200% and $\Delta BOLD_{CO_2}$ from 1% to 5%. The asterisk denotes areas of CBF voids whereas the ‡ symbol indicates an impaired response to hypercapnia. The bottom panel shows the infarction of triphenyltetrazolium chloride (TTC)-stained brain slice at the end of imaging 168 h from the ischemic onset. Arrows point to T1-weighted and TTC-derived lesions. The authors used these data to study the event of spectacular shrinking deficit. *Source*: Reproduced with permission from Ref. (33) (Sprague-Dawley rats, 300 g). (See also color plate section.)

modeling the penumbra. Ultimately, this model remains important in the study of neuropathophysiology relating to cortical infarction.

Rabbit Models
The rabbit model of focal ischemic stroke has been very important to the establishment of thrombolytic therapies that have been brought into clinical practice.

The endogenous thrombotic/thrombolytic profile of the rabbit is the most similar to humans outside of nonhuman primates (44). Moreover, rabbits present a greater similarity with human clot lysis induced by tissue plasminogen activator (t-PA) than there is between human and rat clot lysis (45). This evoked interest in establishing the efficacy of thrombolytics, especially t-PA for experimental cerebral ischemia, primarily using the clot cerebral embolism model in rabbits (46).

Using similar techniques that have been historically employed in the canine model, Zhang et al. (47) described a reproducible experimental model of cerebral infarction without craniotomy in New Zealand white rabbits. This technique uses a silicone rubber cylinder embedded in a nylon suture delivered to the MCA through the ICA. The attachment of the suture allows withdrawal of the silicone embolus to enable the study of reperfusion. Rabbit MCA occlusion has also been performed surgically by ligation or clipping of the MCA through a retro-orbital approach, as well as using the suture model previously discussed in the rodent section. However, like the suture or microsphere embolism models used to create stroke in the rat, these methods do not permit the study of drug or device recanalization strategies.

Although different models have been described using a variety of methods to occlude the large arteries of the cerebrovasculature, here we focus on the small or the large clot embolism model. The key advantage of both of these models is the induction of cerebral ischemia in an awake, intact, normothermic white New Zealand rabbit. The small clot embolism model induces a heterogenous stroke, whereas the large clot model produces a more homogenous stroke. Unfortunately, rabbits like the rodent models have brains that are lissencephalic and thus do not accurately represent the anatomy of the human brain.

The Small Clot Embolism Model

Zivin and his group have used and thoroughly documented the rabbit small clot embolism model (RSCEM) for over two decades (selected from numerous publications (46,48–50)). Blood is derived from a donor rabbit and allowed to clot for 2 h of incubation at 37°C. The clot is suspended in an isotonic solution containing bovine serum albumin and fragmented with a Polytron homogenizer. Subsequently, the solution is filtered to collect emboli that range between 100 and 250 µm in maximum diameter and then centrifuged and weighed. A predetermined weight of emboli are then collected and diluted in phosphate buffered saline for injection into the ICA. Often, the solution containing these microemboli may be seeded with radiolabeled particles to quantify the amount of emboli that make it to the brain and their distribution.

After anesthetizing the rabbits, one of the carotid bifurcations is exposed, and the external carotid artery is ligated. A catheter is then introduced and secured in the common carotid artery. After closing the incision leaving the distal end of the catheter extracorporeal, the animals are allowed to recover for a minimum of 3 h. Thereafter, the solution containing the emboli is injected, and the animals are observed at various points following the induction of cerebral ischemia.

The typical endpoint that is used in this model is a neurological exam that is simplified to a binary outcome, namely noting whether the animal is normal or abnormal. Abnormal animals are those that do not survive the ischemia or present with a variety of neurological deficits including nystagmus, ataxia, leaning, circling, or paralysis. The simplicity of this grading system allows for low to no intraobserver variability and as such is very reproducible. Small weights of clots injected result in no abnormal rabbit behavior, whereas large clot weights produce

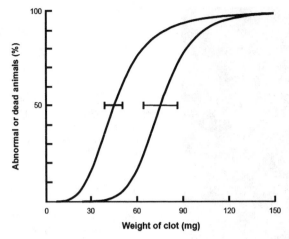

FIGURE 3 The plot shows the percent of neurologically abnormal or dead rabbits versus the weight of small emboli that are released into the intracranial circulation. The control curve is found on the left and those animals treated with tPA are represented in the right curve. These data show that the average weight of clot leading to death or neurological deficit in 50% of the population was significantly higher when tPA was introduced. These data along with data from other studies led to the successful clinical use of tPA. *Source*: From Ref. (46), reprinted with permission from AAAS.

death or encephalopathy. This allows a quantal analysis to be performed typically comparing the results of a thrombolytic or neuroprotective therapy to a control group (Fig. 3).

The advantages of the RSCEM include tracing the emboli with small quantities of radiolabeled material allowing direct visual inspection for documenting thrombosis and thrombolyis if thrombolytic agents are used. This avoids the use of angiography and thus eliminates the risk of repeated injections of contrast dye, which has been demonstrated quite toxic for animals with brain infarction (51). Moreover, the very well established quantal dose analysis method for evaluating the results in using this model is elegant, simple, and repeatable. The disadvantages of the RSCEM involve the administration of blood microclots that result in random infarcts throughout the brain, including the cortical and subcortical structures. This does not model the majority of strokes that occur in humans. Furthermore, a significant variation of the rabbit cervical ICA has been described, which may lead to misdirection of the emboli (52).

The Large Clot Embolism Model

The rabbit large clot embolism model (RLCEM) uses either autologous or allogenic blood that is incubated for 3–4 h at 37°C for later use as a thromboembolus (53–57). Under anesthesia, a catheter is placed into the common carotid artery and the external carotid artery is ligated, as described previously in the RSCEM. The clot is injected in either awake or anesthetized animals depending on the endpoint of the study. Some studies use invasive CBF and intracranial pressure measurements, in which cases the animals remain under anesthesia for the duration of the experiment (53). The clot may be seeded with radiolabeled microparticles to verify that the clot becomes lodged in the brain. It is important when using this model to confirm clot placement and resulting ischemia by (i) CBF measurements, (ii) neurological evidence of cerebral ischemia in awake animals, or (iii) measurement of radioactivity in the brain from the radiolabeled clot. If no occlusion results based on the confirmation method, a second clot may be injected. It is important to note that if inadvertently the clot becomes lodged in

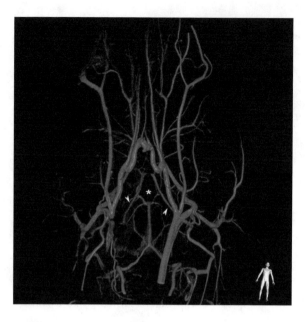

FIGURE 4 3D rotational angiogram (*frontal view*) of the rabbit intra- and extracranial circulations, acquired and reconstructed using Philips Allura FD20 and workstations in our laboratories. Noteworthy are the clear depiction of the internal carotid arteries (*arrowheads*) and the circle of Willis (*asterisk*). Note the absence of the right common carotid artery, which was sacrificed previously, however having no impact on the circulation to the brain or head (White New Zealand rabbit, 3.5 kg). (See also color plate section.)

the ICA, no ischemic stroke will ensue in this model due to the complete circle of Willis in the rabbit (57) (Fig. 4).

Benes et al. (54) developed a reliable model of embolic stroke using autologous arterial thrombus, which may more closely parallel the clinical situation of embolic stroke in humans. The day before the embolization, the rabbits are anesthetized and the auricular arteries of both ears are cannulated with a modified spinal needle. This needle is used to damage a 2-cm segment of the arterial endothelium by mechanical disruption of the vessel lumen. After withdrawing the needle, a ligature is loosely placed proximal to the injured segment of the vessel to diminish blood flow and to enhance thrombus formation. The day after, the rabbits are reanesthetized, the injured segment of the auricular artery is resected and the thrombus separated from the vessel wall. This thrombus may then be injected into the ICA where blood flow carries it to the MCA.

The advantages of the RLCEM include the relative simplicity of the procedure and the use of a larger animal model that is easily managed and monitored/controlled physiologically while under anesthesia as compared with rodents. Moreover, the resulting stroke is more homogenous than the previously described RSCEM. The primary disadvantage in using the RLCEM is the relatively low reproducibility of the infarct. In fact, it has been reported that only about 65% of the animals will incur a stroke as determined by measuring the radioactivity following the injection of radiolabeled large emboli (56).

Cat Models

The cat model is one of the smallest gyrencephalic animal models that has been used in the study of acute stroke. The transorbital approach to occlude the MCA, described in the late 1960s and early 1970s (58,59), has been very important in the study of stroke and imaging of stroke. The larger brain of the cat enables the use of clinical imaging equipment, rather than the specialized scanners that have since been developed for rodents. The most common method for inducing a focal ischemic stroke in cats is to either clipped or ligate the MCA for either permanent or temporary occlusion. An obvious disadvantage of this model is the complete loss of vision in one eye. Not only does this have ethical consideration (Category E, unrelieved distress to the animal), but the absence of ipsilateral visual input affects the neurological assessment of the MCA occlusion. For the latter reason, bilateral enucleation to avoid asymmetries has been described (60). These limiting factors were overcome when a postorbital approach was developed by taking advantage of the lack of a bony wall on both the lateral and the inferior sides of the orbit in cats, thus causing a minimal impairment of vision (61). Owing to ethical issues and the variable infarct size due to excellent collateral circulation (62), the cat model of ischemic stroke is not widely used in the United States, with most current reports coming from abroad.

Dog Models

The canine model of focal brain ischemia is historically very important. Hill et al. described the first embolic stroke model in animals using autologous blood clots to occlude the canine MCA, which predictably caused gross hemorrhagic infarction (25). In this model, a relatively large volume of clot was needed to occlude the MCA. As a result, researchers modified the model by injecting a wide variety of foreign bodies into the intracranial arteries, including liquid vinyl acetate (63), microfibrillar collagen (64,65), and silicone plugs (66,67).

The dog model of focal cerebral ischemia is challenging due to an extensive collateral circulation through the maxillo-carotid and meningocerebral anastomoses (Fig. 5), which makes it difficult to obtain reproducible infarction. In the seminal

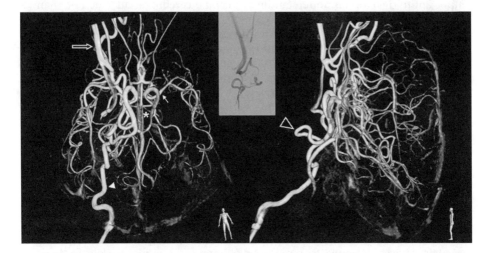

FIGURE 5 3D rotational angiogram (Allura FD20, Philips Healthcare, Best, the Netherlands) from a right internal carotid artery (ICA) (*solid arrowhead*) injection in the dog with contrast perfusing to the left brain hemisphere and posterior circulation, showing a complete circle of Willis in the frontal (*left panel, asterisk*) and lateral projections (*right panel*). Of note is the maxillo-carotid anastomosis (*open arrow*) also shown in a right ICA selective, digitally subtracted angiogram following anterior cerebral artery (ACA) and MCA occlusion with clot (*inset*). The extreme tortuosity is appreciated in the lateral projection (*open arrowhead*) (Mongrel dog, 25 kg).

work of Molinari, infarctions involving the deep ganglia and internal capsule were created by launching a silicone embolus having a diameter of 1.66 mm into the ICA (67). The plug consistently occluded the proximal segment of the MCA despite the size of the dog (the intracranial vasculature was found to have consistent intracranial arterial diameters independent of animal weight). Much later, quantification of the infarct size was performed in this model using creatine kinase BB isoenzyme that was correlated with histological measurements (68), and it was found that the infarct volume is highly variable in this model. This model has been used over the course of nearly four decades to evaluate treatments for stroke in a large animal model, including superficial temporal artery-MCA bypass (69), surgical embolectomy (70,71), and recently prophylactic administration of edaravone (72). In a novel investigation, the model was adapted using a thread that was embedded into the silicone plug, thus allowing removal of the embolus to study the difference between transient and permanent ischemia with calcium 45 autoradiolgraphy (73). In this study dual-isotope single-photon emission computed tomography (SPECT) was used to quantify CBF, thus showing the utility of a large animal model in a clinical imaging system.

The careful characterization of infarct size and distribution, hemodynamics, and clinicopathology as a result of permanently or temporarily clipping combinations of the large intracranial arteries of dogs has been well documented (74–78). Numerous endpoints have been devised when using the canine stroke model, including CBF measurements, MR perfusion/diffusion mismatch, clinical neurological assessment and grading, and somatosensory evoked potential monitoring. Although surgical exposure through a craniotomy and clipping of the cerebrovasculature in the dog is rarely performed today, these experiments have been very important to develop an understanding of canine cerebrovascular hemodynamics and ischemic stroke evolution.

Recent studies have returned to the original canine embolic stroke model, using autologous blood clots injected into the ICA through an angiographic catheter to create an occlusion of the MCA (79). This study demonstrated that the occlusion can be reversed by the intra-arterial administration of t-PA. In this model, both common femoral arteries were cannulated and a catheter was placed in one of the ICAs while a separate catheter was placed in the left atrium of the heart for injection of contrast agent. Four to ten milliliters of arterial blood was drawn, mixed with bovine thrombin, and incubated within a tube at room temperature for 45 min. After rinsing, the clots were injected through a syringe into the catheter located in the ICA. Occlusion of the MCA was confirmed using digital subtraction angiography (DSA). MR perfusion and diffusion-weighted imaging were performed to track the evolution of the infarct. Of note, severe field inhomogeneities resulting in MR artifacts were found due to the large sinuses of the dogs and corrected for by injecting a viscous liquid through burr holes drilled in the sinuses.

Unfortunately, the tortuosity of the ICA is prohibitive for the testing of endovascular devices designed to remove or obliterate the embolus (Fig. 5). For this reason, autologous clots may also be delivered into the posterior cerebral circulation, occluding either the vertebral (80) or the basilar artery (81). The catheter is tracked through the anastamosis between the vertebral and the anterior spinal arteries and then through the vertebrobasilar junction to inject the clot into the basilar artery (Fig. 6). This technique was used to evaluate the safety and efficacy of intra-arterially administered reteplase and intravenous alteplase (81). Levy and

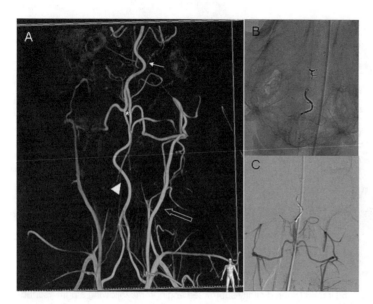

FIGURE 6 Frontal projection of a rotational angiogram (*A*) in a dog with the injection from the left vertebral artery (*open arrow*). The large anterior spinal artery (*arrowhead*) is used to navigate the catheter and subsequent endovascular devices into the basilar artery (*arrow*) through the vertebrobasilar junction (*asterisk*). Tantalum seeded autologous clot (*B*) that was allowed to mature for approximately 15 h produces a basilar top and mid-basilar occlusion (*C*) (Mongrel dog, 25 kg).

colleagues (80) investigated the potential use of intracranial stents in recanalizing large clot embolisms that had occluded the distal vertebral artery.

One of the advantages of the canine model is its compatibility with nonspecialized, clinical imaging equipment, unlike smaller animal models. Additionally, the vessel size and degree of vasospasm in dogs are more similar to humans than rodent models and allow for more targeted arterial embolization. The caliber of the intracranial vasculature is sufficient to permit the investigation of new endovascular devices, an area that in recent years has been gaining traction and discussed with great detail in Part 2, Chapter 7. Vessel occlusion with autologous clots means that this model is useful for studying thrombolytic agents as well.

Canine brains contain less white matter than human brains, which affects the metabolic demands of the brain tissue and thresholds for cell death. This difference could make extrapolating the canine data to human subjects difficult. Moreover, dogs have a strong fibinolytic system (82) which must be taken into consideration as fresh clots have the tendency to autolyse. Finally, like with cats, the sensitivity of the public brings to the forefront ethical considerations when using this model.

Pig and Sheep Models
Both pigs and sheep have an endogenous vascular filter that branches the aberrant blood flow to the brain through a series of small, capillary-like vessels that recoalesce into the ICA (Fig. 7). This vascular structure, the rete mirabile, makes anterior strokes impossible through embolic means. Occlusion of the MCA through vascular

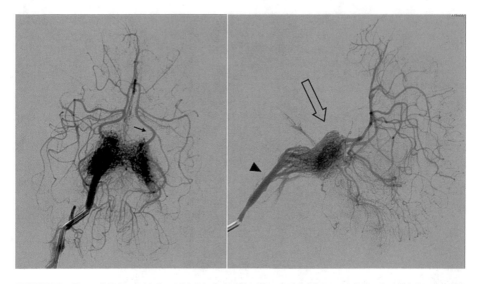

FIGURE 7   Frontal (*left*) and lateral (*right*) digitally subtracted angiograms following a right ascending pharyngeal artery injection (*arrowhead*). The rete-mirabile is the dominant vascular structure (*open arrow*), which with a rapid contrast injection (2.5 ml/s) perfuses both hemispheres (seen clearly in the frontal projection). The internal carotid artery (ICA) arises dorsally from the rete (*arrow*) (Yorkshire pig, 35 kg).

clips by a craniotomy or by a transorbital approach has been described (83,84). Similar to the other gyrencephalic models of stroke, this large animal model allows for the study of stroke with clinical imaging equipment (85–89) and allays some of the public sensitivities posed by cats and dogs.

Despite the inability to stroke the anterior circulation of pigs, endovascular devices intended to recanalize occluded vessels are frequently tested in the extracranial circulation (90–92); however, the impact on infarct size and functional outcomes in terms of stroke may not be evaluated. The rete mirabile in swine (or perhaps sheep) serves to catch distal emboli or fragments that result from endovascular thrombectomy to open occlusions of the ascending pharyngeal artery with autologous clot. Subsequently, the rete may be harvested to quantify the size and number of emboli.

Novel models to induce stroke in pigs include the recently described photothrombosis MCA occlusion model in piglets (93), a lacunar stroke model, wherein the anterior choroidal artery is occluded in minipigs (94) and the use of ethanol to produce contractions of the MCA and basilar artery (95). Unfortunately, these models of stroke in pigs do not enable the study of revascularization drugs or devices.

CONCLUSION

Animal models of focal cerebral ischemia have assisted in the development of (i) understanding the basic pathophysiology of stroke, (ii) the various imaging modalities that are now used clinically to visualize the infarcted and viable tissues as well as the risks associated with revascularization, and (iii) both thrombolytic and thrombectomy devices that improve the quality of life or save the lives of stroke victims everyday. The disappointing results of numerous clinical trials pursuing neuroprotective therapies have generated tremendous controversy surrounding the utility of animal models in acute stroke therapy (96–98). This is not a new phenomenon, as various cancer, myocardial regeneration, or angiogenic therapies have found success in preclinical labs only to be met with failure in large scale clinical trials. The fault lies perhaps not with the inaccuracy of the animal modeling but rather in the interpretation of the data.

Stroke modeling is not a simple endeavor, as a great number of variables including physiological monitoring, thermal control, plasma glucose concentrations, anesthesia maintenance, and experience of the operator all have a dramatic impact on the data collected. Beyond that, like in all areas of science, these variables should be taken into account when proper statistical analyses are performed, and the studies are sufficiently powered. More important are the advantages and limitations posed by each modeling system and asking the appropriate question of that system. This chapter has aimed to provide an overview of the most common animal models of focal ischemia and provide references to more detailed studies, so that the reader may choose the most appropriate model(s) for a given hypothesis.

REFERENCES

1. Sacco RL, Wolf PA, Gorelick PB. Risk factors and their management for stroke prevention: outlook for 1999 and beyond. Neurology 1999; 53(7 suppl 4):S15–S24.
2. del Zoppo GJ, Poeck K, Pessin MS, et al. Recombinant tissue plasminogen activator in acute thrombotic and embolic stroke. Ann Neurol 1992; 32(1):78–86.
3. Hsu CY. Criteria for valid preclinical trials using animal stroke models. Stroke 1993; 24(5):633–636.
4. Yamori Y, Horie R, Handa H, et al. Pathogenetic similarity of strokes in stroke-prone spontaneously hypertensive rats and humans. Stroke 1976; 7(1):46–53.
5. Coyle P. Middle cerebral artery occlusion in the young rat. Stroke 1982; 13(6):855–859.
6. Ginsberg MD, Busto R. Rodent models of cerebral ischemia. Stroke 1989; 20(12):1627–1642.
7. Hoyte L, Kaur J, Buchan AM. Lost in translation: taking neuroprotection from animal models to clinical trials. Exp Neurol 2004; 188(2):200–204.
8. Koizumi J, Yoshida Y, Nakazawa T, et al. Experimental studies of ischemic brain edema. I: a new experimental model of cerebral embolism in rats in which recirculation can be introduced in the ischemic area. Jap J Stroke 1986; 8:1–8.
9. Belayev L, Alonso OF, Busto R, et al. Middle cerebral artery occlusion in the rat by intraluminal suture. Neurological and pathological evaluation of an improved model. Stroke 1996; 27(9):1616–1622; discussion 1623.
10. Takano K, Tatlisumak T, Bergmann AG, et al. Reproducibility and reliability of middle cerebral artery occlusion using a silicone-coated suture (Koizumi) in rats. J Neurol Sci 1997; 153(1):8–11.
11. Longa EZ, Weinstein PR, Carlson S, et al. Reversible middle cerebral artery occlusion without craniectomy in rats. Stroke 1989; 20(1):84–91.
12. Nagasawa H, Kogure K. Correlation between cerebral blood flow and histologic changes in a new rat model of middle cerebral artery occlusion. Stroke 1989; 20(8):1037–1043.
13. Li F, Han S, Tatlisumak T, et al. A new method to improve in-bore middle cerebral artery occlusion in rats: demonstration with diffusion- and perfusion-weighted imaging. Stroke 1998; 29(8):1715–1719; discussion 1719–1720.
14. Li F, Tatlisumak T. Focal brain ischemia models in rodents. In: Tatlisumak T, Fisher M, eds. Handbook of Experimental Neurology: Methods and Techniques in Animal Research. Cambridge: Cambridge University Press, 2006:311–328.
15. Meng X, Fisher M, Shen Q, et al. Characterizing the diffusion/perfusion mismatch in experimental focal cerebral ischemia. Ann Neurol 2004; 55(2):207–212.

16. Kuge Y, Minematsu K, Yamaguchi T, et al. Nylon monofilament for intraluminal middle cerebral artery occlusion in rats. Stroke 1995; 26(9):1655–1657.

17. Zarow GJ, Karibe H, States BA, et al. Endovascular suture occlusion of the middle cerebral artery in rats: effect of suture insertion distance on cerebral blood flow, infarct distribution and infarct volume. Neurol Res 1997; 19(4):409–416.

18. Oliff HS, Weber E, Miyazaki B, et al. Infarct volume varies with rat strain and vendor in focal cerebral ischemia induced by transcranial middle cerebral artery occlusion. Brain Res 1995; 699(2):329–331.

19. Schmid-Elsaesser R, Zausinger S, Hungerhuber E, et al. A critical reevaluation of the intraluminal thread model of focal cerebral ischemia: evidence of inadvertent premature reperfusion and subarachnoid hemorrhage in rats by laser-Doppler flowmetry. Stroke 1998; 29(10):2162–2170.

20. Zhao Q, Memezawa H, Smith ML, et al. Hyperthermia complicates middle cerebral artery occlusion induced by an intraluminal filament. Brain Res 1994; 649(1–2):253–259.

21. Li F, Omae T, Fisher M. Spontaneous hyperthermia and its mechanism in the intraluminal suture middle cerebral artery occlusion model of rats. Stroke 1999; 30(11):2464–2470.

22. Sicard KM, Henninger N, Fisher M, et al. Differential recovery of multimodal MRI and behavior after transient focal cerebral ischemia in rats. J Cereb Blood Flow Metab 2006; 26(11):1451–1462.

23. Sicard KM, Henninger N, Fisher M, et al. Long-term changes of functional MRI-based brain function, behavioral status, and histopathology after transient focal cerebral ischemia in rats. Stroke 2006; 37(10):2593–2600.

24. Futrell N, Watson BD, Dietrich WD, et al. A new model of embolic stroke produced by photochemical injury to the carotid artery in the rat. Ann Neurol 1988; 23(3): 251–257.

25. Hill NC, Millikan CH, Wakim KG, et al. Studies in cerebrovascular disease. VII. Experimental production of cerebral infarction by intracarotid injection of homologous blood clot: preliminary report. Mayo Clin Proc 1955; 30(26):625–633.

26. Kudo M, Aoyama A, Ichimori S, et al. An animal model of cerebral infarction. Homologous blood clot emboli in rats. Stroke 1982; 13(4):505–508.

27. Henninger N, Sicard KM, Schmidt KF, et al. Comparison of ischemic lesion evolution in embolic versus mechanical middle cerebral artery occlusion in Sprague Dawley rats using diffusion and perfusion imaging. Stroke 2006; 37(5):1283–1287.

28. Albers GW. Antithrombotic agents in cerebral ischemia. Am J Cardiol 1995; 75(6):34B–38B.

29. NINDS Study Investigators. Tissue plasminogen activator for acute ischemic stroke. The National Institute of Neurological Disorders and Stroke t-PA stroke study group. N Engl J Med 1995; 333(24):1581–1587.

30. Savitz SI, Fisher M. Future of neuroprotection for acute stroke: in the aftermath of the saint trials. Ann Neurol 2007; 61(5):396–402.

31. Busch E, Kruger K, Hossmann KA. Improved model of thromboembolic stroke and t-PA induced reperfusion in the rat. Brain Res 1997; 778(1):16–24.

32. Takano K, Carano RA, Tatlisumak T, et al. Efficacy of intra-arterial and intravenous prourokinase in an embolic stroke model evaluated by diffusion-perfusion magnetic resonance imaging. Neurology 1998; 50(4):870–875.

33. Henninger N, Sicard KM, Fisher M, et al. Spectacular shrinking deficit: insights from multimodal magnetic resonance imaging after embolic middle cerebral artery occlusion in Sprague-Dawley rats. J Cereb Blood Flow Metab 2007; 27(10):1756–1763.

34. Siegel BA, Meidinger R, Elliott AJ, et al. Experimental cerebral microembolism. Multiple tracer assessment of brain edema. Arch Neurol 1972; 26(1):73–77.

35. Garcia JH. Experimental ischemic stroke: a review. Stroke 1984; 15(1):5–14.

36. Takeda T, Shima T, Okada Y, et al. Pathophysiological studies of cerebral ischemia produced by silicone cylinder embolization in rats. J Cereb Blood Flow 1987; 7(suppl):S66.

37. Fukuchi K, Kusuoka H, Watanabe Y, et al. Correlation of sequential MR images of microsphere-induced cerebral ischemia with histologic changes in rats. Invest Radiol 1999; 34(11):698–703.

38. Gerriets T, Li F, Silva MD, et al. The macrosphere model: evaluation of a new stroke model for permanent middle cerebral artery occlusion in rats. J Neurosci Methods 2003; 122(2):201–211.
39. Watson BD, Dietrich WD, Busto R, et al. Induction of reproducible brain infarction by photochemically initiated thrombosis. Ann Neurol 1985; 17(5):497–504.
40. Dietrich WD, Ginsberg MD, Busto R, et al. Photochemically induced cortical infarction in the rat. 2. Acute and subacute alterations in local glucose utilization. J Cereb Blood Flow Metab 1986; 6(2):195–202.
41. Sugimori H, Yao H, Ooboshi H, et al. Krypton laser-induced photothrombotic distal middle cerebral artery occlusion without craniectomy in mice. Brain Res Brain Res Protoc 2004; 13(3):189–196.
42. Schneider G, Fries P, Wagner-Jochem D, et al. Pathophysiological changes after traumatic brain injury: comparison of two experimental animal models by means of MRI. MAGMA 2002; 14(3):233–241.
43. Carmichael ST. Rodent models of focal stroke: size, mechanism, and purpose. NeuroRx 2005; 2(3):396–409.
44. Heilman CB, Kwan ES, Wu JK. Aneurysm recurrence following endovascular balloon occlusion. J Neurosur 1992; 77(2):260–264.
45. Korninger C, Collen D. Studies on the specific fibrinolytic effect of human extrinsic (tissue-type) plasminogen activator in human blood and in various animal species in vitro. Thromb Haemost 1981; 46(2):561–565.
46. Zivin JA, Fisher M, DeGirolami U, et al. Tissue plasminogen activator reduces neurological damage after cerebral embolism. Science 1985; 230(4731):1289–1292.
47. Zhang SM, Ramirez-Lassepas M, Hernandez LA, et al. A new model of experimental cerebral infarction in New Zealand white rabbits. J Tongji Med Univ 1995; 15(1):5–9.
48. Lapchak PA, Araujo DM, Song D, et al. Neuroprotective effects of the spin trap agent disodium-[(tert-butylimino)methyl]benzene-1,3-disulfonate N-oxide (generic NXY-059) in a rabbit small clot embolic stroke model: combination studies with the thrombolytic tissue plasminogen activator. Stroke 2002; 33(5):1411–1415.
49. Maher P, Salgado KF, Zivin JA, et al. A novel approach to screening for new neuroprotective compounds for the treatment of stroke. Brain Res 2007; 1173:117–125.
50. Lapchak PA, Araujo DM, Pakola S, et al. Microplasmin: a novel thrombolytic that improves behavioral outcome after embolic strokes in rabbits. Stroke 2002; 33(9):2279–2284.
51. Lyden PD, Madden KP, Clark WM, et al. Incidence of cerebral hemorrhage after treatment with tissue plasminogen activator or streptokinase following embolic stroke in rabbits. Stroke 1990; 21(11):1589–1593.
52. Lee JS, Hamilton MG, Zabramski JM. Variations in the anatomy of the rabbit cervical carotid artery. Stroke 1994; 25(2):501–503.
53. Bednar MM, McAuliffe T, Raymond S, et al. Tissue plasminogen activator reduces brain injury in a rabbit model of thromboembolic stroke. Stroke 1990; 21(12):1705–1709.
54. Benes V, Zabramski JM, Boston M, et al. Effect of intra-arterial tissue plasminogen activator and urokinase on autologous arterial emboli in the cerebral circulation of rabbits. Stroke 1990; 21(11):1594–1599.
55. Lapchak PA, Chapman DF, Zivin JA. Pharmacological effects of the spin trap agents N-t-butyl-phenylnitrone (PBN) and 2,2,6, 6-tetramethylpiperidine-N-oxyl (TEMPO) in a rabbit thromboembolic stroke model: combination studies with the thrombolytic tissue plasminogen activator. Stroke 2001; 32(1):147–153.
56. Lapchak PA, Chapman DF, Zivin JA. Metalloproteinase inhibition reduces thrombolytic (tissue plasminogen activator)-induced hemorrhage after thromboembolic stroke. Stroke 2000; 31(12):3034–3040.
57. Russell D, Madden KP, Clark WM, et al. Tissue plasminogen activator cerebrovascular thrombolysis in rabbits is dependent on the rate and route of administration. Stroke 1992; 23(3):388–393.
58. O'Brien MD, Waltz AG. Transorbital approach for occluding the middle cerebral artery without craniectomy. Stroke 1973; 4(2):201–206.

59. Sundt TM, Waltz AG. Experimental cerebral infarction: retro-orbital, extradural approach for occluding the middle cerebral artery. Mayo Clin Proc 1966; 41(3):159–168.
60. Hossmann KA, Mies G, Paschen W, et al. Multiparametric imaging of blood flow and metabolism after middle cerebral artery occlusion in cats. J Cereb Blood Flow Metab 1985; 5(1):97–107.
61. Berkelbach van der Sprenkel JW, Tulleken CA. The postorbital approach to the middle cerebral artery in cats. Stroke 1988; 19(4):503–506.
62. Bose B, Osterholm JL, Berry R. A reproducible experimental model of focal cerebral ischemia in the cat. Brain Res 1984; 311(2):385–391.
63. Davis DO, Rumbaugh CL. Cerebral angiography in the dog. Method for consistent results. Invest Radiol 1967; 2(5):323–325.
64. Purdy PD, Devous MD Sr., Batjer HH, et al. Microfibrillar collagen model of canine cerebral infarction. Stroke 1989; 20(10):1361–1367.
65. Corbett RJ, Purdy PD, Laptook AR, et al. Noninvasive measurement of brain temperature after stroke. AJNR Am J Neuroradiol 1999; 20(10):1851–1857.
66. Molinari GF. Experimental cerebral infarction. II. Clinicopathological model of deep cerebral infarction. Stroke 1970; 1(4):232–244.
67. Molinari GF. Experimental cerebral infarction. I. Selective segmental occlusion of intracranial arteries in the dog. Stroke 1970; 1(4):224–231.
68. Bell RD, Alexander GM, Nguyen T, et al. Quantification of cerebral infarct size by creatine kinase BB isoenzyme. Stroke 1986; 17(2):254–260.
69. Levinthal R, Moseley JI, Brown WJ, et al. Effect of STA-MCA anastomosis on the course of experimental acute MCA embolic occlusion. Stroke 1979; 10(4):371–375.
70. Dujovny M, Osgood CP, Barrionuevo PJ, et al. Middle cerebral artery microneurosurgical embolectomy. Surgery 1976; 80(3):336–339.
71. Laha RK, Israeli J, Dujovny M, et al. Low molecular weight dextran in experimental embolectomy. Stroke 1980; 11(1):59–63.
72. Suzuki T, Kazui T, Yamamoto S, et al. Effect of prophylactically administered edaravone during antegrade cerebral perfusion in a canine model of old cerebral infarction. J Thorac Cardiovasc Surg 2007; 133(3):710–716.
73. Purdy PD, Horowitz MB, Mathews D, et al. Calcium 45 autoradiography and dual-isotope single-photon emission CT in a canine model of cerebral ischemia and middle cerebral artery occlusion. AJNR Am J Neuroradiol 1996; 17(6):1161–1170.
74. Asari S, Kinugasa K, Fujisawa H, et al. Extracranial-intracranial bypass in experimental cerebral infarction in dogs. Stroke 1978; 9(5):461–464.
75. Lawner PM, Laurent JP, Simeone FA, et al. Hemodynamic and clinicopathologic verification of a stroke model in the dog. Stroke 1981; 12(3):313–316.
76. Lawner PM, Laurent JP, Simeone FA, et al. Effect of extracranial-intracranial bypass and pentobarbital on acute stroke in dogs. J Neurosurg 1982; 56(1):92–96.
77. Seki H, Yoshimoto T, Ogawa A, et al. Hemodynamics in hemorrhagic infarction—an experimental study. Stroke 1985; 16(4):647–651.
78. Suzuki J, Tanaka S, Yoshimoto T. Suppression of brain swelling with mannitol and perfluorochemicals. An experimental study. Acta Neurochir (Wien) 1981; 58(3–4):149–160.
79. Shaibani A, Khawar S, Shin W, et al. First results in an MR imaging—compatible canine model of acute stroke. AJNR Am J Neuroradiol 2006; 27(8):1788–1793.
80. Levy EI, Sauvageau E, Hanel RA, et al. Self-expanding versus balloon-mounted stents for vessel recanalization following embolic occlusion in the canine model: technical feasibility study. AJNR Am J Neuroradiol 2006; 27(10):2069–2072.
81. Qureshi AI, Boulos AS, Hanel RA, et al. Randomized comparison of intra-arterial and intravenous thrombolysis in a canine model of acute basilar artery thrombosis. Neuroradiol 2004; 46(12):988–995.
82. Osterman FA, Bell WR, Montali RJ, et al. Natural history of autologous blood clot embolization in swine. Invest Radiol 1976; 11(4):267–276.
83. Imai H, Konno K, Nakamura M, et al. A new model of focal cerebral ischemia in the miniature pig. J Neurosurg 2006; 104(2 suppl):123–132.

84. Zhang L, Cheng H, Shi J, et al. Focal epidural cooling reduces the infarction volume of permanent middle cerebral artery occlusion in swine. Surg Neurol 2007; 67(2):117–121.
85. Rohl L, Sakoh M, Simonsen CZ, et al. Time evolution of cerebral perfusion and apparent diffusion coefficient measured by magnetic resonance imaging in a porcine stroke model. J Magn Reson Imaging 2002; 15(2):123–129.
86. Sakoh M, Gjedde A. Neuroprotection in hypothermia linked to redistribution of oxygen in brain. Am J Physiol Heart Circ Physiol 2003; 285(1):H17–H25.
87. Sakoh M, Ohnishi T, Ostergaard L, et al. Prediction of tissue survival after stroke based on changes in the apparent diffusion of water (cytotoxic edema). Acta Neurochir Suppl 2003; 86:137–140.
88. Sakoh M, Ostergaard L, Gjedde A, et al. Prediction of tissue survival after middle cerebral artery occlusion based on changes in the apparent diffusion of water. J Neurosurg 2001; 95(3):450–458.
89. Sakoh M, Ostergaard L, Røhl L, et al. Relationship between residual cerebral blood flow and oxygen metabolism as predictive of ischemic tissue viability: sequential multitracer positron emission tomography scanning of middle cerebral artery occlusion during the critical first 6 hours after stroke in pigs. J Neurosurg 2000; 93(4):647–657.
90. Culp WC, Porter TR, Lowery J, et al. Intracranial clot lysis with intravenous microbubbles and transcranial ultrasound in swine. Stroke 2004; 35(10):2407–2411.
91. Gralla J, Schroth G, Remonda L, et al. Mechanical thrombectomy for acute ischemic stroke: thrombus-device interaction, efficiency, and complications in vivo. Stroke 2006; 37(12):3019–3024.
92. Gralla J, Burkhardt M, Schroth G, et al. Occlusion length is a crucial determinant of efficiency and complication rate in thrombectomy for acute ischemic stroke. AJNR Am J Neuroradiol 2008; Epub ahead of print:1–6.
93. Kuluz JW, Prado R, He D, et al. New pediatric model of ischemic stroke in infant piglets by photothrombosis: acute changes in cerebral blood flow, microvasculature, and early histopathology. Stroke 2007; 38(6):1932–1937.
94. Tanaka Y, Imai H, Konno K, et al. Experimental model of lacunar infarction in the gyrencephalic brain of the miniature pig: neurological assessment and histological, immunohistochemical, and physiological evaluation of dynamic corticospinal tract deformation. Stroke 2008; 39(1):205–212.
95. Zhang A, Altura BT, Altura BM. Ethanol-induced contraction of cerebral arteries in diverse mammals and its mechanism of action. Eur J Pharmacol 1993; 248(3):229–236.
96. Dirnagl U. Bench to bedside: the quest for quality in experimental stroke research. J Cereb Blood Flow Metab 2006; 26(12):1465–1478.
97. Fisher M, Tatlisumak T. Use of animal models has not contributed to development of acute stroke therapies: con. Stroke 2005; 36(10):2324–2325.
98. Kaste M. Use of animal models has not contributed to development of acute stroke therapies: pro. Stroke 2005; 36(10):2323–2324.

4 Assessment and Management of Vascular Implant Thrombogenecity

Sivaprasad Sukavaneshvar

Medical Device Evaluation Center, Salt Lake City, Utah, U.S.A.

INTRODUCTION

Vascular implants such as stents and coils have been used successfully to treat diseases such as atherosclerosis and aneurysms (1–3). These devices, however, carry the risk of thrombosis, which warrants consideration during device design and during clinical implantation. Device thrombosis and thromboembolism are influenced by surface chemistry, device geometry, inherent blood reactivity, and pharmacological intervention (anticoagulants, antiplatelet agents, etc.). The first two factors influence device design; the latter two factors guide the clinical management of the patient. Both the device design and the clinical management need to account for the flow conditions experienced by the implant. Experimental models and in vitro diagnostic tools have been developed to evaluate device design iterations and to facilitate the clinical management of patients with implants. This chapter will discuss (i) the assessment of the thrombogenic and thromboembolic potential of vascular implants using in vitro and ex vivo experimental models and (ii) the in vitro diagnostic instruments that aid in the assessment of the individual's inherent thrombotic risk and in the assessment of anticoagulant/antiplatelet agent efficacy (Fig. 1).

IN VITRO MODELS

In vitro models for the assessment of device thrombosis and thromboembolism can assume a variety of configurations (4,5). Static models expose a device to blood or blood components (e.g., blood plasma) in a test tube with minimal or no motion and aim to monitor the adsorption of key hemostatic proteins (e.g., fibrinogen) and/or the deposition of cellular elements involved in thrombosis (e.g., platelets) (6). Flow models incorporate blood flow in an attempt to simulate an important aspect of the in vivo situation and generally evaluate the integrated thrombotic process of protein adsorption, platelet adhesion and aggregation, and fibrin consolidation. The discussion in this chapter will be confined to in vitro flow models that utilize fresh mammalian whole blood.

In its most generic form, the in vitro flow model incorporates anticoagulated blood flowing through a test chamber (e.g., polymer tubing) in which the device to be evaluated is deployed (Fig. 2). The thrombus that develops on the device is generally measured after blood has circulated for a desired duration. Blood from the same subject can be divided into as many reservoirs as there are devices to facilitate simultaneous comparisons (e.g., coated vs. uncoated stents). Variations of this basic construct of the model may include different species/sources of blood, methods of anticoagulation, test chamber geometries, hemodynamics (flow rates,

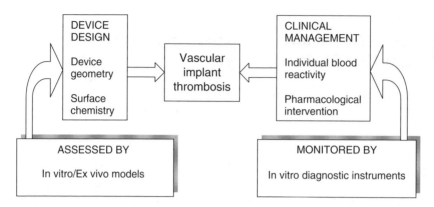

FIGURE 1   Chart depicts the factors that influence vascular implant thrombosis.

flow-inducing mechanisms, etc.), system configurations, experiment duration, and methods to assess thrombosis and thromboembolism. These model parameters are discussed in detail subsequently.

Prior to discussing the specifications of in vitro models, a delineation of the difference between device thrombosis and blood clotting is warranted. The terms "clot" and "thrombus" are often used interchangeably in the literature, and although they are closely related, there are a few essential differences between the thrombosis and clotting that have a bearing on how implants are designed and managed (Table 1). *Device thrombosis* is generally a phenomenon mediated by disturbed flow in which platelets play a major role. Specifically, the presence of (i) high wall shear rates that activate platelets, (ii) reattachment points of increased normal velocity that promote platelet adhesion, and (iii) recirculation zones where activated platelets collide with

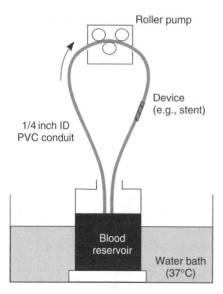

FIGURE 2   A typical dynamic in vitro flow model configuration is illustrated. This schematic shows a single blood reservoir, but multiple devices can be compared with such a model using blood from a single subject divided into separate reservoirs for simultaneous comparisons without cross-over effects.

TABLE 1 Comparison of Thrombosis and Clotting

Thrombosis	Clotting
Requires flow	Does not require flow; occurs in stagnant/ low flow areas (stasis)
Platelets play a major role	Primarily clotting protein mediated
Complex interplay of proteins, platelets, and other blood cells and fluid dynamics	Essentially polymerization of fibrinogen to fibrin

each other to aggregate and fibrin consolidation occurs are required for thrombus formation on devices. Therefore, device thrombosis is a complex interplay of proteins, platelets and other blood cells, and fluid dynamics. In contrast, *clotting* is a phenomenon mediated by plasma-protein and does not require the presence of flow. Blood may clot more readily in regions of low flow and stagnation. Blood clotting, which can be viewed simplistically as the polymerization of fibrinogen to fibrin, does not require platelets or other cellular components (although platelets do participate in-vivo by releasing procoagulant proteins from their granules). The discussion in this chapter will pertain generally to device thrombosis.

Choice of Species
Human, bovine, or porcine blood may be used for in vitro thrombosis studies. Although human blood is preferred intuitively, blood volume limitations may restrict the use of human blood in certain situations. For example, in studies where several devices are to be compared with blood from the same donor at high blood flow rates, large volumes of blood may be required to minimize the impact of extraneous hemostatic component activation on the test and to elicit measurable thrombosis on the devices to improve test sensitivity. As 450–500 ml (1 unit) is considered the maximum volume of blood that can be collected safely from a single human donor, studies that require larger volumes of blood are not served suitably by blood from a single human donor. Blood pooled from several donors may be used, but may be less desirable than blood from a single donor, due to the cost, inconvenience, and absence of data supporting the validity of pooled blood in the context of device thrombosis. In such situations, bovine blood represents an appropriate alternative (7–10). Typically, 5–10 L of blood may be collected from a single large cow in an abattoir through cardiac puncture, which is sufficient for most studies. Although porcine blood is also a suitable alternative to human blood, the volume of blood that can be collected from a single pig is typically less than that obtainable from a cow. Other species such as ovine, canine, primate, murine, and rabbit, which are used for in vivo thrombosis studies, are generally not suitable for in vitro studies due to blood volume limitations, unavailability, and cost.

There have been no comprehensive studies that have compared human blood and blood from various animal species in the context of in vitro device thrombosis to determine whether any particular species approximates human blood more closely than others. However, most in vitro studies are intended to provide *relative* comparisons between multiple devices, and many key hematology parameters for most animals mentioned above overlap with human blood. Thus, the actual species may be less important in the context of comparing thrombosis of various devices in vitro.

Blood Collection and Anticoagulation

Blood is usually collected from the donor by venipuncture (antecubital vein in humans), vascular access (e.g., jugular/femoral vein or artery of animals), or cardiac puncture (animals) into a collection reservoir containing an anticoagulant. One of the important goals during blood collection is to limit the undesirable activation of platelets and the coagulation cascade that can result from blood contact with the needle or other collection components. Owing to more open tissue, trauma, and a potentially greater release of epinephrine (a platelet activator) into bovine blood collected by cardiac puncture in an abattoir compared with human blood collected by venipuncture, hemostatic components may be more activated in bovine blood. In contrast, as it takes less than 5 min to collect 5–10 L of blood from a cow through cardiac puncture (through a 0.5 inch inner diameter (ID) cannula), and it can take longer to collect 450 ml of blood from a human through venipuncture (through a 16-gauge needle), more hemostatic component activation may occur in human blood due to the longer exposure of blood to the needle and other collection components during venipuncture in humans compared with cardiac puncture in cows. In either case, it is prudent to discard some of the initial blood, which may be tainted with tissue factor that activates the hemostatic system.

Owing to the contact of blood with biomaterials (e.g., blood bags, tubing) in in vitro models, which results in the activation of the clotting cascade, anticoagulation is an unavoidable requirement of the in vitro milieu. The anticoagulant is intended to prevent clotting in the system (reservoir, tubing, and so on) but to allow thrombosis on the device of interest. Heparin and sodium citrate are the most commonly used anticoagulants in such models that satisfy this requirement (Table 2). Briefly, heparin deactivates specific clotting proteins (e.g., by binding to antithrombin-III and enhancing antithrombin's ability to neutralize thrombin); citrate binds calcium ions that are required for clotting. A detailed discussion of heparin's mechanism of action can be found elsewhere (11). At the appropriate concentration, heparin can prevent blood clotting while permitting device thrombosis. In contrast, sodium citrate (at the typically used concentration of 0.038%) completely prevents blood clotting and device thrombosis, and recalcification of citrated blood (e.g., with calcium chloride) typically restores coagulation and thrombosis completely. Although partially citrating/recalcifying blood to tune clotting and thrombosis is a theoretical possibility, its practical implementation is challenging, and the citrate–calcium titration for anticoagulation and its reversal is a binary process in reality. Thus, thrombosis and clotting can be delinked and tuned more easily by adjusting heparin concentrations; this is difficult with sodium citrate. A notable ramification of this difference is that heparinized blood facilitates a longer experimental duration (few hours), and citrated blood that is recalcified will allow only short experiments

TABLE 2 Comparison of Heparin and Citrate

Heparin	Citrate
Deactivates specific clotting proteins	Binds calcium ions in the plasma
Allows longer experiment durations	Only short experiments are possible (after recalcification)
Delinks clotting and thrombosis by preventing the former while allowing the latter	Clotting and thrombosis are inextricably intertwined

(<1 h) due to the relatively rapid clotting of this blood. Aside from the logistical advantages of heparin, the fact that it is also the most widely used anticoagulant clinically makes it the preferred anticoagulant for studying device thrombosis in vitro in many situations.

It may be noted that the use of heparin may limit the study of certain device thrombosis situations. One relevant example is platinum coils packed into in vitro models of aneurysms. In such a system, the coils near the neck of the aneurysm will experience disturbed flow and, similar to what is expected in vivo, will foster thrombosis in vitro even with heparinized blood. In contrast, the coils in the fundus of the aneurysm will experience low flow or stagnant blood. Although this is expected to eventually result in clotting in vivo, the presence of heparin restricts (or prevents) clot formation in vitro. The use of recalcified citrated blood will not remedy this problem, due to rapid clotting throughout the system, and such situations expose an important limitation of in vitro models vis-à-vis anticoagulation. Other anticoagulants such as hirudin, acid citrate dextrose (ACD), and ethylene diamine tetraacetic acid (EDTA) are not suitable for in vitro thrombosis studies due to cost or because they completely inhibit clotting and thrombosis.

Test Chamber

The test chamber in which the devices are to be deployed may be configured to mimic the in vivo geometry that the devices experience clinically. For example, a coronary stent may be deployed in a 3.2-mm ID polymer conduit, and additional geometric features may be provided (e.g., in-stent stenosis, residual stenosis) as required (7). Scaled models and flow cells, which attempt to simulate only a few in vivo features in the interest of simplicity, are less desirable because device thrombosis is a complex phenomenon that is influenced by numerous parameters, and scaling the system based on a few parameters is unlikely to be representative in most situations. However, in certain situations, a precise simulation of the in vivo geometry may not be the optimal milieu to compare devices. A pertinent example is the coils packed into the aneurysm model mentioned above. In such situations, a different configuration that circumvents the limitations of the in vitro system may be warranted. Whatever the geometric configuration of the test chamber may be, the system components and the chamber are constructed out of hemocompatible materials. In general, polymers are preferred over metals, and molded components are preferred over machined components due to their smoother surface finish (which is generally less thrombogenic).

Hemodynamics

As mentioned previously, device thrombosis is a flow-mediated phenomenon; a simulation of the appropriate in vivo hemodynamics that the devices experience should be attempted. The relevant flow rate combined with the appropriate chamber geometry usually achieves this objective effectively. For example, pulsatile flow (induced by a peristaltic pump) of 50–120 ml/min in a 3.2-mm ID conduit for a coronary stent simulates the clinical situation. However, in certain high flow rate situations (e.g., hemodialysis catheters), a precise simulation of the clinical flow rates may not be possible due to the differences between in vitro models and the in vivo situation. These differences include the presence of a more dynamic and comprehensive hemostatic system (e.g., the thrombolytic pathway) and less activated platelets and clotting factors in vivo compared with what is achievable in vitro. Some thrombus can develop on other model components (e.g., connectors, tubing) in vitro even if relatively hemocompatible materials are chosen for these components, which can result in circulating thromboemboli that may adversely affect assessment of the target device. This limitation of in vitro blood dictates the use of flow conditions that reduce significant enhancement of platelet and clotting pathway activation by system components. Hence, the flow conditions in the in vitro model may not exactly simulate all of the in vivo conditions but are chosen to strike the appropriate balance between relevance to in vivo conditions and minimizing artifacts to provide reliable results.

System Configuration

Although the simple recirculation configuration shown in Fig. 2 is adequate for many situations, this system has the following limitations: (i) The cumulative platelet activation due to the repeated exposure to the high shear produced by the roller pump and (ii) the possibility of an embolus from the device (or other system components) returning during the next pass and either depositing on the device and affecting the thromboembolic process or continuing to float in-stream (which may be falsely recorded as a new embolus if thromboembolic assessment of the device is being attempted). Recognizing the limitations of the simple recirculation model, a one-pass model may be utilized (6–9). In such a system, approximately 10 L of fresh bovine blood is collected into a container with heparin. Blood is caused to flow by gravity vertically downward (or by a peristaltic pump located distal to the device) through polyvinyl chloride (PVC) tubing containing the device (Fig. 3).

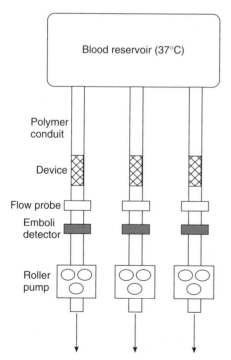

FIGURE 3 An example of a single-pass configuration for the comparison of device thrombogenecity and thromboembolism. A light scattering microemboli detector (LSMD) probe may be placed distal to the devices (the LSMD is discussed later) to quantify emboli released by the devices.

This configuration minimizes the extraneous activation of blood components and prevents the recirculation of emboli, which facilitates a more reliable evaluation of thromboembolism. However, as the blood is not recirculated, this system is limited by blood volume, which narrows the range of the flow rates and experiment durations as well as the number of devices that can be examined simultaneously.

Another limitation of the simple recirculation configuration is that the constant-flow peristaltic pump maintains a steady flow rate, which could result in a significant pressure increase due to the elevation of flow resistance caused by an occlusive device-associated thrombus. Such a pressure increase in the conduit could lead to the artificial embolization of the growing thrombus, which may result in large and unnatural variations of thrombus measurements at the end of the experiment. Such a flow system differs from the in vivo situation where the vascular network and the heart represent a constant pressure system rather than a constant flow system. For example, in patients, thrombus occlusion of the stented vessel reduces the flow rate in that vessel, and the blood flow is routed through other parallel branches. To simulate this in vivo situation, a branched conduit system may be configured. In one example of such a system (12), a 6.4-mm ID PVC conduit is connected to two 3.2-mm ID PVC conduits through a Y-connector to simulate the coronary artery tree (Fig. 4). A stent is deployed in one of the 3.2-mm ID branches, and the blood

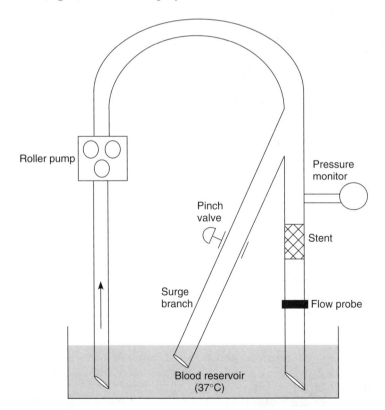

FIGURE 4 A branched in vitro blood flow model is illustrated. The flow rate in the stented branch decreases as occlusive thrombus develops on the stent.

flow rate in this branch is continuously measured using an ultrasonic flow probe. A peristaltic pump is placed on the 6.4-mm ID conduit to perfuse heparinized blood through the system. As the thrombus occludes the conduit with the stent, the flow rate in that conduit decreases, and the rate of flow rate decrease provides a measure of stent thrombosis. Thus, the in vitro system may be configured in a number of ways to address specific objectives and to simulate relevant features of the in vivo vasculature.

Experiment Duration

The inevitable activation of the platelets and the clotting cascade due to blood contact with biomaterials in the in vitro model restricts the duration of in vitro experiments and also dictates that such experiments be conducted within ~8 h of blood collection. The inherent thrombogenecity of the device, the level of anticoagulation, and the blood flow rate are important parameters that influence the length of the experiment. For example, a metallic coronary stent or aneurysm coils tend to be quite thrombogenic in vitro, and a relatively short experiment (~1 h) with a blood flow rate of 75 ml/min in a 3.2-mm ID conduit and 2–3 U/ml of heparin is usually sufficient to detect differences in thrombosis among devices. A polymeric catheter, on the other hand, is usually not as thrombogenic as a stent, and blood circulation generally needs to be maintained longer to detect sufficient thrombus on the device. Such situations, where the thrombogenecity of the device of interest is not substantially greater than that of model components (e.g., connectors, tubing), expose another limitation of in vitro models because the model components may develop thrombi as rapidly as (or more rapidly than) the device, which may adversely affect the development of thrombi on the device. Treating the connectors/tubing with antithrombogenic coatings can minimize this problem, but even with such interventions, the risk of systemic thrombi and thromboemboli cannot be eliminated completely. Thus, the duration of an in vitro experiment is determined usually as the minimum time required to develop detectable thrombi on the device of interest without the development of overwhelming thrombi and thromboemboli from system components. The short duration of in vitro experiments may be viewed as an advantage because such a system represents an accelerated model of acute device thrombosis, and useful information regarding the relative thrombogenecity of devices can be obtained rapidly and inexpensively in the in vitro model.

Assessment of Thrombosis

On completion of the blood circulation for a specified duration, the thrombus on the device may be assessed as follows:

(i) *Qualitative* visual assessment: stereo microscopy, high-resolution digital photography, and scanning electron microscopy as desired. Gamma imaging may also be used to map radiolabeled platelets and fibrinogen incorporated into the thrombi.

(ii) *Quantitative* assessment of thrombosis: radiolabeled platelets. In this technique, prior to the start of the experiment, platelets from a portion of autologous blood are obtained by centrifugation and incubated with indium oxine-111 to allow incorporation of ^{111}In on the platelets (4,13). The labelled platelets are added to the blood reservoir prior to the commencement of the experiment. At the end of the experiment, the device with the thrombus is placed in a gamma counter to quantify the amount of radioactivity, which reflects the amount of thrombus. This is a precise method for measuring thrombosis on a device and is also useful for pinpointing the thrombogenic risk of various locations within a device. In such a case, the device is sectioned as desired, and each section is placed in the gamma counter for quantification. A similar technique may be used to quantify iodine-labeled fibrinogen in the thrombus (14,15). Other techniques such as gravimetric analysis may also be used to quantify thrombosis on devices (6–9).

Assessment of Thromboembolism

Emboli released from devices may be quantified using the Light Scattering Microemboli Detector (LSMD) (16). The LSMD is a unique device that monitors emboli released from devices noninvasively, continuously, and in real time. The LSMD operates by differentiating between the light-scattering patterns of red cells and emboli. A noninvasive probe is placed around the transparent tubing distal to the device of interest. A beam of light illuminates a segment of blood (Fig. 5A), and the difference in the scattering patterns of emboli and red cells (due to differences in size and composition) allows detection of emboli when they traverse the illuminated region (17,18). The light scattered by red cells and emboli is detected by photodiodes, which convert the light into current. The current is amplified and sent to a computer for data processing. A continuous real-time display of the incoming voltages is displayed. The relatively "smooth" baseline represents scattering due to red cells. The appearance of distinct "sharp" peaks indicates the passage of emboli (Fig. 5B).

Data can be analyzed for the number of peaks (reflective of emboli number) and the average peak height (reflective of emboli size) (19,20). The end-point (and/or continuous) assessment of thrombosis combined with the continuous assessment of embolism by the LSMD provides a comprehensive assessment of device thrombosis and thromboembolism. LSMD probes are currently available for conduits 1/8 inch ID or smaller, but probes for larger conduits are being developed.

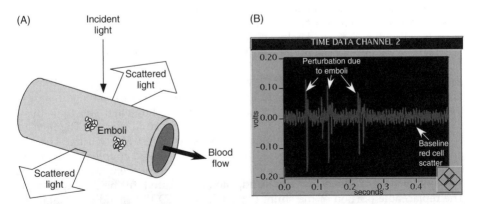

FIGURE 5 (*A*) (left): Schematic of the light scattering microemboli detection concept. (*B*) (right): Sharp peak in an acquisition frame showing the presence of an embolus against a relatively constant background of red cells.

TABLE 3   Merits and Limitations of the in vitro Model

Merits	Limitations
Well-controlled conditions (flow rate, blood donor, anticoagulation)	Does not incorporate device–vessel wall interactions
Ability to compare multiple devices under the same controlled conditions	Platelet and clotting cascade activation by system components (e.g., tubing, connectors, containers)
Economical	Anticoagulation is necessary
Rapid	Limited range of flow rate and experiment duration
Valuable for evaluating device design iterations	

Summary

The in vitro model represents a well-controlled and economical milieu for the study of vascular implant thrombosis and thromboembolism (Table 3). The ability to compare multiple devices under the same conditions is a valuable feature of the in vitro setting. However, such a model does have certain limitations that restrict the ability to extrapolate in vitro results to in vivo situations. In the context of vascular implants, the absence of device–vessel wall interactions in vitro is a major limitation because the vessel wall has thromboresistant and thrombolytic properties that may influence device thrombosis, which are difficult to simulate in vitro. Furthermore, unavoidable platelet and clotting cascade activation occurs in vitro due to the contact of blood with system components (e.g., tubing, connectors, and containers), which also mandates the use of anticoagulants in vitro (which is not always necessary in vivo) and restricts the flow rate as well as the experiment duration. In spite of these limitations, an in vitro test of device thrombosis is a valuable first step in assessing device design iterations and in the preclinical validation of vascular implant safety/efficacy.

EX VIVO SHUNT MODEL

An ex vivo shunt model represents a unique intermediate between in vitro and in vivo studies for assessing the thrombogenecity of certain devices. Multiple devices may be assessed in a live animal for simultaneous comparisons. One configuration of such a system is described below (21).

　　Following anesthesia, the carotid artery of the animal is exposed and a shunt is interposed between the cut ends of the artery. The permanent portion of the shunt consists of woven Dacron grafts attached with adhesive to the ends of polyurethane tubing sections on one end and sutured (end-to-end) to the cut ends of the artery on the other end. The tubing segments are tunnelled subcutaneously with the free ends exiting on the lateral surface of the neck (Fig. 6). The incision is closed, allowing the tubing segments to be accessible from outside. The two open ends of the tubing are connected with a heparin-coated coupler, allowing the blood to flow through the shunt. Some anticoagulation of the animal is required to maintain shunt patency and can be adjusted as required during the experiment. The replaceable portion of the shunt (e.g., a 3.2-mm ID PVC conduit), containing the test devices, is interposed between the externalized tubing segments of the shunt during the experiments. Blood flow through the shunt is monitored using a clamp-on ultrasonic flow probe.

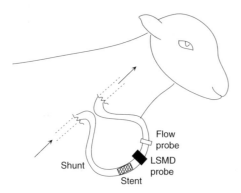

FIGURE 6 Illustration shows an ex vivo arterio-arterial shunt containing a stent, LSMD probe, and flow probe.

Large animals such as calves, sheep, swine, and dogs have been considered for this ex vivo model, because shunt flow rates similar to those in the human coronary artery (i.e., 50–100 ml/min) can be achieved. As this is intended to be a long-term animal model, adult sheep are a good choice because they do not grow, they are relatively docile, and they allow experimental manipulations without restraints or use of sedatives.

Typically, the shunt animals can be used over a 1–2-week period before they develop infection, systemic thrombosis, and so on, allowing the assessment of several devices in the same animal without additional surgical procedures. However, the ex vivo model does share certain limitations of the in vitro model, such as the requirement of anticoagulation and thrombosis of model components (graft, suture, anastamosis, tubing, and connectors) that limit the length of the experiments, and lack of device–vessel wall interactions. A useful feature of this live animal model that distinguishes it from in vitro models is that the effect of pharmacological agents, whose mechanisms depend on in vivo metabolism (e.g., clopidogrel), which cannot be studied in vitro, can be assessed in the ex vivo model. Thromboemboli released from the device are "filtered" by the body, which facilitates the assessment of device thromboembolism. Thus, despite its attendant limitations, the ex vivo model represents a useful and economical intermediate between in vitro and in vivo studies.

Thrombosis and thromboembolism of coronary stents have been assessed in such an ex vivo model (20,22). In these studies, the stents were deployed in 3.2 mm ID PVC tubing and connected to the shunt. Thromboemboli released by the stents was assessed continuously by the LSMD, and thrombus weight was measured at the conclusion of each experiment (typically 1–3 h). The comparison of emboli measurements in the shunt with and without a stent suggested that the stent was the primary source of detectable thromboemboli in this model (20). Such an ex vivo model has also been used to assess the effect of polymer sleeves on stents and was useful in determining those treatments that were relatively resistant to thrombosis and thromboembolism (21). Studies with this model also revealed that a combination of heparin and tirofiban is more effective in mitigating stent thrombosis and thromboembolism compared with either agent alone (23). This synergism is similar to what other researchers have observed clinically (24). Other studies have explored the effect of antiplatelet agents on end-point stent-induced thrombosis using a similar ex vivo model (25), but without the application of the

LSMD system. This suggests that this animal model may help guide the optimization of anticoagulant and antiplatelet strategies directed at mitigating device thrombosis.

IN VITRO DIAGNOSTIC TESTS

The discussion so far has dwelled on the assessment of thrombosis that is governed by the device design (geometry and surface chemistry). The other important parameter that influences device thrombosis is the inherent blood reactivity, specifically platelet and clotting function. Hyper-reactivity of platelets and/or the clotting cascade in specific individuals may lead to thrombosis even if a device is well-designed and generally hemocompatible. Furthermore, as suggested by a growing number of clinical studies, there are individual variations in the efficacy of pharmacological agents (i.e., anticoagulants and antiplatelet agents) administered to mitigate the risk of thrombosis (26–28). For example, "aspirin resistance" (i.e., absence of significant platelet inhibition despite aspirin administration) has been documented in several studies, and adverse outcomes (myocardial infarction, death, etc.) have been correlated with aspirin resistance (29–33). Similar trends are emerging with more potent platelet inhibitors (e.g., clopidogrel) as well. In other cases, anticoagulation to prevent clotting on implants (e.g., warfarin therapy after valve replacement) may lead to bleeding, and the drug dose needs to be adjusted carefully to provide adequate protection against clotting while avoiding bleeding. These concerns have exemplified the need to monitor the hemostatic function in each individual and adjust the drug dosages according to their specific needs. The ensuing discussion delineates in vitro diagnostic tools that monitor clotting and platelet function.

Clotting Time Tests

The coagulation function and the efficacy of anticoagulants are assessed generally by the activated clotting time (ACT), the prothrombin time (PT), or the activated partial thromboplastin time (aPTT). In conducting these tests to determine anticoagulation status, the time of blood collection (after anticoagulant administration), blood collection technique, and delay between blood collection and performing the test must be considered in determining the reliability of the measurements. The following description of the tests is intended to serve as a brief introduction; a more complete discussion of clotting time tests may be found elsewhere (34).

Activated Clotting Time

ACT is a widely used point-of-care clotting test that is most useful for monitoring high-dose heparin anticoagulation. Whole blood is collected into a tube containing a coagulation activator, such as celite (diatomaceous earth), kaolin, or glass particles. These agents activate the intrinsic pathway of coagulation, causing the blood to clot. The tubes are placed into a specialized coagulation analyzer that measures the time it takes for the blood to clot.

The ACT is less precise than aPTT (described below) for low heparin concentrations and lacks high correlation with heparin anti-factor Xa levels. ACT is influenced by a number of variables, including platelet count, platelet function, lupus anticoagulants, factor deficiencies, ambient temperature, hypothermia, and hemodilution. The ACT results from different activators are not standardized;

therefore, results from different methods are not interchangeable. Despite these limitations, ACT is perhaps the most commonly used clinical test to monitor anti-coagulation by heparin in various situations (e.g., bypass, dialysis, percutaneous vascular interventions).

Prothrombin Time

PT measures the clotting time from the activation of factor VII, through the formation of fibrin clot, and is used clinically to monitor patients receiving oral anticoagulant therapy (e.g., warfarin administration after valve replacement) (35). This test measures the integrity of the extrinsic and common pathways of coagulation. Inherent PT prolongations are caused most commonly by factor deficiencies involving fibrinogen or factors II, V, VII, or X.

The PT reagent is called "thromboplastin" (phospholipid with tissue factor and calcium). It is added to patient plasma, and the time until clot formation is measured in seconds. More recently, point-of-care PT test methods that use a single drop of whole blood have become available.

Warfarin (Coumadin) is monitored by the international normalized ratio (INR), which is calculated from PT and is intended to allow valid comparisons of results regardless of the type of PT reagent used among different laboratories (which can result in different PT measurements):

$$INR = \left(\frac{\text{patient PT}}{\text{mean normal PT}} \right)^{ISI}$$

The international sensitivity index (ISI) is a measure of the sensitivity of a particular PT reagent. The ISI for each reagent is determined by the manufacturer and generally ranges between 1 and 3.

During warfarin initiation, the PT-INR typically is checked daily or at least 4–5 times per week until the dose and INR are therapeutic and stable (e.g., INR of 2–3). The interval between PT-INR tests then can be gradually decreased to around once a month, depending on the stability of the dose and the PT-INR result.

Activated Partial Thromboplastin Time

The aPTT measures the clotting time from the activation of factor XII through the formation of fibrin clot and can be used when low heparin doses need to be monitored carefully. This measures the integrity of the intrinsic and common pathways of coagulation. aPTT prolongations are caused by factor deficiencies (especially of factors VIII, IX, XI, and/or XII) or inhibitors (most commonly, lupus anticoagulants or therapeutic anticoagulants such as heparin, hirudin, or argatroban).

aPTT reagent (phospholipid with an intrinsic pathway activator such as silica, celite, kaolin, ellagic acid) and calcium are added to patient plasma, and the time until clot formation is measured in seconds. The phospholipid in the aPTT assay is called "partial thromboplastin" because tissue factor is not present. More recently, point-of-care aPTT test methods that use whole blood have become available. With very high doses of heparin, as used in cardiac bypass surgery, the aPTT is out of range (>150 s) and therefore not useful. ACT is typically used instead in such situations.

Platelet Function Assays

Platelet function and its inhibition by antiplatelet drugs can be assessed by a variety of in vitro assays (36). These assays vary in the method used to measure platelet function and also in the specific aspect of platelet function that is assessed, which is a reflection of the complexity of platelet function as a phenomenon. These assays could assist the clinician in achieving optimal platelet inhibition for each individual and to strike the appropriate balance between thrombosis and hemorrhage in patients receiving vascular implants. The discussion in this section provides an introduction to classical and emerging platelet function assays.

Turbidometric Aggregometer

The optical turbiometric platelet aggregometer is perhaps the most widely used instrument for measuring platelet function in the laboratory (37–39). In this technique, platelet-rich plasma (PRP) is obtained by centrifugation of blood, and a platelet-aggregating agent (e.g., adenosine diphosphate (ADP), arachidonic acid, collagen, or epinephrine) is added to PRP. The ensuing aggregation of platelets changes the turbidity of PRP, which is measured using optical detectors, and usually reported as "percent" aggregation (light transmission). This fluid phase aggregation method has the longest history of all platelet function tests and has been used extensively for the measurement of antiplatelet drug response (40). Some of the early discoveries of aspirin resistance were due to this instrument (41), and it continues to be used as a research tool for exploring various aspects of platelet function. However, due to the labor-intensive and time-consuming nature of the method, it has not been used widely at the point-of-care to monitor patients on antiplatelet agents and consequently has remained a laboratory instrument. The use of PRP rather than whole blood may further limit the clinical relevance of this technique because red cells and leukocytes (present in whole blood but not in PRP) may participate in the thrombotic process (42,43). Also, the centrifugation of blood to obtain PRP may result in the loss of an important platelet subpopulation (44). To address these logistical limitations, several whole blood rapid platelet function assays have been developed recently for point-of-care use.

Impedance Aggregometer (Chronolog)

In the impedance aggregometer, platelets adhere to and aggregate on two electrodes submerged in blood diluted with isotonic saline to which platelet agonists are added (45). The impedance between the two electrodes increases as the platelets aggregate, which is used as a measure of platelet function. This instrument may be credited with revealing the importance of testing platelet function in whole blood, and studies conducted with this instrument have suggested that platelet aggregation in whole blood is quite different from that in PRP (46). Until recently, the electrodes needed to be cleaned very carefully in this instrument, which limited its use at the point-of-care. Disposable electrodes are now available and may increase its clinical utility.

PFA-100 (Dade-Behring)

The PFA-100 simulates platelet-based primary hemostasis in vitro (47). In this instrument, a syringe aspirates citrated whole blood under steady-flow conditions through a small aperture cut into a membrane coated with collagen and epinephrine or collagen and ADP. The instrument records the time necessary for the occlusion of the aperture, defined as the closure time, which is indicative of platelet function.

The PFA-100 has been used in several studies to explore the incidence of aspirin resistance (48–52). One study showed that the PFA-100 indicated a greater incidence of aspirin resistance compared with the PRP aggregometer (9.5% vs. 5.5%) in patients with stable cardiovascular disease, suggesting that the PFA-100 may be a more sensitive test of aspirin resistance than the PRP aggregometer (47). Another study examined patients with cerebrovascular disease and found that the PFA-100 determined as many as 56% of the patients to be aspirin resistant (48). However, the determinations of aspirin resistance by the PFA-100 were found to correlate poorly with long-term clinical outcomes in one study (53), although this may have been due to the small sample size of the study. The PFA-100 has yet to be used for ascertaining excessive platelet inhibition due to antiplatelet drugs (which may lead to bleeding). Its ability to monitor combination therapies (e.g., aspirin and clopidogrel) also is yet to be investigated. Thus, although the PFA-100 is a rapid and convenient test, the breadth of its clinical relevance in the context of predicting prothrombotic states, monitoring antiplatelet drug resistance, and determining coagulopathies is yet to be firmly established.

VerifyNow (Accumetrics)

The VerifyNow (previously known as "Ultegra") optically measures the adhesion of platelets to fibrinogen-coated polymer beads and subsequent agglutination due to platelet agonists (ADP or arachidonic acid or thrombin receptor-activating peptide) (54). This agglutination increases the light transmittance through blood, which is recorded as the response parameter reflective of platelet function.

This rapid and convenient whole blood assay has been useful for measuring the efficacy of GPIIb/IIIa inhibitor (GPI) (e.g., abciximab, tirofiban, and eptifibatide) (55). Studies with the GPI cartridge of the VerifyNow system showed that platelet inhibition measured by this system correlated with a reduced risk of an adverse cardiac event after percutaneous coronary intervention (56). The VerifyNow system has also been used to determine the responsiveness to aspirin in a number of studies (57–62). One study showed that those patients that were aspirin resistant per the VerifyNow system demonstrated a higher incidence of myonecrosis after nonurgent percutaneous coronary intervention despite pretreatment with clopidogrel (58). A cartridge for assessing thienopyridine efficacy has also been recently introduced as part of the VerifyNow system.

One of the limitations of this system as to defining aspirin resistance is that it separates patients into only two categories: sensitive and resistant. A better resolution of the response to aspirin (e.g., into multiple quartiles) may be useful in determining the extent of the problem and also in ascertaining whether a patient is overinhibited (which may enhance the bleeding risk).

Thromboelastograph (Haemoscope)

The Thromboelastograph (TEG) measures the physical property of clots in whole blood using a system that resembles a viscometer and provides a general perspective on hemostasis (63–66). In the TEG, a stationary cylindrical cup holds the blood sample and is oscillated through a specific angle for a specific time. A pin is suspended in the blood by a torsion wire and is monitored for motion. Upon activation of the hemostatic system by agonists such as kaolin and arachidonic acid, the torque of the rotating cup is transmitted to the immersed pin when the fibrin–platelet bonding links the cup and the pin together. The strength of these fibrin–platelet bonds affects the magnitude of the pin motion such that strong clots move the pin directly in phase with the cup motion. Thus, the magnitude of the output is related directly to the strength of the formed clot. As the clot retracts or lyses, these bonds are broken and the transfer of the cup's motion to the pin is diminished. The rotation of the pin is converted by a mechanical-electrical transducer into an electrical signal, which is analyzed by software. The TEG has been used in a number of studies to monitor coagulopathies associated with bypass, artificial heart implantation, and to monitor anticoagulation (67–69). One study showed that the TEG was capable of differentiating between patients with ischemic and hemorrhagic stroke (70). Another study showed that hemorrhagic complications decreased from 81% (using conventional monitoring) to 9% using a multisystem anticoagulation protocol that included the TEG (71).

The TEG measures the integrated hemostatic function, i.e., platelet function and coagulation are not measured separately but monitored in tandem. While it may be argued that such an integrated approach might be more physiologically relevant, it may compromise the ability of the TEG to assess subtle platelet function-related phenomena such as aspirin and thienopyridine resistance. Thus, the value of the TEG for monitoring antiplatelet therapy, especially combination therapy (e.g., aspirin + clopidogrel), is unclear (72,73). Furthermore, the TEG is not designed to identify specific factors, inhibitors, or activators responsible for coagulopathies. Each test with the TEG can take 40 min, which makes it a time-consuming assay. Also, because the instrument is very sensitive, the system has relatively stringent/cumbersome calibration protocols that need to be followed every time the instrument is moved, which limits its portability.

Plateletworks (Helena)

This ICHOR Plateletworks analyzer assesses platelet function by measuring platelet count in whole blood before and after exposure to platelet aggregating agents (74,75). A significant decrease in the platelet count after exposure of blood to aggregating agents suggests normal platelet function, because the platelets would be consumed in aggregates and fewer single platelets will be present. If the platelet count after exposure to aggregating agents is not reduced significantly, platelet inhibition may be indicated (e.g., due to antiplatelet drugs). This technique has been used to assess clopidogrel resistance in patients undergoing coronary stent implantation (76) and revealed that 22% were resistant to clopidogrel. One study suggested that the Plateletworks system was more useful than the TEG in predicting the risk of post-operative bleeding after open-heart surgery (77). One of the limitations of this technique is that it has very stringent time requirements for testing after blood collection (typically within 20 min). Furthermore, the system is somewhat operator intensive because the tube of blood has to be shaken manually to achieve platelet aggregation.

ThromboGuide® (ThromboVision)

The ThromboGuide (T-Guide®) combines the flexibility of the conventional PRP aggregometer with the conveniences of the emerging whole blood rapid platelet function assays (78). In this system, blood is stirred by a magnetic rotor in the disposable sample holder, and platelet aggregating agent ("agonist") is mixed with the blood. The resulting platelet aggregates are detected and characterized using differential light scattering techniques (similar to the principles described above for the LSMD). Briefly, incident laser light is introduced into the transparent sample holder and scattered light is captured by photodetectors. Before blood mixes with the agonist, the red cells elicit a relatively constant light scattering pattern. After blood mixes with the agonist, the resulting aggregates perturb this scattering pattern and are identified as sharp "peaks." The number of these peaks reflects the number of aggregates, and the height of these peaks reflects the aggregate volume.

In preliminary studies, platelet inhibition due to common antiplatelet drugs (aspirin, clopidogrel, and glycoprotein inhibitors) detected by the T-Guide correlated with the PRP aggregometer and with the VerifyNow system (79). Further clinical studies are required to ascertain its utility at the point-of-care.

The aforementioned hemostatic diagnostic tests are also valuable for qualifying the blood to be used in the in vitro models discussed previously in this chapter. The in vitro model is designed to reveal relative thrombogenecities of various devices. Such a comparison is possible only if a measurable amount of thrombus can be generated on the devices, which is contingent upon normal platelet and coagulation function. Thus, measuring the platelet function and clotting time of the collected blood prior to initiating the complex experiments would help select those samples whose hemostatic function is normal and allow the elimination of nonresponsive outliers.

In summary, there are several in vitro diagnostic assays for assessing hemostatic function and its inhibition by anticoagulants/antiplatelet agents. The variety of tests available for determining platelet function and the lack of consensus on a standard test emphasizes the complexity of the platelet aggregation process and our limited understanding of the same as it relates to clinical practice. These limitations notwithstanding, the quest for an economical, rapid, convenient, and reliable point-of-care platelet function assay is an important one to facilitate the elusive balance between thrombosis and bleeding.

SUMMARY

Vascular implant thrombosis is a complex interplay between device geometry, device surface characteristics, an individual's inherent hemostatic response, and the anticoagulation/antiplatelet therapy status. The assessment of vascular implant thrombosis has evolved with our understanding of the underlying cellular and molecular mechanisms, but neither an ideal experimental model nor a perfect in vitro hemostatic function assay exists to precisely simulate physiological and clinical conditions. With that understanding, the salient features, merits, and limitations of state-of-the-art in vitro and ex vivo experimental models for the assessment of vascular implant thrombosis were discussed, and the rationale for the design of such models with their attendant nuances was presented. The relevance of these modes of assessment to the clinical setting and to advancing device design was discussed. Point-of-care blood tests for coagulation and platelet function monitoring were scrutinized to evaluate their role as in vitro diagnostic tools in ascertaining the individual-dependant risk of thrombosis. The relevance of these diagnostic tests in the context of assessing the efficacy of and eventually guiding antiplatelet therapy was discussed. Persistent efforts to better understand vascular implant thrombosis and associated advancements in experimental models and in vitro diagnostic devices will improve device design and clinical management of implant recipients.

REFERENCES

1. Komotar RJ, Mocco J, Wilson DA, et al. Current endovascular treatment options for intracranial carotid artery atherosclerosis. Neurosurg Focus 2005; 18(1):e5.
2. Andaluz N, Zuccarello M. Evidence-based surgical treatment of carotid stenosis. Literature review. J Neurosurg Sci 2004; 48(1):1–9.
3. Bendok BR, Hanel RA, Hopkins LN. Coil embolization of intracranial aneurysms. Neurosurgery 2003; 52(5):1125–1130; discussion 1130.
4. Sukavaneshvar S. In-vitro assessment of device thrombosis and thromboembolism. Proceedings of Roadmap to Successful Development and Regulatory Approval of Medical Devices with Hemocompatible Coatings Workshop, Surfaces in Biomaterials Foundation, Scottsdale, AZ, Aug 2001.
5. Sakariassen KS, Hanson SR, Cadroy Y. Methods and models to evaluate shear-dependent and surface reactivity-dependent antithrombotic efficacy. Thromb Res 2001; 104(3):149–174.
6. International Organization for Standardization. Guideline document for the assessment of blood contacting device hemocompatibility (ISO 10993-4).
7. Sukavaneshvar S, Solen KA, Mohammad SF. An in-vitro model to study device-induced thrombosis and embolism: evaluation of the efficacy of tirofiban, aspirin, and dipyridamole. Thromb Haemost 2000; 83(2):322–326.
8. Sukavaneshvar S, Rosa GM, Solen KA. Enhancement of stent-induced thromboembolism by residual stenoses: contribution of hemodynamics. Ann Biomed Eng 2000; 28(2):182–193.
9. Sukavaneshvar S, Solen KA, Mohammad SF. Device induced thromboembolism in a bovine in vitro coronary stent model. ASAIO J 1998; 44(5):M393–M396.
10. Sukavaneshvar S, Solen KA. Effects of hemodynamics on thromboembolism in coronary stents and prototype flow cells in vitro. ASAIO J 1998; 44(5):M388–M392.
11. Lane DA, Lindahll U. Heparin: Chemical and Biological Properties, Clinical Applications. Boca Raton, FL: CRC Press, 1989.
12. Sukavaneshvar S, Watts M, Bingham J, et al. Assessment of thromboresistance of surface coatings using a novel branched conduit blood flow model. Abstracts of Papers, p. 60, BioInterface 2004 Symposium, Surfaces in Biomaterials Foundation, Baltimore, MD, Oct 27–29, 2004.
13. Thakur ML, Welch MJ, Joist JH, et al. Indium-111 labeled platelets: studies on preparation and evaluation of in vitro and in vivo functions. Thromb Res 1976; 9(4):345–357.
14. Foo RS, Gershlick AH, Hogrefe K, et al. Inhibition of platelet thrombosis using an activated protein C-loaded stent: in vitro and in vivo results. Thromb Haemost 2000; 83(3):496–502.
15. Wabers HD, Hergenrother RW, Coury AJ, et al. Thrombus deposition on polyurethanes designed for biomedical applications. J Appl Biomater 1992; 3(3):167–176.
16. Solen K, Sukavaneshvar S, Zheng Y, et al. Light-scattering instrument to detect thromboemboli in blood. J Biomed Opt 2003; 8(1):70–79.
17. Reynolds LO, Simon T. Size distribution measurements in microaggregates in stored whole blood. Transfusion 1980; 20:669–678.
18. Reynolds LO. Light scattering detection of microemboli. Transactions of the 11th Annual Meeting of the Society for Biomaterials and the 17th International Biomaterials Symposium, Society for Biomaterials, San Diego, CA, Apr 24–28, 1985;8:20.
19. Peng Y. Characterization of microemboli in whole blood by a new laser light-scattering technique (master's thesis). Provo, UT: Brigham Young University, Department of Chemical Engineering, 1994.
20. Zheng Y, Mohammad S, Solen KA. The light-scattering whole blood aggregometer: a novel device for assessment of platelet aggregation in undiluted blood. Arch Pathol Lab Med 1998; 122:880–886.
21. Sukavaneshvar S, Zheng Y, Rosa GM, et al. Thromboembolization associated with sudden increases in flow in a coronary stent ex vivo shunt model. ASAIO J 2000; 46(3):301–304.
22. Sukavaneshvar S, Mohammad F, Herce J, et al. The relative influence of polymer matrices on stent-induced thrombosis and embolism. Abstract#169: Transactions of the 6th World Biomaterials Congress, Kamuela, Hawaii, May 15–20, 2000.

23. Meola S, Burns G, Sukavaneshvar S, Solen K, Mohammad S. Mitigation of device-associated thrombosis and thromboembolism using combinations of heparin and tirofiban. J Extra Corpor Technol. 2006; 38(3):230–234.
24. The Platelet Receptor Inhibition in Ischemic Syndrome Management in Patients Limited by Unstable Signs and Symptoms (PRISM-PLUS) Study Investigators. Inhibition of the platelet glycoprotein IIb/IIIa receptor with tirofiban in unstable angina and non-Q-wave myocardial infarction. N Engl J Med 1998; 338(21):1488–1497.
25. Makkar RR, Eigler NL, Kaul S, et al. Effects of clopidogrel, aspirin and combined therapy in a porcine ex vivo model of high-shear induced stent thrombosis. Eur Heart J 1998; 19(10):1538–1546.
26. Rocca B, Patrono C. Determinants of the interindividual variability in response to antiplatelet drugs. J Thromb Haemost 2005; 3(8):1597–1602.
27. Knoepp SM, Laposata M. Aspirin resistance: moving forward with multiple definitions, different assays, and a clinical imperative. Am J Clin Pathol 2005; 123(suppl):S125–S132.
28. Nguyen TA, Diodati JG, Pharand C. Resistance to clopidogrel: a review of the evidence. J Am Coll Cardiol 2005; 45(8):1157–1164.
29. Eikelboom JW, Hankey GJ. Aspirin resistance: a new independent predictor of vascular events? J Am Coll Cardiol 2003; 41(6):966–968.
30. Eikelboom JW, Hirsh J, Weitz JI, et al. Aspirin-resistant thromboxane biosynthesis and the risk of myocardial infarction, stroke, or cardiovascular death in patients at high risk for cardiovascular events. Circulation 2002; 105(14):1650–1655.
31. Gum PA, Kottke-Marchant K, Poggio ED, et al. Profile and prevalence of aspirin resistance in patients with cardiovascular disease. Am J Cardiol 2001; 88(3):230–235.
32. Gum PA, Kottke-Marchant K, Welsh PA, et al. A prospective, blinded determination of the natural history of aspirin resistance among stable patients with cardiovascular disease. J Am Coll Cardiol 2003; 41(6):961–965.
33. Ajani AE, Cheneau E, Leborgne L, et al. Have we solved the problem of late thrombosis? Minerva Cardioangiol 2002; 50(5):463–468.
34. Van Cott EM, Laposata M. Coagulation. In: Jacobs DS, DeMott WR, Oxley DK, eds. The Laboratory Test Handbook, 5th ed. Cleveland: Lexi-Comp, 2001:327–358.
35. Ezekowitz MD. Anticoagulation management of valve replacement patients. J Heart Valve Dis 2002; 11(suppl 1):S56–S60.
36. Nicholson NS, Panzer-Knodle SG, Haas NF, et al. Assessment of platelet function assays. Am Heart J 1998; 135(5 Pt 2 Su):S170–S178.
37. Marcus AJ. Platelet aggregation. In: Colman RW, Marder VJ, Clowes AW, George JN, Goldhaber SZ, eds. Hemostasis and Thrombosis: Basic Principles and Clinical Practice, 5th ed. Philadelphia, PA: Lippincott Williams & Wilkins, 2005.
38. Born GVR. Platelets: functional physiology. In: Biggs R, ed. Human Blood Coagulation, Haemostasis and Thrombosis. London: Blackwell Scientific Publications, 1972.
39. Breddin HK. Can platelet aggregometry be standardized? Platelets 2005; 16(3–4):151–158.
40. Pongracz E. Measurement of platelet aggregation during antiplatelet therapy in ischemic stroke. Clin Hemorheol Microcirc 2004; 30(3–4):237–242.
41. Helgason CM, Bolin KM, Hoff JA, et al. Development of aspirin resistance in persons with previous ischemic stroke. Stroke 1994; 25(12):2331–2336.
42. Faraday N, Scharpf RB, Dodd-o JM, et al. Leukocytes can enhance platelet-mediated aggregation and thromboxane release via interaction of P-selectin glycoprotein ligand 1 with P-selectin. Anesthesiology 2001; 94(1):145–151.
43. Miller DD, Karim MA, Edwards WD, et al. Relationship of vascular thrombosis and inflammatory leukocyte infiltration to neointimal growth following porcine coronary artery stent placement. Atherosclerosis 1996; 124(2):145–155.
44. Barradas MA, Stansby G, Hamilton G, et al. Diminished platelet yield and enhanced platelet aggregability in platelet-rich plasma of peripheral vascular disease patients. Int Angiol 1994; 13(3):202–207.
45. Zwierzina WD, Kunz F. A method of testing platelet aggregation in native whole blood. Thromb Res 1985; 38(1):91–100.

46. Dyszkiewicz-Korpanty AM, Frenkel EP, Sarode R. Approach to the assessment of platelet function: comparison between optical-based platelet-rich plasma and impedance-based whole blood platelet aggregation methods. Clin Appl Thromb Hemost 2005; 11(1):25–35.

47. Kundu SK, Heilmann EJ, Sio R, et al. Description of an in vitro platelet function analyzer—PFA-100. Semin Thromb Hemost 1995; 21(suppl 2):106–112.

48. von Pape KW, Strupp G, Bonzel T, et al. Effect of compliance and dosage adaptation of long term aspirin on platelet function with PFA-100 in patients after myocardial infarction. Thromb Haemost 2005; 94(4):889–891.

49. Golanski J, Chlopicki S, Golanski R, et al. Resistance to aspirin in patients after coronary artery bypass grafting is transient: impact on the monitoring of aspirin antiplatelet therapy. Ther Drug Monit 2005; 27(4):484–490.

50. Andersen K, Hurlen M, Arnesen H, et al. Aspirin non-responsiveness as measured by PFA-100 in patients with coronary artery disease. Thromb Res 2002; 108(1):37–42.

51. Gum PA, Kottke-Marchant K, Poggio ED, et al. Profile and prevalence of aspirin resistance in patients with cardiovascular disease. Am J Cardiol 2001; 88(3):230–235.

52. Alberts MJ, Bergman DL, Molner E, et al. Antiplatelet effect of aspirin in patients with cerebrovascular disease. Stroke 2004; 35(1):175–178.

53. Steinhubl SR, Varanasi SJ, Goldberg L. Determination of the natural history of aspirin resistance among stable patients with cardiovascular disease. J Am Coll Cardiol 2003; 42(7):1336–1337. Letter to the Editor and Author Reply.

54. Smith JW, Steinhubl SR, Lincoff AM, et al. Rapid platelet-function assay: an automated and quantitative cartridge-based method. Circulation 1999; 99(5):620–625.

55. Wheeler GL, Braden GA, Steinhubl SR, et al. The Ultegra rapid platelet-function assay: comparison to standard platelet function assays in patients undergoing percutaneous coronary intervention with abciximab therapy. Am Heart J 2002; 143(4):602–611.

56. Steinhubl SR, Talley JD, Braden GA, et al. Point-of-care measured platelet inhibition correlates with a reduced risk of an adverse cardiac event after percutaneous coronary intervention: results of the GOLD (AU-Assessing Ultegra) multicenter study. Circulation 2001; 103(21):2572–2578.

57. Lee PY, Chen WH, Ng W, et al. Low-dose aspirin increases aspirin resistance in patients with coronary artery disease. Am J Med 2005; 118(7):723–727.

58. Serebruany VL, Malinin AI, Ziai W, et al. Effects of clopidogrel and aspirin in combination versus aspirin alone on platelet activation and major receptor expression in patients after recent ischemic stroke: for the Plavix Use for Treatment of Stroke (PLUTO-Stroke) trial. Stroke 2005; 36(10):2289–2292.

59. Harrison P, Segal H, Blasbery K, et al. Screening for aspirin responsiveness after transient ischemic attack and stroke: comparison of 2 point-of-care platelet function tests with optical aggregometry. Stroke 2005; 36(5):1001–1005.

60. Malinin A, Spergling M, Muhlestein B, et al. Assessing aspirin responsiveness in subjects with multiple risk factors for vascular disease with a rapid platelet function analyzer. Blood Coagul Fibrinolysis 2004; 15(4):295–301.

61. Wang JC, Aucoin-Barry D, Manuelian D, et al. Incidence of aspirin nonresponsiveness using the Ultegra Rapid Platelet Function Assay-ASA. Am J Cardiol 2003; 92(12):1492–1494.

62. Chen WH, Lee PY, Ng W, et al. Aspirin resistance is associated with a high incidence of myonecrosis after non-urgent percutaneous coronary intervention despite clopidogrel pretreatment. J Am Coll Cardiol 2004; 43(6):1122–1126.

63. Salooja N, Perry DJ. Thrombelastography. Blood Coagul Fibrinolysis 2001; 12(5):327–337. Erratum in: Blood Coagul Fibrinolysis 2002; 13(1):75.

64. Carroll RC, Craft RM, Chavez JJ, et al. A Thrombelastograph whole blood assay for clinical monitoring of NSAID-insensitive transcellular platelet activation by arachidonic acid. J Lab Clin Med 2005; 146(1):30–35.

65. Craft RM, Chavez JJ, Snider CC, et al. Comparison of modified Thrombelastograph and Plateletworks whole blood assays to optical platelet aggregation for monitoring reversal of clopidogrel inhibition in elective surgery patients. J Lab Clin Med 2005; 145(6):309–315.

66. Chavez JJ, Foley DE, Snider CC, et al. A novel thrombelastograph tissue factor/kaolin assay of activated clotting times for monitoring heparin anticoagulation during cardiopulmonary bypass. Anesth Analg 2004; 99(5):1290–1294.

67. Shih RL, Cherng YG, Chao A, et al. Prediction of bleeding diathesis in patients undergoing cardiopulmonary bypass during cardiac surgery: viscoelastic measures versus routine coagulation test. Acta Anaesthesiol Sin 1997; 35(3):133–139.
68. Cherng YG, Chao A, Shih RL, et al. Preoperative evaluation and postoperative prediction of hemostatic function with thromboelastography in patients undergoing redo cardiac surgery. Acta Anaesthesiol Sin 1998; 36(4):179–186.
69. Martin P, Horkay F, Rajah SM, et al. Monitoring of coagulation status using thrombelastography during paediatric open heart surgery. Int J Clin Monit Comput 1991; 8(3):183–187.
70. Handa A, Platts A, Tone S, et al. Vascular surgical society of Great Britain and Ireland: thrombelastography can differentiate ischaemic from haemorrhagic stroke. Br J Surg 1999; 86(5):691.
71. Pavie A, Szefner J, Leger P, et al. Preventing, minimizing, and managing postoperative bleeding. Ann Thorac Surg 1999; 68:705–710.
72. Tantry US, Bliden KP, Gurbel PA. Overestimation of platelet aspirin resistance detection by thrombelastograph platelet mapping and validation by conventional aggregometry using arachidonic acid stimulation. J Am Coll Cardiol 2005; 46(9):1705–1709.
73. Tanaka KA, Szlam F, Kelly AB, et al. Clopidogrel (Plavix) and cardiac surgical patients: implications for platelet function monitoring and postoperative bleeding. Platelets 2004; 15(5):325–332.
74. Carville DG, Schleckser PA, Guyer KE, et al. Whole blood platelet function assay on the ICHOR point-of-care hematology analyzer. J Extra Corpor Technol 1998; 30(4):171–177.
75. Lennon MJ, Gibbs NM, Weightman WM, et al. A comparison of Plateletworks and platelet aggregometry for the assessment of aspirin-related platelet dysfunction in cardiac surgical patients. J Cardiothorac Vasc Anesth 2004; 18(2):136–140.
76. Lau WC, Gurbel PA, Watkins PB, et al. Contribution of hepatic cytochrome P450 3A4 metabolic activity to the phenomenon of clopidogrel resistance. Circulation 2004; 109(2):166–171.
77. Ostrowsky J, Foes J, Warchol M, et al. Plateletworks platelet function test compared to the thromboelastograph for prediction of postoperative outcomes. J Extra Corpor Technol 2004; 36(2):149–152.
78. Zheng Y, Solen KA, Mohammad SF. The light-scattering whole blood aggregometer: a novel device for assessment of platelet aggregation in undiluted blood. Arch Pathol Lab Med 1998; 122(10):880–886.
79. Anderson J, Lappe J, Greene R, et al. Monitoring antiplatelet drug efficacy and resistance with a novel whole blood point-of-care platelet function analyzer. Abstract #615, Cardiovascular Revascularization Therapies, Washington, DC, Mar 2005.

Part 2

Clinical Implications

5

Stroke Imaging (CT, MR, SPECT, PET)

Jens O. Heidenreich and Jeffrey L. Sunshine

Case Western Reserve University and University Hospitals Health System, Cleveland, Ohio, U.S.A.

INTRODUCTION

Stroke is a unifying diagnosis applied to a vast variety of symptoms reflecting a central nervous system dysfunction. The term "stroke" can also represent varied causes of underlying diseases, pathophysiological mechanisms, and patient states. To distinguish among the many possible mechanisms of disease, there is a demand for imaging tools that are easily available and that lead to a clear, fast, and correct diagnosis. Stroke imaging requires speed, as potential recovery is more likely to occur in the early stages. More sophisticated imaging tools can be applied to further aid treatment and follow-up, as patient management does not stop after the initial diagnosis. Many imaging options are currently available for patients presenting with stroke symptoms, as reviewed in this chapter; these are of particular importance in the initial phases to direct the patient toward the most appropriate treatment in the hyperacute phases of the disease.

UNENHANCED CRANIAL COMPUTED TOMOGRAPHY

Computed tomography (CT) is the most commonly available imaging tool in most hospitals in the United States, Europe, and Japan (1). Although often considered relatively insensitive in acute ischemic stroke, a head CT without contrast is the best available and most usual screening imaging tool for patients presenting with acute neurological deficit (2). Head CT without contrast has been used to randomize patients in most major clinical trials on stroke treatment (3–7).

From the differential diagnosis, cranial CT helps to exclude any type of stroke that is related to intracranial hemorrhage. Intracranial hemorrhage accounts for approximately 15%–25% of acute nontraumatic stroke presentations (8,9). Recently, however, there has been an increasing number of reported magnetic resonance imaging (MRI) studies where intracranial hemorrhage in the form of microbleeds were undetected on CT in up to 12% of cases (10–12). On CT intracranial hemorrhage is detectable as a hyperdense area (clot) with attenuation values of 70–90 Hounsfield units (HU) in contrast to gray matter (35–45 HU), white matter (20–30 HU), and cerebrospinal fluid (CSF, 4–8 HU). In cases of a positive finding of intracranial hemorrhage, further differentiation of subtypes follows typical anatomical margins that will follow the tissue compartments from peripheral to central: Epidural and subdural hematomas usually result from trauma and derive blood from meningeal arteries and bridging veins, respectively (Figs. 1 and 2). Epidural hematomas are often associated with fractures of the skull, and CT images should be examined thoroughly for fractures

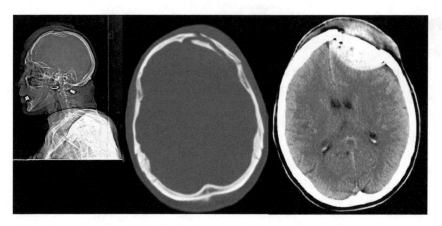

FIGURE 1 A left frontal epidural hematoma is seen associated with a fracture derived from a meningeal artery respecting sutural margins. Note the gas within the blood clot confirming an open skull fracture.

and intracranial gas in the bone window to exclude an open skull fracture. Subdural hematomas occur frequently in elderly patients with minor trauma or idiopathically, as well as in conditions of coagulopathy. The most likely source of a subarachnoid hemorrhage is a ruptured cerebral aneurysm or trauma. Many subarachnoid hemorrhages should be evaluated further in view of a cerebral aneurysm, as trauma potentially may be related to the aneurysm rupture (Fig. 3). Intracerebral or parenchymal hemorrhage is often found in the basal ganglia and thalami due to hypertension and because of the deep perforating arterial supply to these brain regions. Hypertensive hemorrhages may be caused by rhexis bleeding from microaneurysms (13) (Fig. 4). Bleeding in the posterior fossa may involve the brainstem or cerebellum and be caused by hypertension or fill the subarachnoid cisterns as perimesencephalic bleeding that possibly derives from venous stenosis. Other locations of hemorrhage cast suspicion for diverse

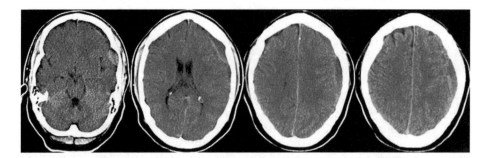

FIGURE 2 Computed tomography (CT) scans of a patient suffering from a subdural hematoma. Note the different densities of the hematoma representing more liquid and organized components of probably different stages, as recurrent bleeding in subdural hematomas is common. The adjacent sulci are narrow, and a midline shift is apparent due to the mass effect.

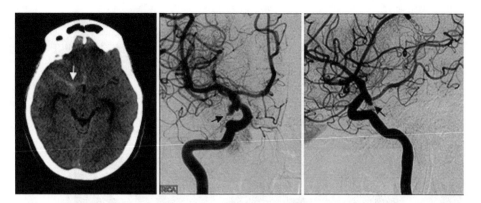

FIGURE 3 Computed tomography (CT) of a patient presenting with a typical subarachnoid hemorrhage (white arrow). The corresponding right internal carotid angiograms (frontal plane in middle panel, and lateral plane in right panel) shows the ruptured posterior communicating artery (PcomA) aneurysm (black arrows).

etiologies such as vascular malformations (associated with prominent vessels), tumors (mass effects and enhancement), mycotic aneurysms (along more distal arteries), amyloidangiopathies (supratentorial cortex in older patients), or other vasculopathies.

Once hemorrhage can be excluded as a cause of stroke symptoms, the image can be interpreted carefully for different discrete signs of cerebral ischemia. The brain tissue can appear unaffected on CT even under symptomatic ischemic conditions, depending on the perfusion pressure, if no vasodilatation or ischemic edema takes place, or if the extent of affected brain tissue does not reach a threshold and become apparent as hypodensity (14). Hypodensity often appears first on CT due to cytotoxic water uptake that initially becomes apparent in gray matter. The lentiform nucleus, in particular, is often affected first because of its threat from lack of collateral blood supply; its appearance degrades through obscured margins. Then, in patients with ischemia involving the central territories of the middle cerebral artery (MCA), the margins of the head of the caudate nuclei will worsen, followed by lost delineation of the insular gray matter ribbon. This principle of diminished gray–white-matter differentiation applies to all brain territories, as water uptake into the cortical gray and, later, also white matter leads to a reduced attenuation. This can lead to mass effect first involving effacement of the cortical sulci and then, depending on the size and region of ischemia, it also may lead to midline shift and ultimately herniation (Fig. 5). Changing the window and center levels may increase the detectability of early hypodensities, obscured margins, or lost gray–white differentiation (15). Level changes may even allow the recognition of increased curvilinear density along the base of the brain in comparison with the contralateral side, the so-called hyperdense MCA sign. The recognition of such a sign implies a poorer outcome, as does the involvement of more than a third of the MCA territory with edema and mass effect (16). A cranial CT may have low sensitivity to very acute brain ischemia; nevertheless, a normal CT (inherently lacking the negative signs described) may be thought to represent a better prognosis among patients presenting with clinical signs of acute stroke.

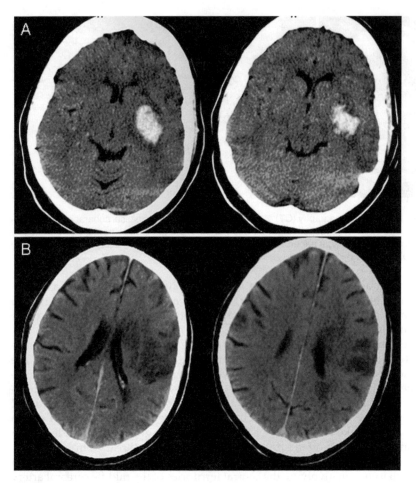

FIGURE 4 (*A*) Intracerebral hemorrhage within the basal ganglia in a patient with arterial hypertension. (*B*) Different patient with a nonhemorrhagic ischemia in the same territory as shown in (*A*). Both patients presented with exactly the same symptoms of a stroke.

CT ANGIOGRAPHY

The advantages of CT angiography (CTA) lie in its accessibility to both extracranial and intracranial arteries for the differentiation of normal, stenotic or occlusive disease, and the characterization of atherosclerotic plaques to allow initiation of the appropriate treatment. The necessity to image the cervical and cerebral vasculature to exclude or detect occlusive disease as cause of ischemia in the acute phase arises from the many ischemic strokes that are of embolic cause and those that may derive from the proximal internal carotid artery (17,18). Modern multidetector CT scanners permit easy coverage of extra- and intracranial vasculature in a single-volume dataset. That data can also show tandem stenoses and other intracerebral vascular malformations that may be present in 13%–50% of cases with primary stenosis (19–21) at the carotid bifurcation. The presence of such additional lesions has a

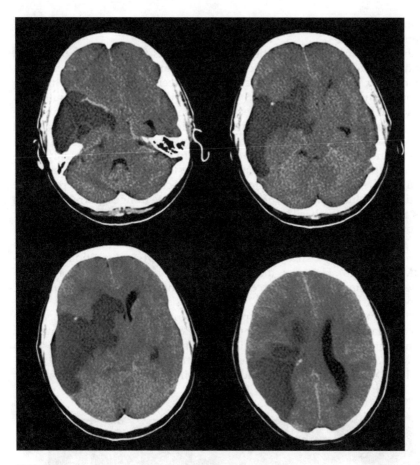

FIGURE 5 Computed tomography (CT) of a patient in a later state of ischemia with diminished gray–white-matter differentiation, narrowing of the adjacent sulci due to water uptake, as well as midline shift and axial herniation. Note the dense right middle cerebral artery (MCA) as cause of the ischemia.

negative predictive value for the outcome of patients undergoing carotid endarterectomy (CEA) and may also change the therapeutic approach to acute stroke treatment.

The technique required for CTA often varies and can depend on the scanner manufacturer, the model, the software level, the type of contrast, physician preference, and individual patient anatomy. CT angiograms require the intravenous administration of contrast; many protocols have been published using, for example, boluses between 75 and 150 ml at injection rates from 1.8 to 5.0 ml/s, with a peak between 2.5 and 3 ml/s. Delay times between 15 and 30 s have proven reliable and reproducible. Automated trigger programs are provided by the manufacturers, which might help to optimize the results of peak enhancement. The current rapid development of multidetector scanners precludes the recommendation of parameters for collimation, pitch, and reconstruction intervals; yet each carries the risk to decrease image quality and increase artifacts or radiation exposure if inappropriate parameters are applied.

Studies have shown a correlation between results from Duplex ultrasound (DUS) and time-of-flight (TOF) magnetic resonance angiography (MRA), raising expectations that CTA could be another alternative screening tool (22). CTA has been found to be helpful in cases where DUS and MRA showed discordant results (23). Also, CTA may allow differentiation between dissected and atherosclerotic arteries by visualizing the intimal flap or atherosclerotic plaque. Data suggest a good interobserver reliability but only a satisfactory correlation with results from digital subtraction angiography (DSA) (24). The same group found CTA to be highly sensitive in the detection of carotid artery stenosis, suggesting it as suitable for screening symptomatic patients (25). Most difficult for CTA detection is the petrous portion of the carotid artery, due to image artifacts from bone; the strongest correlation with DSA was reported in the basilar artery. There is general agreement that, similar to MRI, source images contain the greatest information and should be referred to regularly. The technical justification lies in the limited visualization on maximum intensity projections (MIP), shaded surface displays (SSD), and multiplanar reformations (MPR) (Fig. 6). However, these, as well as the more recently evolved volume rendering technique, remain excellent for screening and very illustrative for demonstration purposes.

Parallel to advances in scanner speed, the postprocessing procedures have improved dramatically and can be performed in less than 20 min. An advantage of CTA lies in its quick availability to examine stenoses in the acute phase of diseases (Fig. 7). There are, however, many issues the interpreter has to attend, i.e., window and level settings, which can lead to a misinterpretation such as over- or

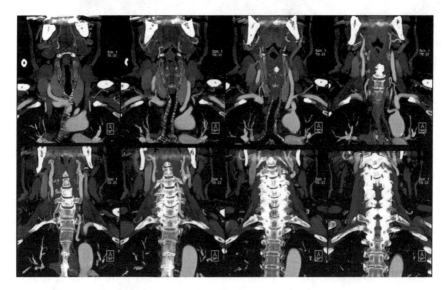

FIGURE 6 A multiplanar reformation (MPR) of the thoracic and cervical vasculature. Note the artifacts at the petrous portion of the internal carotid artery and the V2 segment of the vertebral artery. Stenoses can be overlooked easily, which necessitates the evaluation of source images.

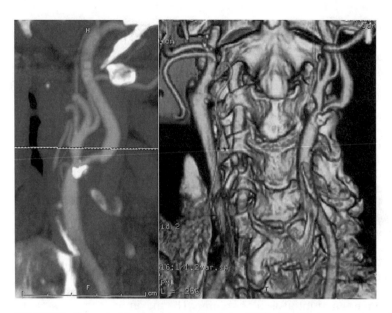

FIGURE 7 Computed tomography angiography (CTA) with 3D reconstruction of the carotid bulb in an 81-year-old man shows a calcified plaque in the carotid bifurcation with extension in to the internal carotid artery with an 80% stenosis. (See also color plate section.)

underestimation of an arterial stenosis. The ulceration of plaque has been analyzed less extensively, but there seems to be a reasonably good correlation between CTA and DSA (26,27). One has to remember that even DSA has a detection rate of only 60%–73% for ulceration, when correlated with results from surgery (28,29). More recent data from bi-plane DSA and, in particular, flat panel technique are not as abundant but do suggest these numbers may be improved (30–33). CTA can serve as a robust additional imaging tool that can be performed in an emergency setting even in severely ill patients or in patients not suitable for MRI, permitting CTA to be used to help triage patients in the very early phase of an anticipated ischemic event.

CT PERFUSION
In recent years CT perfusion has begun to be used as another advanced method to further evaluate cerebral ischemia and its causes by measuring relative cerebral blood flow (CBF), cerebral blood volume (CBV), time-to-peak (TTP), and mean transit time (MTT). CBF is expressed as ml/100 g/min or ml/100 ml/min, and CBV as ml/100 g or as ml/100 ml. TTP describes the time interval in seconds between the first measurable contrast in a major cerebral artery and the local bolus peak in the brain tissue. MTT reflects the time delay between the arrival of contrast in a major cerebral artery and its passage to cortical veins. As this time varies according to anatomical region, MTT is an average of any possible transit time.

The rapid development of helical, multirow, detector CT scanners has made CT perfusion more widely available and accepted as an additional first choice tool in the evaluation of patients presenting with stroke symptoms. Spiral CT imaging is used to sequentially scan the changes in density due to an intravenously injected iodinated contrast agent on its passage through the brain tissue. Postprocessing delivers mathematically reconstructed maps from the time–density curves that are presented as color maps, though these may vary with arterial input function, venous selection, and postprocessing algorithm (Fig. 8). The technique's major restrictions are a limited number of selective slices of brain parenchyma and the radiation of repeated data acquisitions. Future development of scanners with increasing number of detector rows may partially overcome the slice limitation. Although acceptable in the emergency setting, the radiation exposure remains a concern, particularly in comparison with MRI. Further shortcomings of the technique are related to the application of an intravascular contrast agent; a minimum requirement of 18-gage peripheral lines is crucial for some of the patients. Prior to intravenous injection of the contrast material, an impairment of the kidney function has to be ruled out. A simultaneous measurement of all cerebral vessels (i.e., arterial and capillary) leads to a relative overestimation in CBF of regions, including vessels with higher caliber (34), which also impairs the comparison to alternative methods of CBF measurement. Other inherent problems derive from a possible blood–brain barrier breakdown, which may occur in ischemia, and recirculation phenomena that interact with the measured intravascular volume. The maximum slope technique is influenced possibly by the patient's cardiac output function and the technician's choice of the arterial input function.

Depending on the mathematical algorithm used (deconvolution or maximum slope for bolus tracking techniques and slow infusion method), the validity of CT perfusion can be influenced by, among other items, blood–brain barrier disruption, speed of contrast bolus, recirculation, or cardiovascular disease. Despite these influences, both CT perfusion methods have demonstrated to accurately show decreases in CBF and CBV in patients with cerebral ischemia, applying certain thresholds for the different techniques in comparison with MRI (35), MR diffusion (36), and MR perfusion (37), as well as SPECT (38,39). Although CBV can be increased in

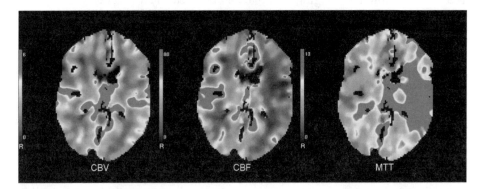

FIGURE 8 CT Perfusion Maps in a patient with acute occlusion of the M1 segment of the left middle cerebral artery (MCA). The cerebral blood volume map (CBV) in this early stage of onset is not altered, yet. The cerebral blood flow (CBF) is already reduced below 20 ml/100 g/min in the left MCA territory, and the mean transit time (MTT) is increased to over 10 s *Source*: Courtesy of Dr. G. Bohner. (See also color plate section.)

cerebral ischemia, it has been shown by CT perfusion and other techniques that a CBV below 2.5 ml/100 g of brain tissue highly correlates with irreversibly damaged brain on follow-up diffusion-weighted MR images (40). Using the maximum slope method, a decrease to 60% of normal CBV values is a strong indicator for irreversible infarction (41).

MTT and TTP have been found to be increased in ischemic brain tissue. Eastwood et al. (35) demonstrated the MTT in patients with acute MCA ischemia to be extended twofold from 3.6 s in unaffected MCA territories to 7.6 s in affected brain areas, so that a TTP of more than 8 s is suspicious for the presence of ischemia. Wintermark and Harrigan (40,42) found MTT and TTP to be affected by ischemia earlier than CBF and CBV and less affected by influences from large vessels. They concluded that the absence of extended TTP and MTT reliably indicated that ischemia was not present.

Measuring CBF using CT perfusion has been found to correlate well with changes shown on DWI (43) and to predict the later infarcted area with high precision. Using the maximum slope algorithm, CBF maps had a high sensitivity (93%) and specificity (98%) to predict later infarct sizes (39). Analogous to MRI, it has been advocated to differentiate the tissue at risk for infarction from infarcted tissue by a mismatch among the regional MTT, CBF, and CBV maps, applying the deconvolution method. With the maximum slope technique, only relative values of CBF and CBV are derived, but they can still be used to distinguish the potentially salvageable tissue as in MRI.

CT and additionally performed CTA and CT perfusion can be obtained at one setting in about 20 min, including postprocessing, and provide the clinician with morphologic and physiologic information about the brain tissue. This adds an excellent alternative to the standards set by MRI, particularly in patients not suitable for MRI and in centers with limited access to MR facilities and trained personnel. Nevertheless, training and equipment should not be traded for this less robust functional tissue imaging method (44). The following paragraphs will describe the arguably superior properties of MRI and some of its future potentials.

MAGNETIC RESONANCE IMAGING

MRI has been established as a research and clinical tool for anatomic imaging for over a decade, and its soft tissue discrimination, in particular, has been recognized to be superior to unenhanced CT. Excellent submillimeter spatial and subsecond temporal resolutions as well as images in multiple orientations are properties that now help to evaluate not only anatomy and pathology but tissue function, metabolism, blood flow, and hemodynamics in normal and diseased tissue. Still, MRI is not as widely available as CT, and access, especially in the emergency situation, is not as easy. Not every patient suffering from stroke symptoms can be examined by means of MRI, due to cardiac pacemakers or other medical implants. Further limitations are related to impaired patient's compliance and risk of aspiration in the emergency situation requiring general anesthesia, possible increased claustrophobia, patient's stiffness, or patient size. Thus, CT remains an important imaging tool to offer a valuable alternative to patients and practitioners.

Even conventional MRI with T1- and T2-weighted spin echo and fluid-attenuated inversion recovery (FLAIR) sequences helps to detect the early signs of ischemia related to interstitial vasogenic edema, leading again to the changes described above for CT, including gyral swelling, diminished gray–white-matter delineation, insular ribbon sign, and mass effect with thinning of sulci and midline shift, all with higher sensitivity (Fig. 9) (45,46). T1-weighted images can be useful to follow the development of ischemia, as signal changes related to vasogenic edema are most prominent 24 h after the onset of the event and disappear within three days from onset (47). Like CT, MRI provides the opportunity to detect hemorrhage reliably by applying T2*-weighted or, even more routine, T2-weighted sequences, as the paramagnetic properties of deoxyhemoglobin cause visible susceptibility artifacts. Fast spin echo (FSE) and turbo spin echo (TSE) sequences are less sensitive to these susceptibility artifacts compared with gradient recalled echo (GRE) sequences, but there has been an increasing number of reports on the reliable detection of hemorrhage with a multimodal MRI protocol (10,12,48–52). More recently, fast FLAIR sequences have been found valuable in the detection of hyperacute subarachnoid hemorrhage (53,54).

DIFFUSION-WEIGHTED MR-IMAGING

Undoubtedly, though, the most advantageous and revolutionary technique in MR for acute stroke imaging is related to the development of high-speed capabilities and enhanced gradient strengths that allow for echo planar imaging (EPI) and spiral imaging, which permit diffusion-weighted Imaging (DWI). In contrast to CT, DWI rapidly detects acute cerebral ischemic changes within minutes after onset. DWI is used to detect the cytotoxic edema in the hyperacute and acute stage of the ischemia with high sensitivity (97%) and specificity (~100%) (55). This occurs as the breakdown of the sodium-potassium ATPase (Na$^+$-K$^+$-ATPase) hinders the

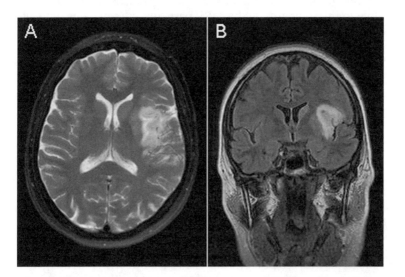

FIGURE 9 (*A*) An axial T2-weighted turbo spin echo (TSE) sequence with early signs of cerebral ischemia. The insular ribbon cannot be recognized, and the gray–white-matter differentiation is impaired due to cortical thickening, with narrow ipsilateral sulci as result of the mass effect. (*B*) Corresponding coronal fluid-attenuated inversion recovery (FLAIR) sequence. Note the zeroed signal from cerebrospinal fluid (CSF) in ventricles and subarachnoid spaces allowing a good visualization of the pathology.

Na$^+$-associated water efflux, resulting in intracellular swelling, decreased interstitial spaces, and restriction of free water diffusion. Signal intensity in DWI relates
to the random (Brownian) movement of water molecules and attenuates with the
degree of displacement. It is generated by applying strong gradients that lead,
initially, to a dephasing and then to a rephasing to sensitize the signal to random
movement of water protons. The phase shift of a moving water proton results in
an imperfect rephasing and, consequentially, signal loss. In other words, areas
with high proton movement are hypointense on DWI, whereas restricted proton
movement leads to relative hyperintensity (Fig. 10).

Hyperintensities on diffusion images, however, can derive from both
T2-effects related to vasogenic edema, often referred to as T2-shine-through, and
regions of truly restricted water diffusion caused by intracellular water uptake.
The diffusion technique allows the differentiation of a cytotoxic from vasogenic
edema by enabling the calculation of trace images and quantitative apparent diffusion coefficient (ADC) maps (56). ADC maps clearly plot zones of restricted
water diffusion found in acute or early subacute ischemia as a dark area. Conversely, ADC maps show zones of increased extracellular free water diffusion
as a bright area, elevated in more chronic stages of cerebral ischemia. The relative diffusion coefficients initially represented in ADC maps start to normalize in
an inhomogeneous matter after a week and end in unrestricted water diffusion
after several weeks, appearing as light tones on ADC maps (57). Interestingly,
on T2-weighted images and DWI, these areas appear homogeneous. It has been
suggested that these differences in degree of homogeneity are caused by different types of infarction and different progression patterns of ischemic evolution.
It may be speculated that these areas of inhomogeneous normalization represent
tissue with a higher resistance to ischemia, similar to areas with prolonged mismatch (58,59). Other authors were able to show a faster development of thrombe-
mbolic infarcts in comparison with watershed infarcts and a slower progression
of lacunar than territorial infarcts in older patients (60,61). More recent studies

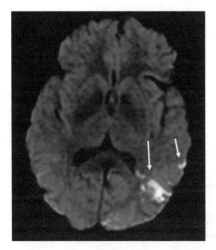

FIGURE 10   Magnetic Resonance diffusion-weighted
image (DWI). The arrows indicate an area of restricted
free water, diffusion clearly visible as a hyperintense
signal.

that evaluate the feasibility of fiber-tracking by diffusion tensor imaging reveal the sensorimotor pathway in stroke patients and find a good correlation with clinical symptoms; yet it is still too early to judge the scientific and clinical impact of this method (62,63). Finally, DWI might permit the separation of irreversibly damaged from potentially salvageable tissue. There is experimental and clinical evidence that ADC normalization within the first hours indicates potential neuronal recovery and correlates with revival of energy metabolism (57,64–67). The absence of normalization at early time points, seen in the majority of ischemic diffusion abnormalities, implies tissue infarction if CBF and perfusion are not restored.

PERFUSION-WEIGHTED MR-IMAGING

The physiological mechanisms and the pathophysiological results of perfusion precede those of diffusion. Early assessment of this information is vital for the patient presenting with ischemic symptoms (68). The main use of perfusion-weighted MR-Imaging (PWI) is to determine whether any hypoperfused tissue exists that can represent the tissue at risk for infarction and thus possibly salvageable tissue: the so-called "penumbra" (Fig. 11). This region of penumbra is characterized by a decreased cerebral perfusion pressure (CPP), a decreased CBF to values of about 20 ml/100 g/min, and a maximally increased oxygen extraction fraction (OEF). The CBV may be either increased due to compensatory vasodilatation and collateral circulation or decreased due to reduced blood flow and/or prolonged blood passage from arteries to veins. Similar to CT perfusion, MTT, and TTP can be evaluated in addition to relative CBF and CBV.

Hemodynamically weighted perfusion MRI can be achieved principally by an intravenous injection of an exogenous tracer agent, i.e., a paramagnetic contrast material, or through endogenous tracer agents, i.e., magnetically labelled blood using arterial spin labeling (ASL). In the former the intravascular gadolinium agent leads to a T2* shortening mainly in the microvasculature on susceptibility-weighted echo planar images (EPI). The T2* shortening can be recognized

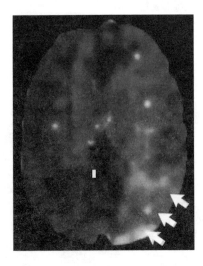

FIGURE 11 Magnetic resonance perfusion-weighted image (PWI) map. The arrows indicate an area of hypoperfused tissue in the distribution of the left middle cerebral artery that is shown as hyperintensity in contrast to the normally perfused tissue.

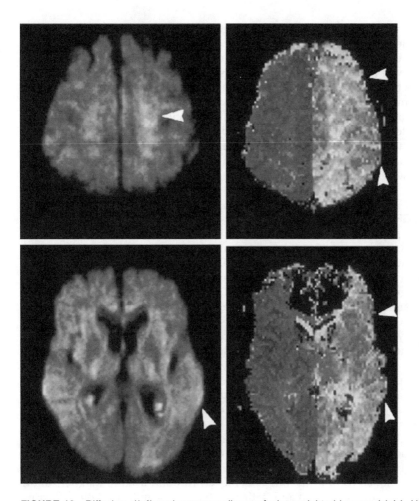

FIGURE 12 Diffusion- (*left*) and corresponding perfusion-weighted images (*right*). Hyperintense signal on diffusion images (*arrowheads*) define the core infarct. The perfusion-weighted image indicates a reduced perfusion of the entire left hemisphere. The mismatch (normal appearing tissue on diffusion images) represents tissue at risk of infarction.

as a short-term signal loss over the entire brain, followed by a return toward baseline values in normal tissue. Rapidly repeated EPI sequences allow the analysis of signal intensities relative to time that represent the regional cerebral perfusion, as expressed in one or more parameter map (regional(r) CBF, rCBV, MTT, TTP). In ASL magnetic tagging is achieved by applying a specifically designed radiofrequency pulse to invert spins of inflowing blood in a thick slab below the region of interest. The differences in baseline signal intensities and intensities from labelled images can be used for qualitative and quantitative assessment of CBF. Theoretically, spin-labeling techniques provide the opportunity to calculate absolute CBF, though practically this is limited by an insufficient signal-to-noise ratio (69).

The consideration of perfusion changes occurring earlier than diffusion changes has led to the concept of perfusion and diffusion mismatch in acute stroke without hemorrhage. Areas that show perfusion deficits, but no diffusion deficits, are believed to represent the potentially salvageable tissue, whereas the DWI defect estimates the core infarct (Fig. 12). As already discussed above, the changes in ADC are more complex and can represent more than just core infarct. It can be suggested that matching perfusion and diffusion deficits represent the final infarct size. A DWI lesion larger than the corresponding PWI lesion may represent a reperfusion situation not yet detectable at PWI. This has helped to triage successfully patients with hyperacute stroke (70–72) and to predict the final infarct volume more accurately.

MR ANGIOGRAPHY

MR angiography (MRA) offers the opportunity to examine the intracranial and extracranial vasculature with high resolution, non-invasively, without iodinated contrast agents, and no ionizing radiation. During the same examination, information on blood flow, flow velocity, and blood volume can be gathered if phase-contrast (PC) angiography techniques are applied (73). The most commonly used MRA techniques are TOF-MRA, PC-MRA, and contrast-enhanced (CE)-MRA, which deliver bright blood vessel images usually displayed as MIP. All MRA techniques are limited by a vulnerability to motion, susceptibility artifacts, slow flow-related signal loss, turbulent flow, or pulsatility. Similar to CTA, all the information is contained in the source images, which should be evaluated carefully in cases of any uncertainty apparent on the projections. If the MRA images or clinical presentation suggest an acute dissection, MRI can provide useful additional information by adding thin slice axial T2-weighted images more quickly or fat saturated T1-weighted images over more time.

TOF techniques are used to show the anatomy of cervical and cerebral vasculature without the addition of intravenous contrast (Fig. 13). The moving blood appears bright, enabling visualization, in contrast to stationary tissue that has a dim saturated look. Technically this is achieved through a large magnetization gradient between moving blood and stationary tissue. The inflowing blood carries a stronger magnetization, leading to a bright signal. The appropriate positioning of saturation pulses prevents inflow phenomena, which may lead to misinterpretation, and allows the imaging of either arterial or venous vasculature. Features such as magnetization transfer (MT); echo time optimization, such that the fat signal is out of phase; application of a ramped tip angle (74); and zero filling to smoothen vessel borders—all help to optimize the contrast-to-noise ratio in three-dimensional (3D) TOF techniques, but they need more time. Increasing magnet field strength and adding multiple channels to allow for parallel imaging techniques can help by significantly reducing the acquisition times and increasing the signal-to-noise ratios.

PC techniques also utilize the movement of blood to yield images. Stationary tissue is magnetized in such a way that the phase is zero, whereas the phase of flowing blood is not. Similar to other angiography, the signal is subtracted from the stationary information to produce flow-sensitive images, and these can be used also to generate various typical projections. As phase measures the distance, magnetization moves out of the transverse plane before detection; images can also

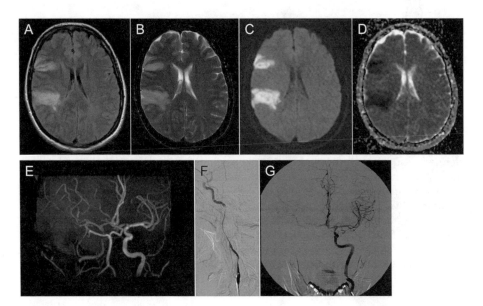

FIGURE 13 Magnetic resonance (MR) images of a 43-year-old female with a right hemispheric stroke. (*A*) Axial fluid-Diffusion-attenuated inversion recovery (FLAIR) image, (*B*) T2-weighted image, (*C*) Diffusion-weighted image (DWI) with (*D*) apparent diffusion coefficient (ADC) map show subacute cortical and subcortical infarctions in the distribution of the right middle cerebral artery (branches of the anterior and posterior divisions). (*E*) Contrast enhanced MR angiography using gradient recalled 3D TOF sequence in coronal plane with maximum-intensity-projection (MIP) reconstructions shows a long segment of tapered narrowing of the proximal portion of the right internal carotid artery. The distal cervical segment is diffusely narrowed and the assessment of its lumen is limited. (*F*) Digital subtraction angiography (DSA) in lateral view shows an extensive dissection of the right internal carotid artery with significant narrowing up to the horizontal segment of the petrous portion and poor antegrade blood flow. (*G*) Angiogram of the left internal carotid artery in frontal view shows collateral blood supply to the right hemisphere through the anterior communication artery.

be expressed in terms of direction, flow rate, and velocity of flow (73). Depending on the information desired, either 2D or 3D images, or one or multiple flow directions, can be encoded with the usual trade-off of expanded acquisition time demands.

CE-MRA, like the two methods described previously, uses the differences in magnetization between moving blood and surrounding tissue to yield a bright signal. Gadolinium is injected intravenously to further shorten the T1 relaxation in flowing blood and enhance the distinction from stationary tissue. For example, on T1-weighted sequences thoracic and cervical arteries can be examined simultaneously with this technique; this allows a reliable interpretation through the typical level of common carotid artery bifurcations (75). For some centers, this method has become the primary and only imaging tool for vascular examinations. Intracranially, the method is limited due to a short time window before venous contamination diminishes the signal clarity. The appropriate timing of the injection of the contrast bolus and the start of the acquisition is crucial for an optimal signal-to-noise ratio. Standard vendor protocols allow the technologist either to calculate the arrival time from a test bolus or to trigger the acquisition upon seeing the initial signal change in a test image or volume. The principal advantages of CE-MRA over the unenhanced MRA methods are its diminished susceptibility to artifacts and shorter acquisition times (76).

MR SPECTROSCOPY

The role of MR spectroscopy (MRS) in the evaluation of acute ischemic stroke is secondary due to its time-consuming planning and postprocessing, limited conspicuity, and decreased availability for most clinicians. Spectroscopy, though, presents the unique potential to examine in vivo and noninvasively the metabolism of a defined tissue. For studies in humans, researchers have concentrated on ^{1}H-proton and ^{31}phosphorous spectroscopy to evaluate the brain metabolism. ^{31}P-spectroscopy allows the analysis of the metabolism of the energy-carrying phosphates and intracellular pH values that can be estimated from the chemical shift of inorganic phos phospho-mono- and di-esters (PME, PDE) can be identified in ^{31}P-spectra (77). At 1.5 T, peaks from N-acetyl-aspartate (NAA), Choline (Ch), and (phospho)-creatine (Cr) can be detected reliably in ^{1}H-proton spectra (78). A duplet signal from lactate can become visible under ischemic conditions due to anaerobic glycolysis. In later phases of ischemia and infarction, the peaks from NAA, which is almost exclusively present in neuronal cells, decrease and disappear with progressive cell death. Areas of elevated lactate and normal NAA levels may indicate ischemic tissue at risk for infarction. In further phases of infarction the Ch-signal increases, possibly reflecting an accelerated membrane metabolism. MRS may add to the understanding of the metabolic basis of ischemia and, some suggest, impact the patient selection process for specific treatments (79); first, however, one must overcome the practical limitations of current MRS.

SINGLE-PHOTON EMISSION COMPUTED TOMOGRAPHY

Since its introduction in the early 1980s, single-photon emission computed tomography (SPECT) has delivered reliable, functional information related to blood flow to brain tissue. SPECT measures the rCBF, which indicates tissue viability, and can be used, for example, in the hyperacute phase of ischemia even before conventional CT and MRI become sensitive (80). Unlike CT and magnetic resonance tomography, the special resolution is less, but desired functional information is still gained. After the intravenous application of the radiotracers ^{99m}Technetium (Tc)-hexamet hylpropylene-amino-oxime (HMPAO), ^{99m}Technetium (Tc)-ethyl-cysteinate-dimer (ECD), or N-isopropyl-p-[^{123}I]iodoamphetamine (^{123}I-IMP) (the latter is not commercially available in the United States), these can cross the blood–brain barrier and bind to central nervous neurons proportionally to the rCBF. Gamma cameras then identify possible perfusion deficits by discriminate relatively diminished or absent radioactivity. However, as measured values are relative and not absolute perfusion values, they do not allow an adequate differentiation of the penumbra. Historically, ^{133}Xenon (^{133}Xe)–SPECT has been an important method to evaluate brain hemodynamics, offering quantitative rCBF measurement. The low photon energy emitted by the ^{133}Xe gamma rays, however, results in low special resolution and abundant scatter (81,82). Nevertheless, SPECT has been used successfully to triage patients for thrombolysis, to help reduce hemorrhagic complications, and to improve neurological outcome (83). The advance of SPECT combined with CT as a single unit may improve further the spatial resolution of the technique.

POSITRON EMISSION TOMOGRAPHY

Positron emission tomography (PET) allows the in vivo examination of blood flow and oxygen metabolism. Much of our pathophysiological understanding of ischemia, particularly the concept of OEF, has been validated by PET (84). A PET camera registers the counts emitted from an isotope while traveling in the circulation through the brain, and these are plotted as a regional image map representing CBF. In day-to-day practice related to acute ischemia, however, PET has not had much impact on diagnosis and management, which is in part due to the limited access to both PET scanners and the most widely applied specific isotope, ^{15}O (which itself requires an onsite or very nearby cyclotron because of its short half-life). Other limitations include long examination times, low spatial resolution, and sensitivity to motion artifacts.

PET scan examinations of the brain vary in output, dependent on the tracer employed and the type of processing applied. Usually, an injection of ^{15}O-labeled water allows one to gain information on brain perfusion in terms of quantifiable CBF. One can then evaluate CBV through the application of ^{15}O carbon monoxide or ^{15}O carbon dioxide. Independent measurement of ^{15}O inhalation scan in comparison to CBF and CBV generates the OEF. OEF, CBF, and arterial oxygen content can be combined to form the cerebral metabolic consumption rate of oxygen ($CMRO_2$). During the aberrant metabolism of ischemia, as a result of falling perfusion pressure, the OEF will increase to a maximum to compensate for the reduced CBF and to restore normal values for $CMRO_2$. This has been described as a characteristic sign for tissue at risk of infarction (85). If the drop in perfusion pressure persists and the circulation is not reestablished, then the OEF compensation may fail, and that may begin a decrease in $CMRO_2$. Plummeting $CMRO_2$ then can spread gradually from central to peripheral parts of the ischemic tissue and represent a completed transition from ischemic to now infarcted parenchyma. To some extent some of the tissue with only moderately reduced $CMRO_2$ may still be salvageable, and this has been referred to as the "dynamic penumbra" (86). In a pre-infarct at risk population, OEF has been a powerful marker for risk of subsequent stroke in patients with occlusive atherosclerotic disease (87,88). These measures already can impact the selection of patients for CEA and/or carotid stenting and may suggest those occluded patients for whom a bypass procedure may be relevant.

FUTURE DIRECTIONS

Current research attempts to investigate the underlying causes of ischemia. One major concern is the visualization of the atherosclerotic inflammatory plaque. This problem has been addressed by utilizing small (SPIO) and ultra small superparamagnetic iron oxide (USPIO) particles as contrast agents in hyperlipidemic rabbits. It has proven feasible to image the atherosclerotic aorta (89,90). Preliminary clinical results suggest that the composition of the plaque rather than the degree of stenosis determines patient outcome (91).

Less promising results come from research at modern CT scanners trying to predict future stroke probability from carotid calcium scores (92), though the method delivers reliable results on the degree of the stenoses (24,93). Cardiologists have put much effort into the visualization of vulnerable plaque in the coronary arteries, and they have worked with the development of intravascular ultrasound (IVUS). Interventional Neuroradiologists have worked similarly with these techniques to evaluate cerebrovascular disease and postinterventional results (94,95). Researchers approached the topic of the characterization of the thrombus/embolus again by applying iron oxide particles and were able to demonstrate promising experimental results (96,97). Clinically, this has been tested in patients with lower limb deep vein thrombosis at high field strength MRI. The thrombus can be visualized as a bright signal if there is a sufficiently suppressed signal from flowing blood, stationary blood, and fat (98). Finally, animal studies at 7.0 T are addressing the different types of infarct evolution as they relate to preconditioned brain tissue, and results suggest a cell death-preventing effect from lipo-polysaccharide-induced tolerance (99).

CONCLUSION

Radiologists and the wider clinical community are offered multiple ways to diagnose patients presenting with symptoms of stroke. All the techniques offered have improved dramatically during the past few years and have become much more available to the daily routine. Still, none of the techniques offer the ultimate solution to examine stroke and target our immediate therapeutic efforts, to triage our patients in the most appropriate way by excluding differential diagnoses and reliably predicting infarction differentiated from penumbra. MRI techniques are currently the most likely to realize this aim for whole brain studies, but CT also has added valuable information and is an excellent alternative in the emergency situation. PET can help researchers and clinicians to understand further the pathophysiology of stroke, to develop new treatment strategies, and to further characterize different phases of ischemia. However, it needs to be emphasized that different imaging modalities are only as good as the person trained to use it. Many multicenter studies have shown a limitation in the training factor and the subsequent confidence with which the diagnosis occurs. Among all the limitations the various methods may have and the efforts undergone to reduce these, continuous education and sharing of knowledge remain the most necessary.

REFERENCES

1. Sunshine JL. CT, MR imaging, and MR angiography in the evaluation of patients with acute stroke. J Vasc Interv Radiol 2004; 15:S47–S55.
2. Kucinski T. Unenhanced CT and acute stroke physiology. Neuroimaging Clin N Am 2005; 15:397–407, xi–xii.
3. Hacke W, Kaste M, Fieschi C, et al. Intravenous thrombolysis with recombinant tissue plasminogen activator for acute hemispheric stroke. The European Cooperative Acute Stroke Study (ECASS). JAMA 1995; 274(13):1017–1025.
4. von Kummer R, Bourquain H, Bastianello S, et al. Early prediction of irreversible brain damage after ischemic stroke at CT. Radiology 2001; 219:95–100.
5. The National Institute of Neurological Disorders and Stroke t-PA Stroke Study Group. Tissue plasminogen activator for acute ischemic stroke. N Engl J Med 1995; 333:1581–1587.
6. del Zoppo GJ, Higashida RT, Furlan AJ, et al. PROACT: a phase II randomized trial of recombinant pro-urokinase by direct arterial delivery in acute middle cerebral artery stroke. PROACT investigators. Prolyse in acute cerebral thromboembolism. Stroke 1998; 29:4–11.
7. Furlan A, Higashida R, Wechsler L, et al. Intra-arterial prourokinase for acute ischemic stroke. The PROACT II study: a randomized controlled trial. Prolyse in acute cerebral thromboembolism. JAMA 1999; 282:2003–2011.
8. Stroke–1989. Recommendations on stroke prevention, diagnosis, and therapy. Report of the WHO task force on stroke and other cerebrovascular disorders. Stroke 1989; 20:1407–1431.

9. Qureshi AI, Tuhrim S, Broderick JP, et al. Spontaneous intracerebral hemorrhage. N Engl J Med 2001; 344:1450–1460.

10. Kidwell CS, Saver JL, Villablanca JP, et al. Magnetic resonance imaging detection of microbleeds before thrombolysis: an emerging application. Stroke 2002; 33:95–98.

11. Fiebach JB, Schellinger PD, Gass A, et al. Stroke magnetic resonance imaging is accurate in hyperacute intracerebral hemorrhage: a multicenter study on the validity of stroke imaging. Stroke 2004; 35:502–506.

12. Fiebach JB, Schellinger PD, Geletneky K, et al. MRI in acute subarachnoid haemorrhage; findings with a standardised stroke protocol. Neuroradiology 2004; 46:44–48.

13. Lee J, Berry CL. Cerebral micro-aneurysm formation in the hypertensive rat. J Pathol 1978; 124:7–11.

14. von Kummer R. Imaging the cerebral parenchyma in ischemic stroke, computed tomography. In: Latchaw RE, Kucharczyk J, Moseley ME, eds. Imaging of the Nervous System. Philadelphia: Elsevier Mosby, 2005;199.

15. Lev MH, Farkas J, Gemmete JJ, et al. Acute stroke: improved nonenhanced CT detection—benefits of soft-copy interpretation by using variable window width and center level settings. Radiology 1999; 213:150–155.

16. Larrue V, von Kummer RR, Müller A, et al. Risk factors for severe hemorrhagic transformation in ischemic stroke patients treated with recombinant tissue plasminogen activator: a secondary analysis of the European-Australasian Acute Stroke Study (ECASS II). Stroke 2001; 32:438–441.

17. Brant-Zawadzki M, Heiserman JE. The roles of MR angiography, CT angiography, and sonography in vascular imaging of the head and neck. AJNR Am J Neuroradiol 1997; 18:1820–1825.

18. Leblang SD, Fukui MB. Helical CT angiography for stroke. In: Latchaw RE, Kucharczyk J, Moseley ME, eds. Imaging of the Nervous System. Philadelphia: Elsevier Mosby, 2005:357.

19. Simonetti G, Bozzao A, Floris R, et al. Non-invasive assessment of neck-vessel pathology. Eur Radiol 1998; 8:691–697.

20. Griffiths PD, Worthy S, Gholkar A. Incidental intracranial vascular pathology in patients investigated for carotid stenosis. Neuroradiology 1996; 38:25–30.

21. Barnett HJ, Meldrum HE, Eliasziw M. The appropriate use of carotid endarterectomy. CMAJ 2002; 166:1169–1179.

22. Schwartz RB, Jones KM, Chernoff DM, et al. Common carotid artery bifurcation: evaluation with spiral CT. Work in progress. Radiology 1992; 185:513–519.

23. Cinat ME, Pham H, Vo D, et al. Improved imaging of carotid artery bifurcation using helical computed tomographic angiography. Ann Vasc Surg 1999; 13:178–183.

24. Zhang Z, Berg M, Ikonen A, et al. Carotid stenosis degree in CT angiography: assessment based on luminal area versus luminal diameter measurements. Eur Radiol 2005; 15:2359–2365.

25. Berg M, Zhang Z, Ikonen A, et al. Multi-detector row CT angiography in the assessment of carotid artery disease in symptomatic patients: comparison with rotational angiography and digital subtraction angiography. AJNR Am J Neuroradiol 2005; 26:1022–1034.

26. Cumming MJ, Morrow IM. Carotid artery stenosis: a prospective comparison of CT angiography and conventional angiography. AJR Am J Roentgenol 1994; 163:517–523.

27. Anderson GB, Ashforth R, Steinke DE, et al. CT angiography for the detection and characterization of carotid artery bifurcation disease. Stroke 2000; 31:2168–2174.

28. Edwards JH, Kricheff II, Riles T, et al. Angiographically undetected ulceration of the carotid bifurcation as a cause of embolic stroke. Radiology 1979; 132:369–373.

29. Eikelboom BC, Riles TR, Mintzer R, et al. Inaccuracy of angiography in the diagnosis of carotid ulceration. Stroke 1983; 14:882–885.

30. Hankey GJ, Warlow CP, Molyneux AJ. Complications of cerebral angiography for patients with mild carotid territory ischaemia being considered for carotid endarterectomy. J Neurol Neurosurg Psychiatry 1990; 53:542–548.

31. Buskens E, Nederkoorn PJ, Buijs-Van Der Woude T, et al. Imaging of carotid arteries in symptomatic patients: cost-effectiveness of diagnostic strategies. Radiology 2004; 233:101–112.

32. Anzalone N, Scomazzoni F, Castellano R, et al. Carotid artery stenosis: intraindividual correlations of 3D time-of-flight MR angiography, contrast-enhanced MR angiography, conventional DSA, and rotational angiography for detection and grading. Radiology 2005; 236:204–213.

33. Derdeyn CP. Conventional angiography remains an important tool for measurement of carotid arterial stenosis. Radiology 2005; 235:711–712, author reply 712–713.

34. Roberts H. Neuroimaging techniques in cerebrovascular disease: computed tomography angiography/computed tomography perfusion. Semin Cerebrovasc Dis Stroke 2001; 1:303–316.

35. Eastwood JD, Lev MH, Azhari T, et al. CT perfusion scanning with deconvolution analysis: pilot study in patients with acute middle cerebral artery stroke. Radiology 2002; 222:227–236.

36. Wintermark M, Fischbein NJ, Smith WS, et al. Accuracy of dynamic perfusion CT with deconvolution in detecting acute hemispheric stroke. AJNR Am J Neuroradiol 2005; 26:104–112.

37. Eastwood JD, Lev MH, Wintermark M, et al. Correlation of early dynamic CT perfusion imaging with whole-brain MR diffusion and perfusion imaging in acute hemispheric stroke. AJNR Am J Neuroradiol 2003; 24:1869–1875.

38. Koenig M, Klotz E, Luka B, et al. Perfusion CT of the brain: diagnostic approach for early detection of ischemic stroke. Radiology 1998; 209:85–93.

39. Mayer TE, Hamann GF, Baranczyk J, et al. Dynamic CT perfusion imaging of acute stroke. AJNR Am J Neuroradiol 2000; 21:1441–1449.

40. Wintermark M, Reichhart M, Thiran JP, et al. Prognostic accuracy of cerebral blood flow measurement by perfusion computed tomography, at the time of emergency room admission, in acute stroke patients. Ann Neurol 2002; 51:417–432.

41. Koenig M, Kraus M, Theek C, et al. Quantitative assessment of the ischemic brain by means of perfusion-related parameters derived from perfusion CT. Stroke 2001; 32:431–437.

42. Harrigan MR, Leonardo J, Gibbons KJ, et al. CT perfusion cerebral blood flow imaging in neurological critical care. Neurocrit Care 2005; 2:352–366.

43. Wintermark M, Reichhart M, Cuisenaire O, et al. Comparison of admission perfusion computed tomography and qualitative diffusion- and perfusion-weighted magnetic resonance imaging in acute stroke patients. Stroke 2002; 33:2025–2031.

44. Hacke W, Warach S. Diffusion-weighted MRI as an evolving standard of care in acute stroke. Neurology 2000; 54:1548–1549.

45. Bryan RN, Levy LM, Whitlow WD, et al. Diagnosis of acute cerebral infarction: comparison of CT and MR imaging. AJNR Am J Neuroradiol 1991; 12:611–620.

46. Yuh WT, Crain MR, Loes DJ, et al. MR imaging of cerebral ischemia: findings in the first 24 hours. AJNR Am J Neuroradiol 1991; 12:621–629.

47. Rydberg JN, Hammond CA, Grimm RC, et al. Initial clinical experience in MR imaging of the brain with a fast fluid-attenuated inversion-recovery pulse sequence. Radiology 1994; 193:173–180.

48. Linfante I, Llinas RH, Caplan LR, et al. MRI features of intracerebral hemorrhage within 2 hours from symptom onset. Stroke 1999; 30:2263–2267.

49. Kidwell CS, Alger JR, Saver JL. Beyond mismatch: evolving paradigms in imaging the ischemic penumbra with multimodal magnetic resonance imaging. Stroke 2003; 34:2729–2735.

50. Linfante I. Editorial comment—can MRI reliably detect hyperacute intracerebral hemorrhage? Ask the medical student. Stroke 2004; 35:506–507.

51. Hjort N, Butcher K, Davis SM, et al. Magnetic resonance imaging criteria for thrombolysis in acute cerebral infarct. Stroke 2005; 36:388–397.

52. Hjort N, Christensen S, Solling C, et al. Ischemic injury detected by diffusion imaging 11 minutes after stroke. Ann Neurol 2005; 58:462–465.

53. Bakshi R, Kamran S, Kinkel PR, et al. Fluid-attenuated inversion-recovery MR imaging in acute and subacute cerebral intraventricular hemorrhage. AJNR Am J Neuroradiol 1999; 20:629–636.

54. Wiesmann M, Mayer TE, Yousry I, et al. Detection of hyperacute subarachnoid hemorrhage of the brain by using magnetic resonance imaging. J Neurosurg 2002; 96:684–689.
55. Mullins ME, Schaefer PW, Sorensen AG, et al. CT and conventional and diffusion-weighted MR imaging in acute stroke: study in 691 patients at presentation to the emergency department. Radiology 2002; 224:353–360.
56. Provenzale JM, Sorensen AG. Diffusion-weighted MR imaging in acute stroke: theoretic considerations and clinical applications. AJR Am J Roentgenol 1999; 173:1459–1467.
57. Schlaug G, Siewert B, Benfield A, et al. Time course of the apparent diffusion coefficient (ADC) abnormality in human stroke. Neurology 1997; 49:113–119.
58. Heiss WD, Huber M, Fink GR, et al. Progressive derangement of periinfarct viable tissue in ischemic stroke. J Cereb Blood Flow Metab 1992; 12:193–203.
59. Darby DG, Barber PA, Gerraty RP, et al. Pathophysiological topography of acute ischemia by combined diffusion-weighted and perfusion MRI. Stroke 1999; 30:2043–2052.
60. Huang IJ, Chen CY, Chung HW, et al. Time course of cerebral infarction in the middle cerebral arterial territory: deep watershed versus territorial subtypes on diffusion-weighted MR images. Radiology 2001; 221:35–42.
61. Copen WA, Schwamm LH, Gonzalez RG, et al. Ischemic stroke: effects of etiology and patient age on the time course of the core apparent diffusion coefficient. Radiology 2001; 221:27–34.
62. Lee JS, Han MK, Kim SH, et al. Fiber tracking by diffusion tensor imaging in corticospinal tract stroke: topographical correlation with clinical symptoms. Neuroimage 2005; 26:771–776.
63. Yamada K, Ito H, Nakamura H, et al. Stroke patients' evolving symptoms assessed by tractography. J Magn Reson Imaging 2004; 20:923–929.
64. Fiehler J, Foth M, Kucinski T, et al. Severe ADC decreases do not predict irreversible tissue damage in humans. Stroke 2002; 33:79–86.
65. Fiehler J, Kucinski T, Knudsen K, et al. Are there time-dependent differences in diffusion and perfusion within the first 6 hours after stroke onset?. Stroke 2004; 35:2099–2104.
66. Fiehler J, Knudsen K, Thomalla G, et al. Vascular occlusion sites determine differences in lesion growth from early apparent diffusion coefficient lesion to final infarct. AJNR Am J Neuroradiol 2005; 26:1056–1061.
67. Fiehler J, Remmele C, Kucinski T, et al. Reperfusion after severe local perfusion deficit precedes hemorrhagic transformation: an MRI study in acute stroke patients. Cerebrovasc Dis 2005; 19:117–124.
68. Bammer R, Moseley ME. Perfusion magnetic resonance and the perfusion/diffusion mismatch in stroke. In: Latchaw RE, Kucharczyk J, Moseley ME, eds. Imaging of the Nervous System. Philadelphia: Elsevier Mosby, 2005; 303.
69. Petrella JR, Provenzale JM. MR perfusion imaging of the brain: techniques and applications. AJR Am J Roentgenol 2000; 175:207–219.
70. Sunshine JL, Tarr RW, Lanzieri CF, et al. Hyperacute stroke: ultrafast MR imaging to triage patients prior to therapy. Radiology 1999; 212:325–332.
71. Sunshine JL, Bambakidis N, Tarr RW, et al. Benefits of perfusion MR imaging relative to diffusion MR imaging in the diagnosis and treatment of hyperacute stroke. AJNR Am J Neuroradiol 2001; 22:915–921.
72. Fiehler J, von Bezold M, Kucinski T, et al. Cerebral blood flow predicts lesion growth in acute stroke patients. Stroke 2002; 33:2421–2425.
73. Korosec F, Turski P. Velocity and volume flow rate measurements using phase contrast magnetic resonance imaging. Int J Neuroradiology 1997; 3:293–318.
74. Nagele T, Klose U, Grodd W, et al. The effects of linearly increasing flip angles on 3D inflow MR angiography. Magn Reson Med 1994; 31:561–566.
75. Leclerc X, Gauvrit JY, Nicol L, et al. Contrast-enhanced MR angiography of the craniocervical vessels: a review. Neuroradiology 1999; 41:867–874.
76. Korosec FR, Turski PA. Magnetic resonance angiography. In: Latchaw RE, Kucharczyk J, Moseley ME, eds. Imaging of the Nervous System. Philadelphia: Elsevier Mosby, 2005:385.

77. Michaelis T, Merboldt KD, Hanicke W, et al. On the identification of cerebral metabolites in localized 1H NMR spectra of human brain in vivo. NMR Biomed 1991; 4:90–98.
78. Bruhn H, Frahm J, Gyngell ML, et al. Cerebral metabolism in man after acute stroke: new observations using localized proton NMR spectroscopy. Magn Reson Med 1989; 9:126–131.
79. Saunders DE. MR spectroscopy in stroke. Br Med Bull 2000; 56:334–345.
80. De Roo M, Mortelmans L, Devos P, et al. Clinical experience with Tc-99m HM-PAO high resolution SPECT of the brain in patients with cerebrovascular accidents. Eur J Nucl Med 1989; 15:9–15.
81. Obrist WD, Thompson HK Jr, King CH, et al. Determination of regional cerebral blood flow by inhalation of 133-xenon. Circ Res 1967; 20:124–135.
82. Wintermark M, Sesay M, Barbier E, et al. Comparative overview of brain perfusion imaging techniques. Stroke 2005; 36:e83–e99.
83. Ueda T, Sakaki S, Yuh WT, et al. Outcome in acute stroke with successful intra-arterial thrombolysis and predictive value of initial single-photon emission-computed tomography. J Cereb Blood Flow Metab 1999; 19:99–108.
84. Derdeyn CP. Positron emission tomography imaging of cerebral ischemia. Neuroimaging Clin N Am 2005; 15:341–350, x–xi.
85. Baron JC. Mapping the ischaemic penumbra with PET: implications for acute stroke treatment. Cerebrovasc Dis 1999; 9:193–201.
86. Heiss WD, Graf R, Wienhard K, et al. Dynamic penumbra demonstrated by sequential multitracer PET after middle cerebral artery occlusion in cats. J Cereb Blood Flow Metab 1994; 14:892–902.
87. Grubb RL Jr., Derdeyn CP, Fritsch SM, et al. Importance of hemodynamic factors in the prognosis of symptomatic carotid occlusion. JAMA 1998; 280:1055–1060.
88. Yamauchi H, Fukuyama H, Nagahama Y, et al. Significance of increased oxygen extraction fraction in five-year prognosis of major cerebral arterial occlusive diseases. J Nucl Med 1999; 40:1992–1998.
89. Schmitz SA, Taupitz M, Wagner S, et al. Magnetic resonance imaging of atherosclerotic plaques using superparamagnetic iron oxide particles. J Magn Reson Imaging 2001; 14:355–361.
90. Schmitz SA, Taupitz M, Wagner S, et al. Iron-oxide-enhanced magnetic resonance imaging of atherosclerotic plaques: postmortem analysis of accuracy, inter-observer agreement, and pitfalls. Invest Radiol 2002; 37:405–411.
91. Corti R. Noninvasive imaging of atherosclerotic vessels by MRI for clinical assessment of the effectiveness of therapy. Pharmacol Ther 2006; 110:57–70.
92. Fanning NF, Walters TD, Fox AJ, et al. Association between calcification of the cervical carotid artery bifurcation and white matter ischemia. AJNR Am J Neuroradiol 2006; 27:378–383.
93. Bartlett ES, Walters TD, Symons SP, et al. Quantification of carotid stenosis on CT angiography. AJNR Am J Neuroradiol 2006; 27:13–19.
94. Benndorf G, Singel S, Proest G, et al. The Doppler guide wire: clinical applications in neuroendovascular treatment. Neuroradiology 1997; 39:286–291.
95. Hayashi K, Kitagawa N, Morikawa M, et al. A case of intimal hyperplasia induced by stenting for vertebral artery origin stenosis: assessed on intravascular ultrasound. Neurol Res 2003; 25:357–360.
96. Schmitz SA, Winterhalter S, Schiffler S, et al. USPIO-enhanced direct MR imaging of thrombus: preclinical evaluation in rabbits. Radiology 2001; 221:237–243.
97. Schmitz SA, Winterhalter S, Schiffler S, et al. USPIO-enhanced direct thrombus MRI. Acad Radiol 2002; 9(suppl 2):S339–S340.
98. Schmitz SA, O'Regan DP, Gibson D, et al. Magnetic resonance direct thrombus imaging at 3T field strength in patients with lower limb deep vein thrombosis: a feasibility study. Clin Radiol 2006; 61:282–286.
99. Furuya K, Zhu L, Kawahara N, et al. Differences in infarct evolution between lipopolysaccharide-induced tolerant and nontolerant conditions to focal cerebral ischemia. J Neurosurg 2005; 103:715–723.

6

Pharmacology and Clot: Immediate and Chronic Interventions

Michael A. Kurz

MA Consulting Services, Wayne, Pennsylvania, U.S.A.

INTRODUCTION

Stroke is the third cause of death in the United States and the leading cause of disability in terms of cost of care and loss of productivity. According to the newest data from the American Stroke Association, each year ~700,000 individuals experience a new or recurrent stroke and 160,000 of these events are fatal. In terms of care and disability, it is estimated that the annual cost of stroke totals approximately $56.8 billion. Acute ischemic stroke (AIS) accounts for approximately 85% of all strokes (1,2). The human brain is exquisitely sensitive to ischemia. Irreversible cell damage may begin to occur within minutes in profoundly ischemic tissue, so rapid treatment is paramount. It has been estimated that in patients with a large vessel AIS, 120 million neurons, 830 billion synapses, and 714 km (447 miles) of myelinated fibers are lost every hour. In each minute, 1.9 million neurons, 14 billion synapses, and 12 km (7.5 miles) of myelinated fibers are destroyed (3). A great many unsuccessful attempts have been made to develop "neuroprotective" agents that might prevent or delay the onset of irreversible injury. Systematic reviews found no evidence that calcium channel antagonists, gamma-amino butyric acid (GABA) agonists, tirilazad, glycine antagonists, lubeluzole, or N-methyl D-aspartate (NMDA) antagonists improved clinical outcomes in people with AIS (4–11). The lack of success at improving clinical outcomes with this approach likely is attributable to one inescapable fact: human tissue dies if deprived of nutrients and oxygen for a sufficient period of time. Even if such an agent or therapy were to be discovered, delivering it to the ischemic tissue would be extraordinarily difficult while the offending vascular obstruction were in place. Thus it is not surprising that current data suggest that the most critical and immediate goal during an evolving cerebral infarction is to restore blood flow to the ischemic vascular bed. Because AIS, like acute myocardial infarction (AMI), is caused most often by blood clot(s) obstructing conduit blood vessel(s), pharmacological treatment approaches focus on enhancing thrombolysis, inhibiting platelet activity, and inhibiting the coagulation cascade. Fig. 1 depicts the sites of action of several commonly used agents in the process of pathological thrombosis.

"BRAIN ATTACK" VERSUS "HEART ATTACK"

Recombinant tissue plasminogen activator (t-PA, alteplase), developed originally for treatment of AMI, is the only treatment for AIS approved by the Food and Drug Administration (FDA) in the United States. Because of the strict inclusion criteria and 3-hour time window, it has been estimated that only 2%–5% of patients are eligible for treatment. To improve public awareness of the need to seek emergency

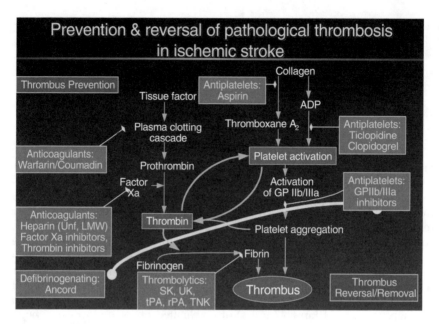

FIGURE 1 The sites of action of agents used in the treatment and prevention of acute ischemic stroke (AIS). (See also color plate section.)

medical attention, we often describe acute stroke as a "brain attack" to encourage comparison to the more common, better publicized, and better understood heart attack. Initial attempts at developing reperfusion therapies for AIS logically were based on successful and well-studied AMI therapies. However, investigators quickly learned that two critical differences between AIS and AMI profoundly limited their ability to translate successful AMI approaches into successful AIS therapies.

First, while myocardial infarctions (MI) almost always are caused by an occlusive thrombus formed locally at the site of rupture of an unstable atherosclerotic plaque, the etiology of AIS is variable and less predictable. There are several well-established causes of cerebral artery occlusion, such as (i) local atherothrombotic events (as with AMI), (ii) artery to artery embolism (e.g., carotid disease, vertebral artery disease), and (iii) thromboembolism of cardiogenic origin. This variable etiology likely will impact the ability of a chosen pharmacological therapy to produce the desired result of rapid and complete tissue reperfusion.

In most cases of cardiogenic embolism, the offending embolus is a gelatinous "red clot," formed from locally stagnant blood, which has escaped the heart and lodged in a cerebral artery. Such clots tend to be very rich in fibrin, are packed with erythrocytes, and are relatively platelet-poor. Pharmacologically, the most logical acute treatment choice for such a clot would be a fibrinolytic agent, and the most logical preventative strategy would be anticoagulation. In contradistinction, as a consequence of the high-blood-flow environment in which they form, thromboemboli from locally ruptured arterial plaques tend to have much higher concentrations of platelets and, at least in the early stages of their formation, relatively less fibrin. It is logical to assume that t-PA would be relatively less effective at lysing this type of clot, but a potent antiplatelet agent might be of some benefit if it were capable of reversing platelet aggregation.

A second significant difference between AMI and AIS is the intuitively obvious, yet frequently overlooked, difference in sensitivity of the target organ to hemorrhage. In addition to parenchymal damage, profound ischemia inevitably also injures the distal vasculature itself. Microvascular permeability is increased (12), and the weakened vessel wall is susceptible to rupture upon reperfusion. In the heart, compressive forces within contracting myocardium help to confine hemorrhage to the site of leakage, but no such advantage exists in the brain. Neurons also are much more sensitive than myocytes to direct contact with blood, so local hemorrhagic events that are of little consequence (and likely go unnoticed) in reperfused myocardium represent a very serious complication of reperfusion therapy for AIS. The potential for disaster is exacerbated greatly by the use of antithrombin or antiplatelet agents.

A vast body of evidence clearly supports the use of heparin for suspected AMI. Heparin likely does not improve significantly the rate or extent of pharmacological lysis; rather, it helps prevent reocclusion of the infarct-related vessel—whether reperfusion is accomplished by pharmacological or mechanical means. It would be reasonable to assume that heparin should provide similar benefit in AIS; however, heparin is a difficult medication to titrate and use safely. The data seem to indicate a marginal benefit with increased risk of intracerebral hemorrhage (13). Nevertheless, the use of heparin in AIS is still the subject of debate. Because of this experience, concurrent heparin use is contraindicated when treating AIS with t-PA. On the other hand, trials such as the Warfarin-Aspirin Recurrent Stroke Study (WARSS) and Warfarin-Aspirin Symptomatic Intracranial Disease (WASID) showed good results with aspirin in the secondary prevention of stroke.

THROMBOLYTIC AGENTS

The indications for the use of antithrombotic agents have evolved from initial empirical use based on anecdotal evidence to current recommendations following multicenter trials. Based on these data intravenous (IV) t-PA has been approved in the United States, Canada, Australia, and the European Union for the treatment of AIS within 3 hours after symptom onset. The following sections address the different agents used in the treatment of stroke and also elaborate on those used for primary or secondary prevention.

The success of thrombolytic therapy for patients presenting within 3 hours of acute stroke onset has demonstrated that neurological outcome can be improved with timely treatment (14,15). IV t-PA in acute stroke patients who meet the inclusion/exclusion criteria of the National Institute of Disorders and Stroke (NINDS) is associated with a 6%–8% risk of symptomatic intracranial hemorrhage. Such risk is higher in protocol violators or in patients treated beyond the 3-hour window. Case reports are suggestive that IV t-PA may be useful also in selected patients presenting 3 hours after symptom onset; however, it remains unclear which patients are most likely to benefit from this treatment.

Tissue Plasminogen Activator (t-PA)

Thrombolytic therapy with t-PA is the only FDA-approved agent for the treatment of patients presenting within 3 hours of stroke onset after assessment of inclusion/exclusion criteria (15). Reperfusion within a few hours of stroke onset appears to be effective in preventing neuronal damage. Early treatment (i.e., within 90 min) may be more likely to result in a favorable outcome (evidence level II). Later treatment, at 90–180 min, is also beneficial (evidence level I; for more details see Part 2, Chapter 8).

In a systematic review (17 randomized clinical trials; 5216 patients; primary sources: Cochrane Collaboration Stroke Group, Medicine, Embase, the Ottawa Stroke Trials registry, hand searches of references quoted in thrombolysis papers, direct contact with principal investigators of trials, colleagues, and pharmaceutical companies), the authors compared thrombolysis with placebo given soon after the onset of stroke (15,16). All trials used computed tomography (CT) or magnetic resonance scanning before randomization to exclude intracranial hemorrhage or other nonstroke disorders. Results for three different thrombolytic agents (streptokinase, urokinase, and t-PA) were included, but direct comparison of different thrombolytic drugs was not possible. Two trials used intra-arterial (IA) administration and the remainder used the IV route. The IA administration of fibrinolytics through superselective catheterization is an alternative option that may offer advantages in certain settings (e.g., angiography suite, intraoperatively); however, intracerebral hemorrhage with neurological deterioration continues to be a risk (17). Thrombolysis reduced the risk of death or dependency at the end of the studies (adjusted relative risk (ARR)=4.2%; 95% confidence interval (CI)=1.2%–7.2%; relative risk reduction (RRR)=7%; 95% CI=3%–12%; number needed to treat (NNT)=24; 95% CI=14%–83%). Although there was no significant heterogeneity of treatment effect overall, a heterogeneity of results was noted for the outcomes of death, and death or dependency at final follow-up among the eight trials of IV t-PA. Explanations may include the combined use of antithrombotic agents (aspirin or heparin within the first 24 hours of thrombolysis), stroke severity, the presence of early ischemic changes on CT scan, and the time from stroke onset to randomization. A subgroup analysis suggested that thrombolysis may be more beneficial if given within 3 hours of symptom onset, but the duration of the "therapeutic time window" could not be determined reliably. Most of the trial results were of outcomes at 3 months; only one trial reported 1-year outcome data (15).

In the subset of trials that assessed IV t-PA, the findings were similar (ARR=5.7%; 95% CI=2.0%–9.4%; RRR=10%; 95% CI=4%–16%; NNT=18; 95% CI=11%–50%). In contrast to results with t-PA, one meta-analysis (four randomized clinical trials, individual results of 1292 people with AIS treated with streptokinase or placebo) found that streptokinase versus placebo had no clear effect on the proportion of people dead or dependent at 3 months and included the possibility of both substantial benefit or substantial harm (RRR=+1%; 95% CI=–6% to +8%) (18). People allocated to streptokinase were more likely to be dead after 3 months (RR interval (RRI)=46%; 95% CI=24%–73%). Although the combination of aspirin plus streptokinase significantly increased mortality at 3 months (p=0.005), this did not affect the combined risk of death or severe disability. In the systematic review detailed above (16), thrombolysis increased fatal intracranial hemorrhage, compared with placebo (autoregulatory index (ARI)=4.4%; 95% CI=3.4%–5.4%; RRI=396%; 95% CI=220%–668%; number needed to harm (NNH)=23; 95% CI=19%–29%). In the subset of trials that assessed intravenous t-PA, the findings were similar (ARI=2.9%; 95% CI=1.7%–4.1%; RRI=259%; 95% CI=102%–536%; NNH=34; 95% CI=24%–59%).

The strict NINDS inclusion/exclusion criteria on the use of IV t-PA have reinforced the need to develop alternative and complementary therapies. Fibrinogen, the soluble plasma–protein precursor of fibrin, also has been studied as a target for AIS therapy. In this respect, it should be mentioned that the Stroke Treatment with Ancrod Trial (STAT) showed that infusion with the defibrinogenating agent ancrod, started 30 min to 3 hours after onset of AIS, was associated with better functional status at 3 months compared with placebo (19). However, ancrod therapy resulted in an *increase in the rate of asymptomatic intracranial hemorrhage* and a trend toward an increase in the rate of symptomatic intracranial hemorrhage, without affecting total mortality. Patients who achieved early controlled defibrinogenation had a greater benefit from therapy (19).

ANTIPLATELET AGENTS

Several clinical trials have shown that antiplatelet agents are effective in secondary stroke prevention. The trials usually define secondary stroke prevention such as recurrent stroke and/or other major vascular events in patients who have undergone a transient ischemic attack (TIA) or stroke. Aspirin is used the most widely, although its effect is very modest (RRR 20%), and most physicians use between 100 and 325 mg daily as a maintenance dose. Randomized trials have shown that anticoagulants and aspirin are safe in patients with nonvalvular atrial fibrillation, leading to 70% and 22% risk reduction of strokes, respectively. For patients who develop stroke on aspirin treatment, the options are either to increase the dose of aspirin or to administer another antiaggregate. In patients who cannot tolerate aspirin, the options are clopidogrel 75 mg once daily or dipyridamole 400 mg combined with 50 mg aspirin (Aggrenox, Boehringer Ingelheim Pharmaceuticals, Ingelheim Germany; aspirin/extended-release dipyridamole 25mg/200mg). A proposed approach is to combine different antiplatelet drugs with different modes of action, such as aspirin and clopidogrel, to achieve a better and more effective antithrombotic effect. Several trials such as Prevention Regimen For Effectively Avoiding Second Strokes (PRoFESS) and Clopidogrel for High Atherothrombotic Risk and Ischemic Stabilization, Management, and Avoidance (CHARISMA) are addressing these issues in a controlled setting.

Although antiplatelet and anticoagulant drugs are of proven usefulness in secondary prevention of stroke, the value of many of them in improving outcome after AIS has not been established. Potentially effective drugs include aspirin, coumadin, heparin, low-molecular-weight heparins (LMWH) and heparinoids, direct thrombin inhibitors, thienopyridines (clopidogrel and ticlopidine), dipyridamole, and the glycoprotein IIb/IIIa platelet receptor antagonists, among others. Because its value is established, aspirin has been used as a control to evaluate other antiplatelet agents in the prevention of complications in cerebrovascular disease. The opinions of physicians regarding the efficacy of these agents in indirect comparisons and the differences in their safety profiles, availability, and cost will influence the choice of agent for the individual patient.

Aspirin

Mechanism of Action

Aspirin affects platelet aggregation by irreversibly inhibiting platelet prostaglandin cyclooxygenase, an effect that lasts for the life of the platelet and prevents the formation of the platelet-aggregating factor thromboxane (Tx) A2. Aspirin inhibits platelets by inhibiting the conversion of arachidonic acid to prostaglandin H_2 mediated by cyclooxygenase (COX)-1 or -2 (Fig. 2). Mature platelets contain predominantly COX-1, and nucleated cells such as monocytes or endothelial cells that line the blood vessels produce prostaglandin H_2 through COX-2.

COX-1 and -2 catalyze the formation of prothrombotic and antithrombotic eicosanoids, respectively. Aspirin, conventional nonsteroidal anti-inflammatory drugs (NSAIDs), and COX-2-specific inhibitors exhibit different patterns of inhibition of

Arachidonic acid

$$\blacktriangledown \quad \blacktriangleleft \text{ Cyclooxygenase } \blacktriangleleft \textbf{Aspirin}$$

Prostaglandin H_2

$$\blacktriangledown \quad \blacktriangleleft \text{ Thromboxane synthase}$$

Thromboxane A_2

$$\blacktriangledown$$

Thromboxane B_2

$$\blacktriangledown \quad \blacktriangleleft \text{ 11-hydroxy thromboxane dehydrogenase}$$

11–dehydrothromboxane B_2

FIGURE 2   Flow chart showing how aspirin inhibits cyclooxygenase.

COX-1-mediated Tx biosynthesis and COX-2-mediated prostacyclin biosynthesis. COX-1 catalyzes the synthesis of Tx-A2, which causes platelet activation, vasoconstriction, and smooth muscle proliferation. Tx-A2 levels are elevated in conditions associated with platelet activation, including unstable angina and cerebral ischemia. Conversely, COX-2 controls the synthesis of prostacyclin (PGI2), a local platelet regulator with an effect opposite to that of Tx-A2. PGI2 is produced as a compensatory response to increases in Tx-A2 during ischemic events. Aspirin is a more potent inhibitor of COX-1 than of COX-2, unlike other NSAIDs, which have limited selectivity. Aspirin at low doses selectively inhibits the formation of Tx-A2 without inhibiting the basal biosynthesis of cardioprotective PGI2. Aspirin causes complete enzyme inhibition, without the recovery of enzyme activity at trough drug levels associated with conventional NSAIDs. Even low-dose aspirin (81 mg) completely and permanently inhibits COX-1.

Aspirin also has nonplatelet-mediated effects that contribute to its efficacy in the primary and secondary prevention of vascular events. These include antiarrhythmic effects, as shown in animal studies, and antiatherosclerotic effects related to an increase in nitric oxide synthesis/activity and a reduction in inflammatory mediators. Increasing evidence supports a central role for inflammation in the cascade of events that results in fissuring of the vulnerable atherosclerotic plaque that underlies the development of thrombotic ischemic stroke and AMI. Lesion macrophages synthesize matrix metalloproteinases (MMPs); in particular, 72-kDa (MMP-2) and 92-kDa (MMP-9) gelatinase, which are proteolytic enzymes capable of degrading plaque constituents. The enhanced MMP-2 and MMP-9 production by macrophages in vulnerable plaques may be related to the enhancement of prostaglandin E2 (PGE2) synthesis as a result of the induction of COX-2.

Clinical Studies

Aspirin has been proposed for treatment of AIS. In a review, authors report that antiplatelet treatment with aspirin started within 48 hours of AIS reduces the risk of death and dependence (20). Most people had a CT scan to exclude hemorrhage before treatment was started. A subgroup analysis of two large randomized clinical trials found evidence that aspirin should not be delayed if a CT scan is not readily available within 48 hours; people given aspirin who subsequently were found to have a hemorrhagic rather than an ischemic stroke had similar outcomes to people who were given placebo (21,22).

One systematic review (eight randomized clinical trials; 41,325 people with definite or presumed ischemic stroke; primary sources Cochrane Collaboration Stroke Group, Register of the Antiplatelet Trialists' Collaboration, MedStrategy, and contact with pharmaceutical companies marketing antiplatelet drugs) compared antiplatelet treatment started within 14 days of the stroke versus placebo (20). Of the data in the systematic review, 98% came from two large randomized clinical trials of aspirin 160–300 mg daily started within 48 hours of stroke onset (21,22). Most people had an ischemic stroke confirmed by CT scan before randomization, but people who were conscious could be randomized before CT scan if the stroke was very likely to be ischemic on clinical grounds. The duration of treatment varied from 10 to 28 days. Aspirin started within the first 48 hours of AIS reduced death or dependency at 6-month follow-up and increased the number of people making a complete recovery.

A prospective combined analysis (23) of two large randomized controlled trials (21,22) found a significant reduction in the outcome of further stroke or death with aspirin versus placebo. The effect was similar across subgroups (older vs. younger; male vs. female; impaired consciousness or not; atrial fibrillation or not; blood pressure; stroke subtype; timing of CT scanning). For the 773 people subsequently found to have had a hemorrhagic stroke rather than an ischemic stroke, the subgroup analysis found no difference in the outcome of further stroke or death between those who were randomized to aspirin versus placebo (16% vs. 18%). One recent metaregression analysis of the dose–response effect of aspirin on stroke found a uniform effect of aspirin in a range of doses from 50 to 1500 mg daily.

In clinical trials of subjects with TIAs due to fibrin platelet emboli or ischemic stroke, aspirin has been shown to reduce significantly the risk of the combined endpoint of stroke or death and the combined endpoint of TIA, stroke, or death by about 13%–18%. Atherosclerotic plaques in the carotid arteries are important contributors to TIAs and strokes. Experiments by two groups demonstrated local prevention of thrombosis in the dog and rabbit carotid arteries by using magnetically concentrated autologous erythrocytes that had been loaded with aspirin and a ferromagnetic colloid compound (24).

Adverse Events

Although aspirin is used for the prevention of ischemic stroke, it may also increase the risk of hemorrhagic stroke, especially in women. As is the case with other antiplatelet treatments, bleeding is the most important adverse effect of aspirin treatment. A review published in 1994 found that the excess risk of intracranial bleeding with aspirin treatment was small (at most, 1 or 2 bleeds per 1000 people per year) in trials of long-term treatment (25). Aspirin treatment produced a small but significant excess of nonfatal major extracranial bleeds (3 bleeds per 1000 people), but there was no clear excess of fatal extracranial bleeds (25). In the acute phase of stroke, the aspirin-associated risk of hemorrhagic complications was higher compared with treatment in the stable phase after stroke. For the first 4 weeks after stroke, 0.48 (95% CI=0.13%–0.83%) fatal or severe bleeds per 100 treated patients were observed in the Chinese Acute Stroke Trial and 0.41 (95% CI=0.05%–0.77%) in the International Stroke Trial. Still, there was a net benefit with the prevention of about one death or nonfatal ischemic stroke per 100 treated patients. In one randomized clinical trial directly comparing two different doses of aspirin, 1200 mg daily was associated with more gastrointestinal bleeding than 325 mg daily. The latter observations of increased adverse events with higher aspirin doses are supported by several studies.

Thienopyridines (Clopidogrel, Ticlopidine)
Clinical Studies

Ticlopidine, a unique inhibitor of platelet aggregation, was approved for clinical use in the early 1990s by the US FDA to reduce the risk of fatal or nonfatal thrombotic stroke precursors and in patients who have had a completed thrombotic stroke. Two large randomized trials, the Ticlopidine Aspirin Stroke Study (TASS) and the Canadian American Ticlopidine Study (CATS), demonstrated that ticlopidine reduces the risk of subsequent stroke in patients presenting with a TIA or stroke. A subgroup analysis of TASS showed that these conclusions extended to patients with reversible ischemic disease. Although the CATS intention-to-treat analysis showed that ticlopidine was more effective than aspirin for stroke prevention, it was less well tolerated than aspirin and was associated with severe but reversible neutropenia in almost 1% of patients and diarrhea in 2% of cases. In vitro experiments on platelets from normal volunteers and in animal models showed that the addition of aspirin to treatment with ticlopidine improves their antiplatelet activity, and better results could be obtained in arterial thrombotic prevention strategies. However, the African-American Antiplatelet Stroke Prevention Study (AAASPS), a randomized, double-blind, investigator-initiated, multicenter trial of 1809 black men and women who recently had a noncardioembolic ischemic stroke found no statistically significant difference between ticlopidine and aspirin in the prevention of recurrent stroke, MI, or vascular death (26). There was a nonsignificant trend for a reduction of fatal or nonfatal stroke among those in the aspirin group. The investigators concluded that, because of these data and the risk of serious adverse events with ticlopidine, aspirin is a better treatment for aspirin-tolerant black patients with noncardioembolic ischemic stroke (26). Because of the incidence of thrombocytopenia, the use of ticlopidine is currently extremely limited.

Clopidogrel is a more recently available thienopyridine, and it has displaced ticlopidine almost completely because of its more favorable safety profile and similar or better efficacy. The cornerstone in clinical evidence of the relative efficacy of thienopyridines (clopidogrel, ticlopidine) versus aspirin in the secondary prevention of vascular disease is the Clopidogrel versus Aspirin in Patients at Risk of Ischemic Events (CAPRIE) trial (27). This trial showed a modest benefit in the reduction of vascular events by clopidogrel. The results differed according to qualifying disorder: MI, −3.7%; ischemic stroke, +7.3%; and peripheral arterial disease, +23.8%. Similar results were found for ticlopidine after brain ischemia. The safety of clopidogrel appears to be similar to that of aspirin and, as mentioned above, better than that of ticlopidine. However, the recent reports of rare cases of thrombotic thrombocytopenic purpura in association with clopidogrel should be kept in mind. Although both aspirin (300 mg daily) and ticlopidine (500 mg daily) are effective in the secondary prevention of cerebral ischemic accidents associated with atherosclerosis, with a 20% and 30%, respectively, reduction of risk, the 1994 Antiplatelet Trialists' Collaboration review (25) found no evidence that any antiplatelet regimen was more effective than medium dose aspirin in the prevention of vascular events.

MATCH Trial

The Management of Atherothrombosis with Clopidogrel in High-risk Patients with Recent Transient Ischemic Attack or Ischemic Stroke (MATCH) trial was designed to investigate the safety and efficacy profile of clopidogrel versus aspirin and in combination (28). Investigators randomly assigned 7599 patients who had had a recent stroke or TIA and at least one additional vascular risk factor to clopidogrel (75 mg daily)+aspirin (75 mg daily) or clopidogrel (75 mg daily)+placebo. The duration of treatment and follow-up was 18 months. Primary endpoint was ischemic stroke, MI, vascular death (including hemorrhagic death of any origin), or rehospitalization for an acute ischemic event. Combination therapy was only minimally and nonsignificantly more effective than clopidogrel alone for both primary and secondary vascular events; A small but nonsignificant effect on event rates was seen for aspirin+clopidogrel over clopidogrel alone in most patient subgroups. However, for the secondary endpoint of ischemic stroke, the RRR of 7.1% for combination therapy versus clopidogrel alone was not significant (95% CI$=-8.5$ to 20.4; $p=0.353$) nor was significance found for the 2.0% RRR noted for clopidogrel+aspirin versus monotherapy for any stroke (95% CI$=-13.8$ to 15.6; $p=0.790$).

The main finding of MATCH was that combination therapy was associated with a significantly greater incidence of both major and minor bleeding complications compared with clopidogrel alone. Although the combination and clopidogrel-only treatment arms had similar rates of fatal bleeding events, almost twice as many patients taking clopidogrel+aspirin experienced life-threatening bleeding, including symptomatic intracranial hemorrhage. In consideration of these findings, using clopidogrel+aspirin as secondary prevention in the stroke and TIA population is not currently recommended.

Adverse Events

A systematic review of randomized trials of the thienopyridines versus aspirin found that thienopyridines produced significantly less gastrointestinal hemorrhage and upper gastrointestinal upset than aspirin (29). Nevertheless, they increased the odds ratio of skin rash and diarrhea: ticlopidine by about twofold and clopidogrel by about a third. Ticlopidine (but not clopidogrel) increased the odds of neutropenia (29). Observational studies also have found that ticlopidine is associated with thrombocytopenia and thrombotic thrombocytopenic purpura (30,31). There is no clear evidence, however, of an excess of hematological adverse side effects with clopidogrel (32,33). The results of two randomized clinical trials (about 1700 people undergoing coronary artery stenting) of clopidogrel plus aspirin versus ticlopidine plus aspirin suggested clopidogrel to be superior to ticlopidine in terms of safety and tolerability (34,35).

Dipyridamole

Dipyridamole inhibits platelet activation and adhesion. Its mechanism of action has not been fully elucidated, but the primary beneficial effects likely are adenosine mediated. Dipyridamole inhibits cellular reuptake and catabolism of adenosine by red blood cells and endothelial cells, which may increase local extracellular adenosine concentrations sufficiently to inhibit platelet activation. Dipyridamole also inhibits phosphodiesterase (PDE-5), which may increase cGMP concentrations in platelets and vascular smooth muscle cells, thus promoting improved blood flow by inhibiting both platelet activation and local vasospasm.

Safety and efficacy of dipyridamole had been the object of several trials. The European Stroke Prevention Trial (ESPS-2) data showed superiority of the combination of aspirin plus extended release dipyridamole in secondary stroke prevention (36). ESPS-2 was a randomized, placebo-controlled, double-blind trial conducted in 6602 patients and which assessed the efficacy of combination therapy—aspirin+extended-release dipyridamole (25+200 mg) versus extended-release dipyridamole alone (200 mg twice a day), aspirin alone (25 mg twice a day), or matched placebo. Primary endpoints were stroke, death, or both stroke and death. Secondary end-points were TIA, MI, ischemic events, and other vascular events. As compared with placebo, the risk of recurrent stroke was significantly reduced by 18.1% ($p=0.013$) with aspirin alone (odds ratio OR=0.79; 95% CI=0.65%–0.97%), by 16.3% ($p=0.039$) with extended-release dipyridamole alone (OR=0.81; 95% CI=0.67%–0.99%), and by 37.0% ($p< 0.001$) with combination therapy (OR=0.59; 95% CI=0.48%–0.73%). A comparison of combination therapy with each of the other two active agents demonstrated efficacy as well, with a significant 23.1% ($p=0.006$) reduction in risk of stroke for the combination therapy over aspirin alone and a significant 24.7% ($p=0.002$) reduction over extended-release dipyridamole alone. Bleeding occurred significantly more often in both aspirin-containing regimens. However, the difference between the risk associated with aspirin alone and that associated with combination therapy was not significant.

Since the publication of those data, results from randomized controlled trials of dipyridamole, given with or without aspirin, have given conflicting results. To elucidate these discrepancies, The Dipyridamole in Stroke Collaboration (DISC) Trial Investigators performed a meta-analysis using individual patient data from relevant randomized controlled trials such as the Cochrane Library, other electronic databases, references lists, earlier reviews, and contact with the manufacturer of dipyridamole (37). Data were merged from 5 of 7 relevant trials involving 11,459 patients. Recurrent stroke was reduced by dipyridamole as compared with control (OR=0.82; 95% CI=0.68–1.00%) and by combined aspirin and dipyridamole versus aspirin alone (OR=0.78; 95% CI=0.65%–0.93%), dipyridamole alone (OR=0.74; 95% CI=0.60%–0.90%), or control (OR=0.61;95% CI=0.51%–0.71%). Similar findings were observed for nonfatal stroke. The combination of aspirin and dipyridamole also significantly reduced the composite outcome of nonfatal stroke, nonfatal MI, and vascular death as compared with aspirin alone (OR=0.84; 95% CI=0.72%–0.97%), dipyridamole alone (OR=0.76; 95% CI=0.64%–0.90%), or control (OR=0.66; 95% CI=0.57%–0.75%). Vascular death was not altered in any group. The authors concluded that dipyridamole, given alone or with aspirin, reduces stroke recurrence in patients with previous ischemic cerebrovascular disease. The combination of aspirin and dipyridamole also reduces the composite of nonfatal stroke, nonfatal MI, and vascular death as compared with aspirin alone (37).

GPIIb/IIIa Inhibitors
The efficacy and safety of treatment with inhibitors of the platelet surface glycoprotein IIb/IIIa (GPIIb/IIIa, fibrinogen) receptor in AIS have been examined in clinical trials. GPIIb/IIIa inhibitors were proposed to work as treatment for AIS because they might enhance endogenous fibrinolysis, prevent acute primary and secondary thrombosis, and prevent microvascular injury. The most promising and closely studied of the latter agents in this context has been abciximab (13). The phase III Abciximab Emergent Stroke Treatment Trial (AbESTT-2) was stopped in May 2005, because of an increased risk of intracranial hemorrhage in the studied population (38).

ANTICOAGULANTS
Coumadin (Warfarin)

As detailed below, coumadin (warfarin) therapy has proved safe and effective in a number of randomized controlled trials of stroke prophylaxis in patients with non-valvular atrial fibrillation, reducing the risk of stroke in these patients by two thirds. One trial concluded that after an ischemic, noncardioembolic stroke, both warfarin and aspirin are acceptable therapeutic alternatives (39).

Atrial fibrillation, with a prevalence of 6% in those over 65 years, is responsible for 75,000–100,000 strokes each year in the United States. Almost one in ten patients with nonrheumatic atrial fibrillation is at risk of stroke. These strokes are more severe and have less favorable long-term prognosis than strokes due to other mechanisms. Although the average annual stroke rate among atrial fibrillation patients is about 4%–5%, considerable risk heterogeneity exists, and warfarin is not recommended in all cases.

Four large, prospective, randomized trials examined the risks and benefits of warfarin therapy for stroke prophylaxis in patients with nonvalvular atrial fibrillation. All four studies showed a substantially reduced incidence of stroke and a low incidence of significant bleeding in patients treated with warfarin (40). One of these studies also showed that aspirin reduced the incidence of stroke. From a review (search of Cochrane Stroke Group Specialized Register of Trials and the database of the Antithrombotic Trialists' Collaboration, as well as reference lists of relevant articles), the investigators concluded that, considering all the randomized data, aspirin modestly (by about 20%) reduces stroke and major vascular events in patients with nonvalvular atrial fibrillation (41). The investigators also concluded that, for primary prevention among atrial fibrillation patients with an average stroke rate of 4.5% per year, about 10 strokes would be prevented yearly for every 1000 given aspirin.

In contrast to the results described above, a review of randomized trials with concealed treatment allocation on long-term (more than 6 months) secondary prevention after recent (less than 6 months) TIA or minor ischemic stroke of presumed arterial origin (last search date; June 2000) concluded that for the secondary prevention of further vascular events after TIA or minor stroke of presumed arterial origin, there is, despite some enthusiasm, insufficient evidence to justify the routine use of low intensity oral anticoagulants (international normalized ratio (INR) 2.0–3.6). More intense anticoagulation (INR 3.0–4.5) is not safe and should not be used in this setting.

Based on the findings described above, risk stratification is important to differentiate patients with a risk high enough to justify warfarin from those whose risk is so low that they are better off on aspirin or even no antithrombotic therapy (42). The subgroups that appear to be at high risk for embolic events include patients with hypertension, previous embolic events, structural heart disease (enlarged left atrial size, previous MI, left ventricular dysfunction), and older age. Young patients with no evidence of structural heart disease or hypertension (lone atrial fibrillation) have a low embolic rate and may not warrant anticoagulation. Anticoagulation is also recommended for patients undergoing elective cardioversion (recent onset of atrial fibrillation greater than two days in duration) and for patients with atrial fibrillation and hyperthyroidism, because of studies suggesting a higher rate of embolism if these patients are not anticoagulated. Therefore, ideal antithrombotic therapy is individualized, balancing the risks of thromboembolism versus bleeding on antithrombotic therapy and considering the preferences of patients as well as the potential benefits of surgery.

Patients with atrial fibrillation and mitral stenosis who are not given warfarin are in an extremely hypercoagulable state; even some patients with atrial fibrillation without mitral stenosis who are not given antithrombotic agents are also moderately hypercoagulable. A study revealed that increased levels of plasma thrombin–antithrombin III complex (TAT) and prothrombin fragment 1+2 (PTF) were observed more frequently in patients with atrial fibrillation and associated mitral stenosis than in patients with atrial fibrillation alone (43). In cases of atrial fibrillation without mitral stenosis, plasma levels of TAT and PTF were significantly lower in those patients receiving antithrombotic agents (aspirin or warfarin) than in those receiving no antithrombotic agents. Plasma levels of PTF were also significantly lower in patients receiving warfarin than in those receiving aspirin.

Elderly patients with ischemic stroke and atrial fibrillation are at an especially increased risk for recurrent stroke. Warfarin sodium is highly effective in reducing this risk. A study determined the use of warfarin among a population sample of elderly patients with atrial fibrillation hospitalized in 1994 for ischemic stroke. Among 635 patients (402 women; 585 white; 218 patients 85 years or older; 147 patients with a new diagnosis of atrial fibrillation), 334 patients had stroke as a principal diagnosis (44). Among those discharged alive after a stroke, only 147 (53%) of 278 patients were prescribed warfarin at discharge. Among 130 (47%) of 278 patients not prescribed warfarin at discharge, 81 (62%) of 130 patients also were not prescribed aspirin. The increased potential benefit (additional vascular risk factors) was not associated with a higher rate of warfarin use. The low risk for anticoagulation (lack of risk factors for bleeding) was associated with a slightly higher rate of warfarin use. Among those with an increased risk of stroke and a low risk for bleeding (ideal candidates), 124 (62%) of 278 patients were discharged on a regimen of warfarin. The investigators concluded that the anticoagulation of elderly stroke patients with atrial fibrillation, even among ideal candidates, is underused, a conclusion they had reached in a previous study published in 1997 (45). The increased use of warfarin among these patients represents an excellent opportunity for reducing the risk of recurrent stroke in this high-risk population. Other investigators found a low percentage of use of warfarin or aspirin in patients with atrial fibrillation, and they attributed this finding to the reluctance by physicians driven by fears of bleeding complications.

The WARSS (Warfarin Aspirin Recurrent Stroke Study) trial revealed no differences in outcome, including mortality, recurrent stroke, or major hemorrhage between patients treated with warfarin and aspirin after ischemic noncardioembolic stroke. The investigators concluded that both aspirin and warfarin are acceptable therapeutic modalities (39).

Unfractionated Heparin, Low-Molecular-Weight Heparins, Thrombin Inhibitors, and Inhibitors of Factor Xa

Antithrombin therapies, thrombin antagonists and inhibitors as well as inhibitors of Factor Xa, have also been studied; however, bleeding and other adverse events associated with antithrombin therapy have largely negated their potential benefit.

As detailed below, one systematic review found no short- or long-term improvement in AIS with immediate systemic anticoagulants (unfractionated heparin, LMWH, heparinoids, or specific thrombin inhibitors) versus usual care without systemic anticoagulants. Immediate systemic anticoagulants reduce the risk of deep venous thrombosis and pulmonary embolus, but this benefit is offset by a dose-dependent risk of intracranial and extracranial hemorrhage. In people with AIS and atrial fibrillation, one randomized clinical trial found no evidence that LMWH is superior to aspirin alone.

There is one systematic review (21 randomized clinical trials; 23,427 people; primary sources: Cochrane Collaboration Stroke Group, MedStrategy, Antithrombotic Trialists' Collaboration Trials Register, and contact with manufacturers of anticoagulants) (46) and two subsequent randomized clinical trials (47,48). The systematic review compared unfractionated heparin, LMWH, heparinoids, oral anticoagulants, or specific thrombin inhibitors versus usual care with systemic anticoagulants. Over 80% of the data came from one trial, which randomized people with any severity of stroke to either subcutaneous heparin or placebo, usually after exclusion of hemorrhage by CT scan (22). The systematic review found no significant difference in the proportion of people dead or dependent in the treatment and control groups at the end of follow-up (3–6 months after the stroke: ARR+0.4%, 95% CI−0.9% to+1.7%; RRR 0%, 95% CI−2% to+3%). There was no clear short- or long-term benefit of anticoagulants in any prespecified subgroups (stroke of presumed cardioembolic origin vs. others; different anticoagulants). The first subsequent randomized clinical trial (449 people with acute stroke and atrial fibrillation) found no significant difference between dalteparin (a LMWH) versus aspirin for the primary outcome of recurrent ischemic stroke during the first 14 days (ARI+1.0%, 95% CI−3.6% to 6.2%) or for secondary outcomes, including functional outcome at 3 months (47). The second randomized clinical trial allocated 404 people to one of four different doses of the LMWH certoparin within 12 hours of stroke onset (48). There was no difference in neurological outcome between the four groups 3 months after treatment.

The systematic review detailed above (46) found that anticoagulation slightly increased symptomatic intracranial hemorrhages within 14 days of starting treatment, compared with control (ARI 0.93%, 95% CI 0.68%–1.18%; RRI 163%, 95% CI 95%–255%; NNH 108, 95% CI 85%–147%). The large trial of subcutaneous heparin found that this effect was dose-dependent (symptomatic intracranial hemorrhage by using medium-dose compared with low-dose heparin for 14 days; RRI 143%, 95% CI 82%–204%; NNH 97, 95% CI 68%–169%) (22). The review also found a dose-dependent increase in major extracranial hemorrhages after 14 days of treatment with anticoagulants (ARI 0.91%, 95% CI 0.67%–1.15%; RRI 231%, 95% CI 136%–365%; NNH 109, 95% CI 87%–149%). The subsequent randomized clinical trial of dalteparin versus aspirin for people with AIS and atrial fibrillation found no difference in adverse events, including symptomatic or asymptomatic intracerebral hemorrhage, progression of symptoms, or early or late death (47). As in the systematic review (46), the more recent randomized clinical trial comparing different doses of the LMWH certoparin found that intracranial hemorrhage occurred more often in those receiving a higher dose of anticoagulant (48). However, the overall number of patients experiencing hemorrhagic complications in the randomized clinical trial may have been lowered artificially because the study protocol was changed during the trial period so as to exclude patients with early ischemic changes on CT scan.

A randomized, double-blind, aspirin-controlled trial tested the safety and efficacy of treatment with high-dose tinzaparin (175 anti-Xa IU/kg daily; 487 patients), medium-dose tinzaparin (100 anti-Xa IU/kg daily; 508 patients), or aspirin (300 mg daily; 491 patients) started within 48 hours of AIS and given for up to 10 days (49). This trial showed that treatment with tinzaparin, at high or medium dose, within 48 hours of AIS did not improve functional outcome compared with aspirin.

Although high-dose tinzaparin was superior in preventing deep-vein thrombosis, it was associated with a higher rate of symptomatic intracranial hemorrhage. Similarly, the Heparin in Acute Embolic Stroke Trial (HAEST), a multicenter, randomized, double-blinded, and double-dummy trial on the effect of LMWH (dalteparin 100 IU/kg subcutaneously twice a day) or aspirin (160 mg every day) for the treatment of 449 patients with AIS and atrial fibrillation did not provide evidence that LMWH is superior to aspirin for the treatment of AIS in patients with atrial fibrillation (47).

The SPORTIF II (Stroke Prevention by Oral Thrombin Inhibitors in Atrial Fibrillation) trial assessed the tolerability and safety of three doses (20, 40, or 60 mg twice a day) of ximelagatran (an oral direct thrombin inhibitor) versus warfarin in patients with nonvalvular atrial fibrillation (50). The study found that they were tolerated well without the need for either anticoagulation monitoring or for dose adjustment. Although the intensity of anticoagulation was not monitored or regulated in patients receiving ximelagatran (an advantage of this agent), these patients had less bleeding than those receiving warfarin (51).

Experimentally, hirudin, hirulog, D-Phe-L-Pro-L-Arg-CH2Cl (PPACK), and argatroban are clearly more effective than heparin in inhibiting platelet deposition and thrombus formation and also show promise in preventing reocclusion after thrombolysis for both experimental thrombotic and embolic stroke. However, the risk of hemorrhage in patients with cerebrovascular disease is unknown for these agents (52). A study examined the pharmacodynamic and pharmacokinetic effects of the thrombin inhibitor, argatroban, alone and in combination with aspirin in normal male volunteers.

Argatroban induced a dose-dependent prolongation of the thrombin time and the activated partial thromboplastin time (aPTT). aPTT returned to its pretreatment value 1 hour after terminating argatroban infusion (53). Six male subjects received an infusion of 1 µg/kg/min argatroban after the administration of two doses of 162.5 mg aspirin or a matching placebo. Using this dose, aspirin decreased serum thromboxane B2 by a mean of 99% and prolonged the bleeding time (230 ± 52 s vs. 320 ± 113 s, $p < 0.01$). Argatroban given alone increased thrombin time by $454 \pm 18\%$ and aPTT by $160 \pm 3\%$. Steady-state plasma concentrations were achieved at 1 hour and declined exponentially with an elimination half-life of 24 ± 4 min. Aspirin altered neither the anticoagulant effects nor the plasma concentrations of argatroban. Argatroban did not increase the bleeding time when given alone and did not prolong further the bleeding time when combined with aspirin.

Another recently developed oral anticoagulant, which directly inhibits factor Xa (see Chapter 1, Part 1) is rivaroxaban (Xarelto, Bayer, and Johnson & Johnson). The drug is being evaluated in more than 40,000 patients (phase III development). Data from the pivotal RECORD 3 (Regulation of Coagulation in major Orthopaedic surgery reducing the Risk of deep venous thrombosis (DVT) and pulmonary embolism (PE)) trial presented by Lassen M et al. (54) support its use for prevention of DVT and PE after surgery. A total of 2531 patients underwent total knee replacement surgery; DVT, nonfatal PE, and all-cause mortality (composite primary endpoint) occurred in 9.6% of rivaroxaban-treated patients compared with 18.9% of enoxaparin-treated patients (RRR 49%; p < 0.001). A significantly greater reduction in risk of developing major venous thromboembolism (VTE)-the composite of proximal DVT, nonfatal PE, and VTE-related death-was also observed in this trial: 1.0% of rivaroxaban-treated patients versus 2.6% of enoxaparin-treated patients (RRR 62%; p = 0.01).The frequency of major bleeding events was similar to enoxaparin

A. Initiation (capture, adhesion, activation)

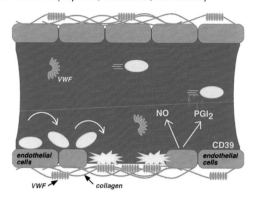

B. Extension (cohesion, secretion)

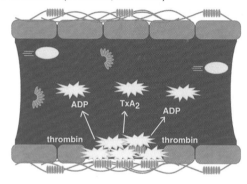

C. Perpetuation (stabilization)

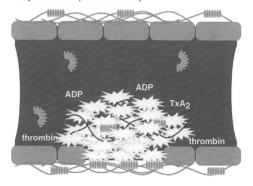

FIGURE 1.1 Steps in platelet plug formation. Prior to vascular injury, platelet activation is suppressed by endothelial cell-derived inhibitory factors. These include prostaglandin (PG) I_2 (prostacyclin), nitric oxide, and CD39, an ADPase on the surface of endothelial cells that can hydrolyze trace amounts of ADP that might otherwise cause inappropriate platelet activation. (*A*) Initiation. The development of the platelet plug is initiated by thrombin and by the collagen–vWF complex, which captures and activates moving platelets. Platelets adhere and spread, forming a monolayer. (*B*) Extension. The platelet plug is extended as additional platelets are activated via the release or secretion of thromboxane A_2 (TXA$_2$), ADP, and other platelet agonists, most of which are ligands for G protein-coupled receptors on the platelet surface. Activated platelets stick to each other via bridges formed by the binding of fibrinogen, fibrin, or vWF to activated αIIbβ3. (*C*) Perpetuation. Finally, close contacts between platelets in the growing hemostatic plug, along with a fibrin meshwork (shown in red), help to perpetuate and stabilize the platelet plug. *Source*: Reproduced with permission from Ref. (2). (See p. 4.)

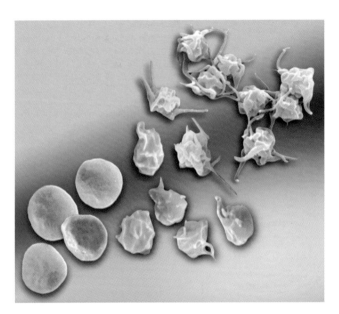

FIGURE 1.2 Platelet shape change and aggregation. Scanning electron micrographs of resting (*lower left*), partially activated (*lower middle*), and fully activated platelets (*upper right*), showing the accompanying shape changes, formation of filopodia and lamellipodia, and platelet aggregation. *Source*: Reproduced with permission from Ref. (2). (See p. 5.)

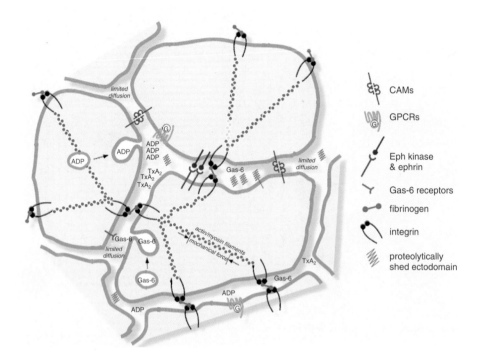

FIGURE 1.3 Contact-dependent and contact-facilitated events during thrombus formation. The onset of aggregation brings platelets into sufficiently close contact for integrins and other cell adhesion molecules to interact and for the activation of Eph receptor kinases by their cell surface ligands known as "ephrins." The space between platelets also provides a protected environment in which soluble agonists for G protein-coupled receptors (ADP, thrombin, and TXA$_2$) and receptor tyrosine kinases (Gas-6), and the proteolytically shed bioactive ectodomains of platelet surface proteins (CD40L) can accumulate. The mechanical forces generated by the contraction of actin/myosin filaments help to compress the space between platelets, improving contacts and possibly increasing the concentration of soluble agonists. *Abbreviations*: ADP, adenosine diphosphate; CAMs, cell adhesion molecules; Gas-6, growth-arrest specific gene 6; GPCRs, G protein-coupled receptors; TXA$_2$, thromboxane A$_2$. *Source*: Reproduced with permission from Ref. (2). (See p. 8.)

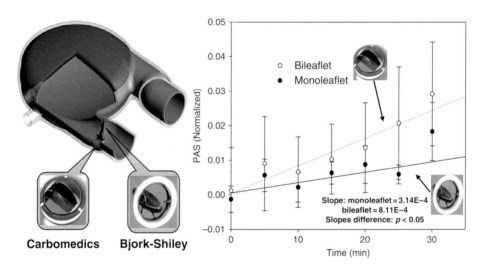

FIGURE 2.5 In vitro platelet activity measurements in left ventricular assist devices: the bileaflet mechanical heart valve (MHV) generated higher platelet activity than the monoleaflet MHV ($p < 0.05$). *Abbreviation*: PAS, platelet activity state. *Source*: Adapted from Ref. (41) with permission of Future Drugs Ltd. (See p. 26.)

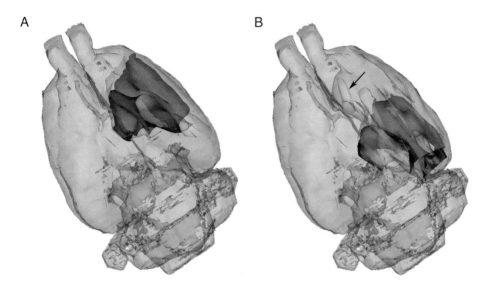

FIGURE 3.1 Comparison of the suture (*A*) and the thromboembolic (*B*) middle cerebral artery (MCA) occlusion models acquired 30 min after the onset of ischemia. 3D renderings of the evolving stroke with superimposed apparent diffusion coefficient (red) and cerebral blood flow (green) lesion volumes are shown. Note the increased perfusion–diffusion mismatch and the presence of a smaller perfusion lesion in the anterior component of the MCA territory (*arrow*). The authors hypothesize that this second lesion could be the result of clot fragmentation and migration. Finally, the lesion volume of the thromboembolic model extends further into the posterior aspect of the cerebrum. *Source*: Reproduced with permission from Macmillan Publishers Ltd: Ref. (27) (Sprague-Dawley rats, 300 g). (See p. 41.)

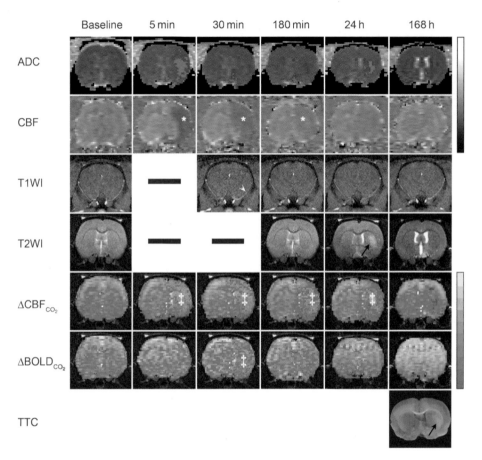

FIGURE 3.2 This montage shows magnetic resonance and histology images before and at various points after the onset of ischemic stroke using the rat thromboembolic model. In the case shown here, the middle cerebral artery (MCA) spontaneously recanalized within 15 min after injection of the clot. Shown are the results of apparent diffusion coefficient (ADC), cerebral blood flow (CBF), T1-weighted, T2-weighted, and changes to CBF and blood oxygenation level-dependent (BOLD) signal in response to hypercapnia (ΔCBF_{CO_2} and $\Delta BOLD_{CO_2}$, respectively) imaging. The gray scale bar provides the range of ADC values from 0 to 0.001 mm^2/s and CBF from 0 to 3 ml/g per min; and the color scale gives the ΔCBF_{CO_2} range from 0% to 200% and $\Delta BOLD_{CO_2}$ from 1% to 5%. The asterisk denotes areas of CBF voids whereas the ‡ symbol indicates an impaired response to hypercapnia. The bottom panel shows the infarction of triphenyltetrazolium chloride (TTC)-stained brain slice at the end of imaging 168 h from the ischemic onset. Arrows point to T1-weighted and TTC-derived lesions. The authors used these data to study the event of spectacular shrinking deficit. *Source*: Reproduced with permission from Ref. (33) (Sprague-Dawley rats, 300 g). (See p. 43.)

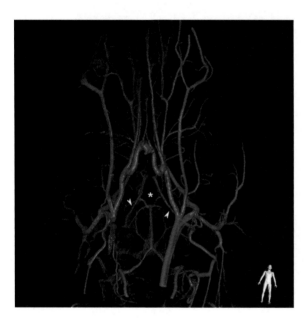

FIGURE 3.4 3D rotational angiogram (*frontal view*) of the rabbit intra- and extracranial circulations, acquired and reconstructed using Philips Allura FD20 and workstations in our laboratories. Noteworthy are the clear depiction of the internal carotid arteries (*arrowheads*) and the circle of Willis (*asterisk*). Note the absence of the right common carotid artery, which was sacrificed previously, however having no impact on the circulation to the brain or head (White New Zealand rabbit, 3.5 kg). (See p. 46.)

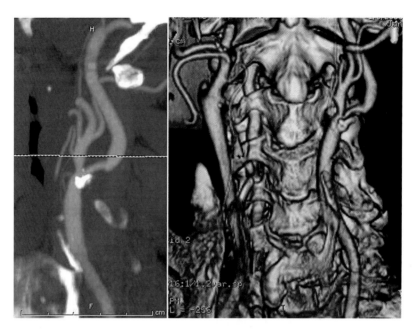

FIGURE 5.7 Computed tomography angiography (CTA) with 3D reconstruction of the carotid bulb in an 81-year-old man shows a calcified plaque in the carotid bifurcation with extension in to the internal carotid artery with an 80% stenosis. (See p. 87.)

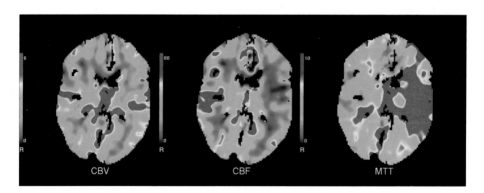

FIGURE 5.8 CT Perfusion Maps in a patient with acute occlusion of the M1 segment of the left middle cerebral artery (MCA). The cerebral blood volume map (CBV) in this early stage of onset is not altered, yet. The cerebral blood flow (CBF) is already reduced below 20 ml/100 g/min in the left MCA territory, and the mean transit time (MTT) is increased to over 10 s *Source*: Courtesy of Dr. G. Bohner. (See p. 88.)

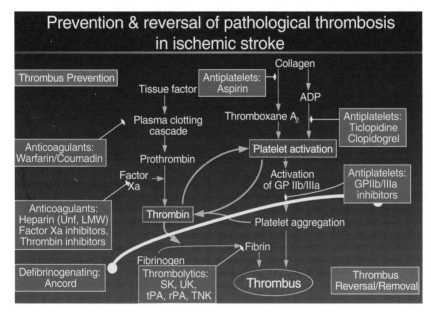

FIGURE 6.1 The sites of action of agents used in the treatment and prevention of acute ischemic stroke (AIS). (See p. 104.)

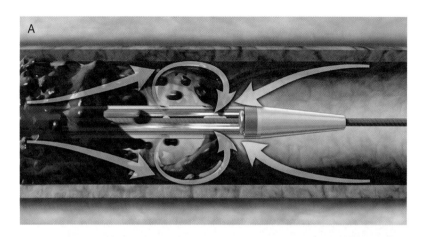

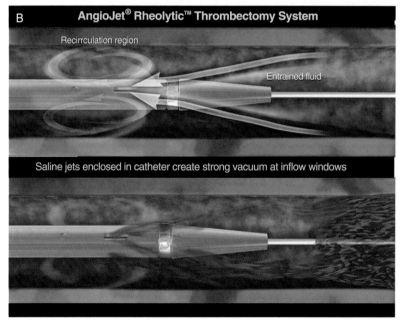

FIGURE 7.8 (*A*) Illustrative view of the distal tip of the AngioJet Rheolytic Thrombectomy device (Possis Medical, Inc., Minneapolis, MN) as it is advanced using the over-the-wire technique in to the clot, prior to activation of the device. (*B*) Illustration of the Bernoulli Principle involved that drives the AngioJet suction-thrombectomy device. The saline jets within the tip of the catheter and forces high pressure saline retrograde back into the catheter lumen, which then creates a low pressure recirculation region. This draws the entrained fluid, with blood clot, from the arterial lumen into the device lumen. *Source*: Permission from Possis Medical, Inc., Minneapolis, MN. (See p. 134.)

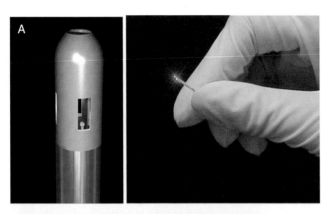

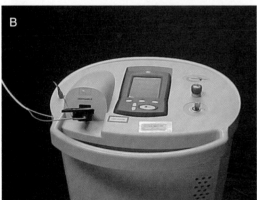

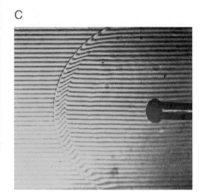

FIGURE 7.10 (*A*) View of the distal flexible tip of the 3 Fr EPAR (Endovascular PhotoAcoustic Recanalization) device based on laser technology. The hydrophilic coated catheter is placed over a standard 0.014-inch microwire into the clot (EndoVasix, Inc.). (*B*) Catheter attached to the EPAR laser energy source. The energy is delivered through fiberoptics to the tip of the catheter. (*C*) Absorption of laser light by darkly pigmented material (i.e., clot) converts the photo energy to acoustic energy, which emulsifies clot inside the catheter tip (EndoVasix, Inc.). (See p. 137.)

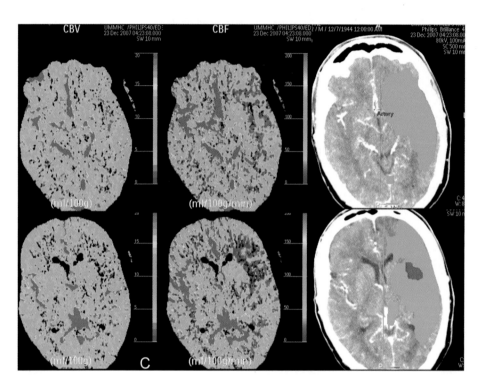

FIGURE 7.14 (*C*) CT perfusion studies show a mismatch (*right*) between cerebral blood volume (*left*) and cerebral blood flow (*center*) indicating the penumbra (*green*). Note red represents the dead tissue. (See p. 144.)

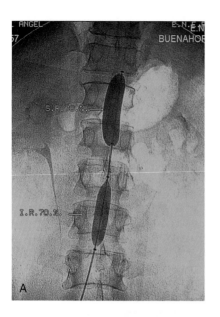

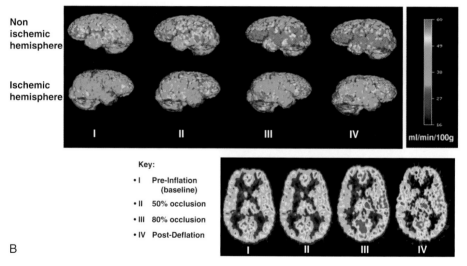

Key:
- I   Pre-Inflation (baseline)
- II   50% occlusion
- III   80% occlusion
- IV   Post-Deflation

FIGURE 7.17 (*A*) Cerebral perfusion augmentation with a partial aortic occlusion. NeuroFlo System (Coaxia, Maple Grove, MN) has been inflated in the abdominal aorta of a patient. (*B*) A 38-year-old male (NIHSS = 11) presenting with a hemiplegia associated with a thromboembolic middle cerebral artery occlusion as shown on an MRA study. The patient was treated 10 h after the acute ischemic stroke with a NeuroFlo system. Images represent a sequence of PET images on the patient. The scale indicates the level of perfusion (ml/min/100 g) (*upper right*). The individual panels are as follows: I (baseline, before treatment), II (approximately 30%–50% balloon occlusion), III (70%–80% balloon occlusion), and IV Deflation (after both balloons are deflated, 60 min of inflation time). A progressive and significant increased perfusion (30%) is seen with a maximum in the cortical rim; reduction of the penumbra. Follow-up MRA showed no recanalization (not shown). Final MRI showed a small basal ganglia infarct. At 30 days the patient presented with a NIHSS of 5 and mRs = 2. *Source*: Permission from Dr. WD Heiss, Max-Planck-Institute, Germany. (See p. 151.)

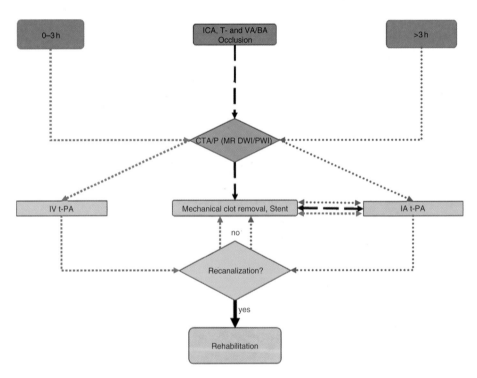

FIGURE 9.1   Imaging-based paradigm for acute stroke treatment. (See p. 168.)

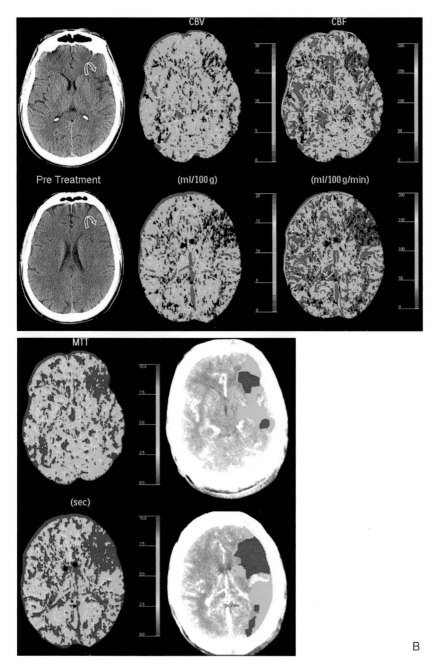

FIGURE 9.2 (*B*) CT perfusion maps of cerebral blood flow (CBF), cerebral blood volume (CBV), mean transit time (MTT), and time-to-peak (TTP) after injection of 40 ml of Isovue-370. There is evidence of changes in the CBV images in the left frontal lobe and slightly larger area of increased MTT and TTP in the left frontal lobe as well as parieto-temporal areas. A "mismatch" between CBF and CBV is seen (*right image*). (See p. 170.)

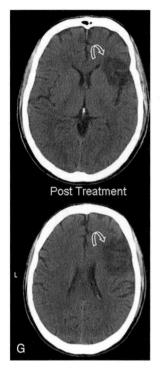

FIGURE 9.2 (*G*) Follow-up CT 24 h after admission shows an ischemic area within the insula and operculum (*curved arrow*) corresponding to changes seen on the initial CBF map. (See p. 172.)

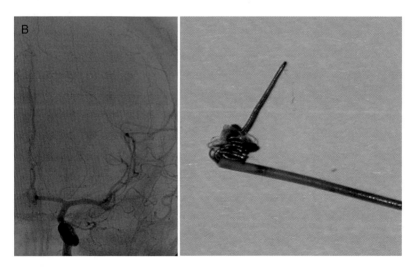

FIGURE 9.7 (*B*) Successful recanalization of the occluded MCA is achieved (*left panel*). Multiple opercular MCA branches are occluded because of clot fragments. Photograph of the clot removed from the MCA with the retriever (*right panel*). (See p. 195.)

(0.6% vs. 0.5% respectively, ns). Filing for regulatory approval in the US is expected in 2008. Clinical trials are also ongoing to evaluate rivaroxaban for cardioembolic stroke prevention in patients with atrial fibrillation and acute coronary syndrome.

STENTS AND ANTIPLATELET THERAPY

Since its first description, percutaneous transluminal angioplasty (PTCA) with stent placement has revolutionized the care of patients with acute myocardial ischemia (AMI). However, it is well-known that PTCA and, in particular, stent placement can induce endothelial damage and platelet activation, ultimately resulting in acute and/or delayed stent thrombosis. It has been reported that platelet aggregation at the site of vascular injury occurs in 3.5%–8.6% incidence of acute and subacute thrombosis after stent implantation (55). For these reasons, anti-platelet medications have assumed a major role in the prevention of endothelial activation and damage after the procedure (55–59).

The safety and efficacy of the combination of aspirin plus dipyridamole and clopidogrel or ticlopidine plus aspirin after PTCA has been the object of clinical trials. The data show that the combination of aspirin plus dipyridamole does not result in an additional prevention of stent thrombosis events compared with aspirin alone. On the other hand, the combination of clopidogrel and aspirin decreases significantly the incidence of acute and/or chronic stent thrombosis. The CURE trial enrolled 2658 patients with non-ST elevation acute coronary syndromes (55). All patients were treated with aspirin and then were randomized to a combination of aspirin plus clopidogrel (300 mg bolus, 75 mg daily) or aspirin plus placebo. Patients on the combination treatment of aspirin with clopidogrel had a 30% risk reduction of AMI, death, and need for revascularization within 30 days from stent implantation. After CURE and other clinical trials, a regimen of aspirin 325 mg and clopidogrel 75 mg once a day for 8 months was part of the guidelines for prevention of thromboembolic complications after coronary stent placement. Subsequently, the data from the Clopidogrel for the Reduction of Events During Observation (CREDO) trial showed that the combination of aspirin plus clopidogrel for 12 months resulted in a sustained reduction of recurrent AMI or cardiac death (56).

LIMITATIONS OF ANTIPLATELET MEDICATIONS
Aspirin Resistance and Clinical Nonresponders

As previously discussed, undoubtedly antiplatelet medications are effective in the prevention of stroke and AMI as well as in the prevention of thromboembolic complications after stent implantation in the coronary system or in the cerebral circulation. However, 10%–20% of patients with a thrombotic event will have a second event even if they are treated with aspirin. Such variability has been termed "aspirin resistance" (60). It has been argued by many authors that the term "aspirin resistance" is not appropriate because the failure of aspirin to prevent recurrent events is multifactorial, such as noncompliance, bleeding complications, and poor control of other significant risk factors. As suggested by several investigators, a more appropriate term is probably "clinical non-responders." As tested by clinical laboratory methods, there is variability among patients' response to aspirin. Some authors report that variability in platelet aggregation tests among individuals varies between 6% and 40% (57,58,60). As previously described, aspirin is an effective antithrombotic agent because of the different response of the endothelial cells and platelets to the inhibition of COX-1. In fact, aspirin irreversibly acetylates serine 529 of COX-1, resulting in the inhibition of Tx A2 release from platelets and prostacycline from the endothelium (57). Although the endothelium recovers by generating new COX, the platelets cannot. Therefore, it was intuitive to hypothesize that genotypic variation in the COX-1 gene may be the base of aspirin resistance. Hillarp et al. (61) found that such genetic variability was not associated with the variation in response present in the laboratory. In contrast, several other authors found that five types of single-nucleotide polymorphisms (SNPs) in COX-1 were significantly associated with different response to aspirin on platelet function testing (62–67). Therefore, currently, the heterogeneity in the genotype of COX-1 is considered the main reason behind the variability in platelet response to aspirin. On the basis of these data, several authors proposed altering the aspirin dosage in patients based on in vitro platelet function tests. However, the International Society on Thrombosis and Haemostasis (ISTH) Working Group on Aspirin Resistance recently concluded that "other than in research trials, it is not currently appropriate to test for aspirin resistance in patients or to change therapy based on such tests." Similar conclusions have been published by both the American College of Chest Physicians' 7th Consensus Conference on Antithrombotic Therapy and the Consensus Task Force on the Use of Antiplatelet Agents in Patients with Atherosclerotic Cardiovascular Disease of the European Society of Cardiology (ESC) (68–71). Some potential reasons for aspirin "resistance" are listed in Table 1.

Clopidogrel Resistance and Clinical Nonresponders

Clopidogrel effectively inhibits adenosine diphosphate (ADP)-induced platelet activation and aggregation by selectively and irreversibly blocking the P2Y12 receptor. A standardized laboratory method that simulates the in vivo platelet response to antiplatelet therapy is still lacking. As clopidogrel specifically inhibits one of two ADP receptors, ex vivo measurement of ADP-induced maximum platelet aggregation by light transmittance aggregometry (LTA) has been the most commonly used laboratory method to evaluate clopidogrel responsiveness and is considered the gold standard (68).

Since this initial description, multiple investigators have confirmed the phenomenon of clopidogrel resistance (72). Several authors report the prevalence of clopidogrel nonresponsiveness at 5%–44%. Such large variation likely is secondary to dosing, different laboratory methods of clopidogrel-induced platelet

---

TABLE 1 Mechanisms Implicated in "Aspirin Resistance"

- Increased cyclooxygenase production
- Concurrent use of nonsteroidal anti-inflammatory drugs
- Platelet genetic defects
- Elevated cholesterol levels
- Patient noncompliance with aspirin therapy
- Inadequate blockade of erythrocyte-induced platelet activation
- Biosynthesis of F2-isoprostane 8-iso-prostaglandin (PGF2alpha), a bioactive product of arachidonic acid peroxidation
- Stimulation of platelet aggregation by cigarette smoking
- Aspirin-resistant platelet aggregability by increased levels of norepinephrine, as seen during excessive exercise or periods of mental stress
- Increased platelet sensitivity to collagen.

activation, and timing of blood sampling (73,74). Numerous possible mechanisms have been hypothesized to explain the mechanism of clopidogrel resistance (57,72,75). Those include poor bioavailability (noncompliance, under-dosing, poor absorption, interference by atorvastatin with cytochrome P450), accelerated platelet turnover (with the introduction into the bloodstream of newly formed, drug-unaffected platelets), and SNPs in the *P2Y* gene. In addition, even without clopidogrel, there is large interindividual variation in the platelet response to ADP (57–67,75).

Interestingly, recently, the higher resistance estimates are present following the 300 mg loading dose, and the lower estimates occur after the 600 mg loading dose. Subsequent investigations have unequivocally demonstrated that clopidogrel nonresponsiveness is dependent on dose. In the largest pharmacodynamic study comparing 300 and 600 mg clopidogrel loading doses, treatment with a 600 mg loading dose during elective percutaneous coronary interventions (PCI) and subsequent stenting reduced clopidogrel nonresponsiveness to 8% compared with 28%–32% after a 300 mg loading dose (73). Moreover, the study demonstrated a narrower response profile following treatment with 600 mg compared with 300 mg clopidogrel. Müller et al. (74) also observed a time- and dose-dependent effect of clopidogrel in patients undergoing stenting. A similar increased responsiveness was also observed in the Intracoronary Stenting and Antithrombotic Regimen: Choose Between 3 High Oral Doses for Immediate Clopidogrel Effect (ISAR-CHOICE) study, where a ceiling effect of platelet inhibition was observed with a 600 mg clopidogrel loading dose, whereas a nonsignificant increase in platelet inhibition was observed with a 900 mg loading (76).

REFERENCES

1. Bonita R. Epidemiology of stroke. Lancet 1992; 339(8789):342–344.
2. Bamford J, Dennis M, Sandercock P, et al. A prospective study of acute cerebrovascular disease in the community: the Oxfordshire community stroke project, 1981–1986. 2. Incidence, case fatality rates and overall outcome at one year of cerebral infarction, primary intracerebral and subarachnoid hemorrhage. J Neurol Neurosurg Psychiatry 1990; 53(1):16–22.
3. Saver JL. Time is brain—quantified. Stroke 2006; 37(1):263–266.
4. Albers GW, Goldstein LB, Hall D, et al. Aptiganel hydrochloride in acute ischemic stroke. A randomized controlled trial. JAMA 2001; 286(21):2673–2682.
5. Diener HC, Cortens M, Ford G, et al. for the LUBINT-13 investigators. Lubeluzole in acute ischemic stroke treatment. A double-blind study with an 8-hour inclusion window comparing a 10-mg daily dose of lubeluzole with placebo. Stroke 2000; 31(11):2543–2551.
6. Horn J, Limburg M. Calcium antagonists for acute ischemic stroke. In: The Cochrane Library, Issue 3,2000. Oxford.
7. Horn J, Limburg M. Calcium antagonists for ischemic stroke: a systematic review. Stroke 2001; 32(2):570–576.
8. Ricci S, Celani MG, Canisani AT, et al. Piracetam for acute ischaemic stroke. In: The Cochrane Library, Issue 3,2000. Oxford.
9. Sacco RL, DeRosa JT, Haley EC Jr, et al. for the GAIN Americas Investigators. Glycine Antagonist in Neuroprotection for Patients with Acute Stroke. GAIN Americas: a randomized controlled trial. JAMA 2001; 285(13):1719–1728.
10. Tirilazad International Steering Committee. Tirilazad mesylate in acute ischemic stroke: a systematic review. Stroke 2000; 31(9):2257–2265.
11. Wahlgren NG, Ranasinha KW, Rosolacci T, et al. Clomethiazole acute stroke study (CLASS): results of a randomized, controlled trial of clomethiazole versus placebo in 1360 acute stroke patients. Stroke 1999; 30(1):21–28.

12. Kassner A, Roberts T, Taylor K, et al. Prediction of hemorrhage in acute ischemic stroke using permeability MR imaging. AJNR Am J Neuroradiol 2005; 26(9):2213–2217.
13. Sherman DG. Antithrombotic and hypofibrinogenetic therapy in acute ischemic stroke: what is the next step? Cerebrovasc Dis 2004; 17(suppl 1):138–143.
14. Clark WM, Wissman S, Albers GW. Recombinant tissue-type plasminogen activator (alteplase) for ischemic stroke 3 to 5 hours after symptom onset. The ATLANTIS study: a randomized controlled trial. Alteplase Thrombolysis for Acute Noninterventional Therapy in Ischemic Stroke. JAMA 1999; 282(21):2019–2026.
15. Kwiatkowski TG, Libman RB, Frankel M, et al. Effects of tissue plasminogen activator for acute ischemic stroke at one year. National Institute of Neurological Disorders and stroke recombinant tissue plasminogen activator stroke study group. N Engl J Med 1999; 340(23):1781–1787.
16. Wardlaw JM, del Zoppo G, Yamaguchi T. Thrombolysis for acute ischaemic stroke. In: The Cochrane Library, Issue 3,2000, Oxford.
17. Furlan A, Higashida R, Wechsler L, et al. Intra-arterial prourokinase for acute ischemic stroke. The PROACT II study: a randomized controlled trial. Prolyse in Acute Cerebral Thromboembolism. JAMA 1999; 282(21):2003–2011.
18. Comu C, Boutitie F, Candelise L, et al. Streptokinase in acute ischemic stroke: an individual patient data meta-analysis: the Thrombolysis in Acute Stroke Pooling Project. Stroke 2000; 31(7):1555–1560.
19. Sherman DG, Atkinson MP, Chippendale T, et al. Intravenous ancrod for treatment of acute ischemic stroke. The STAT study: a randomized controlled trial. JAMA 2000; 283(18):2395–2403.
20. Gubtiz G, Sandercock P, Counsell C. Antiplatelet therapy for acute ischemic stroke. In: The Cochrane Library, Issue 3,2000a. Oxford.
21. CAST. Randomised placebo-controlled trial of early aspirin use in 20,000 patients with acute ischaemic stroke. CAST (Chinese Acute Stroke Trial) collaborative group. Lancet 1997; 349(9066):1641–1649.
22. International Stroke Collaborative Group. The international stroke trial (IST): a randomized trial of aspirin, heparin, both or neither among 19,435 patients with acute ischaemic stroke. Lancet 1997; 349(9065):1569–1581.
23. Chen ZM, Sandercock P, Pan HC, et al. Indication for early aspirin use in acute ischemic stroke: a combined analysis of 40,000 randomized patients from the Chinese Acute Stroke Trial and the International Stroke Trial. Stroke 2000; 31(6):1240–1249.
24. Orekhova NM, Akchurin RS, Belyaev AA, et al. Local prevention of thrombosis in animal arteries by means of magnetic targeting of aspirin-loaded red cells. Thromb Res 1990; 57(4):611–616.
25. Antiplatelet Trialists' Collaboration. Collaborative overview of randomised trials of antiplatelet therapy—I: prevention of death, myocardial infarction, and stroke by prolonged antiplatelet therapy in various categories of patients. BMJ 1994; 308(6921):81–106.
26. Gorelick PB, Richardson D, Kelly M, et al. Aspirin and ticlopidine for prevention of recurrent stroke in black patients: a randomized trial. JAMA 2003; 289(22):2947–2957.
27. CAPRIE Steering Committee. A randomised, blinded trial of clopidogrel versus aspirin in patients at risk of ischaemic events. Lancet 1996; 348(9038):1329–1339.
28. Diener HC, Bogousslavsky J, Brass LM, et al. Aspirin and clopidogrel compared with clopidogrel alone after recent ischaemic stroke or transient ischaemic attack in high-risk patients (MATCH) randomized, double-blind, placebo-controlled trial. Lancet 2004; 364(9431):331–337.
29. Hankey GJ, Sudlow CLM, Dunbadin DW. Thienopyridine derivatives (ticlopidine, clopidogrel) versus aspirin for preventing stroke and other serious vascular events in high vascular risk patients. In: The Cochrane Library, Issue 1,2001. Oxford.
30. Bennett CL, Davidson CJ, Raisch DW, et al. Thrombotic thrombocytopenic purpura associated with ticlopidine in the setting of coronary artery stents and stroke prevention. Arch Intern Med 1999; 159(21):2524–2528.
31. Moloney BA. An analysis of the side effects of ticlopidine. In: Hass WK, Easton JD, eds. Ticlopidine, Platelets and Vascular Disease. New York: Springer, 1993:117–139.

32. Bennett CL, Connors JM, Carwile JM, et al. Thrombotic thrombocytopenic purpura associated with clopidogrel. N Eng J Med 2000; 342(24):1773–1777.
33. Hankey GJ. Clopidogrel and thrombotic thrombocytopenic purpura. Lancet 2000; 356(9226):269–270.
34. Bertrand ME, Rupprecht H-J, Urban P et al. Double-blind study of the safety of clopidogrel with and without a loading dose in combination with aspirin compared with ticlopidine in combination with aspirin after coronary stenting. The Clopidogrel Aspirin Stent International Cooperative Study (CLASSICS). Circulation 2000; 102(6):624–629.
35. Müller C, Büttner HJ, Petersen J, et al. A randomized comparison of clopidogrel and aspirin versus ticlopidine and aspirin after the placement of coronary artery stents. Circulation 2000; 101(6):590–593.
36. Diener HC, Cunha L, Forbes C, et al. European secondary prevention study 2: dipyridamole and acetylsalicylic acid in the secondary prevention of stroke. J Neurol Sci 1996; 143(1–2):1–13.
37. Leonardi-Bee J, Bath PM, Bousser MG, et al. Dipyridamole for preventing recurrent ischemic stroke and other vascular events: a meta-analysis of individual patient data from randomized controlled trials. Stroke 2005; 36(1):162–168.
38. Ringleb PA. Thrombolytics, Anticoagulants, and Antiplatelet Agents. Stroke 2006; 37(2):312–313.
39. Mohr JP, Thompson JL, Lazar RM, et al. A comparison of warfarin and aspirin for the prevention of recurrent ischemic stroke. N Engl J Med 2001; 345(20):1444–1451.
40. Benavente O, Hart RG, Koudstaal PJ, et al. Oral anticoagulants for preventing stroke in patients with non-valvular atrial fibrillation and no previous history of stroke or transient ischemic attacks. In: The Cochrane Library, Issue 1,2001a. Oxford.
41. Benavente O, Hart RG, Koudstaal PJ, et al. Antiplatelet therapy for preventing stroke in patients with non-valvular atrial fibrillation and no previous history of stroke or transient ischemic attacks. In: The Cochrane Library, Issue 1,2001b. Oxford.
42. Hellemons BS, Langenberg M, Lodder J, et al. Primary prevention of arterial thromboembolism in non-rheumatic atrial fibrillation in primary care: randomised controlled trial comparing two intensities of coumarin with aspirin. BMJ 1999; 319(7215):958–964.
43. Asakura H, Hifumi S, Jokaji H, et al. Prothrombin fragment F1+2 and thrombin-antithrombin III complex are useful markers of the hypercoagulable state in atrial fibrillation. Blood Coagul Fibrinolysis 1992; 3(4):469–473.
44. Brass LM, Krumholz HM, Scinto JD, et al. Warfarin use following ischemic stroke among medicare patients with atrial fibrillation. Arch Intern Med 1998; 158(19):2093–2100.
45. Brass LM, Krumholz HM, Scinto JM, et al. Warfarin use among patients with atrial fibrillation. Stroke 1997; 28(12):2382–2389.
46. Gubitz G, Sandercock P, Counsell C, et al. Anticoagulants for acute ischaemic stroke. In: The Cochrane Library, Issue 3,2000b. Oxford.
47. Berge E, Abdelnoor M, Nakstad PH, et al. Low-molecular-weight heparin versus aspirin in people with acute ischaemic stroke and atrial fibrillation: a double-blind randomised study. HAEST Study Group. Heparin in Acute Embolic Stroke Trial. Lancet 2000; 355(9211):1205–1210.
48. Diener HC, Ringelstein EB, von Kummer R, et al. Treatment of acute ischemic stroke with the low-molecular-weight heparin certoparin: results of the TOPAS Trial. Stroke 2001; 32(1):22–29.
49. Bath PM for the TAIST Investigators. Tinzaparin in acute ischaemic stroke trial (TAIST). Cerebrovasc Dis 2000; 10(suppl 2):81.
50. Peterson P, Grind M, Adler J, et al. Ximelagatran vs. warfarin for stroke prevention in patients with nonvalvular atrial fibrillation. SPORTIF II. A dose-guiding tolerability, and safety study. J Am Coll Cardiol 2003; 41(9):1445–1451.
51. Olsson SB on behalf of the Executive Steering Committee on behalf of the SPORTIF III Investigators. Stroke prevention with the oral direct thrombin inhibitor ximelagatran compared with warfarin in patients with nonvalvular atrial fibrillation (SPORTIF III): randomized controlled trial. Lancet 2003; 362(9397):1691–1698.
52. Albers GW. Antithrombotic agents in cerebral ischemia. Am J Cardiol 1995; 75(6):34B–38B.
53. Clarke RJ, Mayo G, FitzGerald GA, et al. Combined administration of aspirin and a specific thrombin inhibitor in man. Circulation 1991; 83(5):1510–1518.

54. Lassen MR, Turpie AG, Rosencher N, et al. Late breaking clinical trial: rivaroxaban an oral, direct factor Xa inhibitor for the prevention of venous thromboembolism in total knee replacement surgery: results of the RECORD 3 study. J Thromb Hemost 2007; 5(suppl 1):OS–006B.

55. Mehta SR, Yusuf S, Peters RJ, et al. Clopidogrel in unstable angina to prevent recurrent events trial (CURE) Investigators. Effects of pretreatment with clopidogrel and aspirin followed by long-term therapy in patients undergoing percutaneous coronary intervention: the PCI-CURE study. Lancet 2001; 358(9281):527–533.

56. Steinhubl SR, Berger PB, Mann JT III, et al. Early and sustained dual oral antiplatelet therapy following percutaneous coronary intervention. A randomized controlled trial. JAMA 2002; 288(19):2411–2420.

57. Michelson AD, (ed). Platelets, 2nd ed. New York: Academic Press/Elsevier Science; 2007:1–1387.

58. Patrono C, Coller B, FitzGerald GA, et al. Platelet-active drugs: the relationships among dose, effectiveness, and side effects. Chest 2004; 126:234S–264S.

59. Tang WH, Steinhubl SR, van Lente F, et al. Risk stratification for patients undergoing nonurgent percutaneous coronary intervention using N-terminal pro-B-type natriuretic peptide: a Clopidogrel for the Reduction of Events During Observation (CREDO) substudy. Am Heart J. 2007; 153(1):36–41.

60. Patrono C. Aspirin resistance: definition, mechanisms and clinical read-outs. J Thromb Haemost 2003; 1(8):1710–1713.

61. Hillarp A, Palmqvist B, Lethagen S, et al. Mutations within the cyclooxygenase-1 gene in aspirin non-responders with recurrence of stroke. Thromb Res 2003; 112(5–6):275–283.

62. Ruggeri ZM. Platelets in atherothrombosis. Nature Med 2002; 8(11):1227–1234.

63. Halushka MK, Walker LP, Halushka PV. Genetic variation in cyclooxygenase 1: effects on response to aspirin. Clin Pharmacol Therap 2003; 73(1):122–130.

64. Maree AO, Curtin RJ, Chubb A, et al. Cyclooxygenase-1 haplotype modulates platelet response to aspirin. J Thromb Haemost 2005; 3(10):2340–2345.

65. Jefferson BK, Foster JH, McCarthy JJ, et al. Aspirin resistance and a single gene. Am J Cardiol 2005; 95(6):805–808.

66. Andrioli G, Minuz P, Solero P, et al. Defective platelet response to arachidonic acid and thromboxane A(2) in subjects with Pl(A2) polymorphism of beta(3) subunit (glycoprotein IIIa). Br J Haematol 2000; 110(4):911–918.

67. Michelson AD, Furman MI, Goldschmidt-Clermont P, et al. Platelet GP IIIa Pl(A) polymorphisms display different sensitivities to agonists. Circulation 2000; 101(9):1013–1018.

68. Michelson AD. Platelet function testing in cardiovascular diseases. Circulation 2004; 110(19):e489–e493.

69. Michelson AD, Cattaneo M, Eikelboom JW, et al. Aspirin resistance: position paper of the Working Group on Aspirin Resistance. J Thromb Haemost 2005; 3(6):1309–1311.

70. Michelson AD. Aspirin Resistance. Pathophysiol Haemost Thromb 2006; 35(1–2):5–9.

71. Patrono C, Bachmann F, Baigent C, et al. Expert consensus document on the use of antiplatelet agents. The task force on the use of antiplatelet agents in patients with atherosclerotic cardiovascular disease of the European Society of Cardiology. Eur Heart J 2004; 25(2):166–181.

72. Gurbel PA, Lau WC, Bliden KP, et al. Clopidogrel resistance: implications for coronary stenting. Curr Pharm Des 2006; 12(10):1261–1269.

73. Jaremo P, Lindahl TL, Fransson SG, Richter A. Individual variations of platelet inhibition after loading doses of clopidogrel. J Intern Med 2002; 252(3):233–238.

74. Müller I, Besta F, Schulz C, et al. Prevalence of clopidogrel non-responders among patients with stable angina pectoris scheduled for elective coronary stent placement. Thromb Haemost 2003; 89(5):783–787.

75. Michelson AD, Linden MD, Furman MI et al. Evidence that pre-existent variability in platelet response to ADP accounts for clopidogrel resistance. J Thromb Haemost 2007; 5(1):75–81.

76. von Beckerath N, Taubert D, Pogatsa-Murray G, et al. Absorption, metabolization, and antiplatelet effects of 300-, 600-, and 900-mg loading doses of clopidogrel: results of the ISAR-CHOICE (Intracoronary Stenting and Antithrombotic Regimen: Choose Between 3 High Oral Doses for Immediate Clopidogrel Effect) Trial. Circulation 2005; 112(19):2946–2950.

7

Acute Ischemic Stroke: Endovascular Revascularization and Reperfusion

Ajay K. Wakhloo[1], Matthew J. Gounis[2], and Robert A. Mericle[3]

[1]*Department of Radiology, Neurology and Neurosurgery, University of Massachusetts Medical School, Worcester, Massachusetts, U.S.A.*

[2]*Department of Radiology, New England Center for Stroke Research, University of Massachusetts Medical School, Worcester, Massachusetts, U.S.A.*

[3]*Department of Neurosurgery, Vanderbilt University, Vanderbilt University Medical Center, Nashville, Tennessee, U.S.A.*

INTRODUCTION

At this time, intravenous (IV) recombinant tissue plasminogen activator (t-PA) is the only Food and Drug Administration (FDA)-approved medical management for recanalization of a thromboembolic acute stroke in the United States. Approximately 50% of patients with a moderate stroke show a good recovery. However, only 8% of patients with a severe stroke have a chance of significant neurological improvement. Thus, other alternatives are being explored for a more effective treatment. Since its first publication by Zeumer et al. in 1983 (1), intraarterial (IA) thrombolysis has evolved gradually from a superselective and local application of the fibrinolytic agents such as urokinase and t-PA for the treatment of posterior circulation stroke to an accepted endovascular treatment for selected patients presenting with a major stroke within the 6-h window associated with a middle cerebral artery (MCA) occlusion (Class I, Level of Evidence B) (Table 1) (2–4). Furthermore, IA thrombolysis is recommended for stroke patients who have contraindications for an IV use of thrombolytics, such as after a recent surgery (Class IIa, Level of Evidence C). However, the availability of IA thrombolysis should not preclude the use of IV administration of t-PA in otherwise eligible patients (Class III, Level of Evidence C) (2). More recent developments in endovascular technology for the treatment of acute ischemic stroke, such as use of angioplasty or stenting, mechanical thrombectomy, or clot disruption, are providing fragmented evidence that a safe and effective revascularization can be achieved. Endovascular mechanical intervention can be combined with no or small amounts of IV or IA thrombolytics. The Mechanical Embolus Removal in Cerebral Ischemia (MERCI) clot retriever is the first of its kind used for a clot extraction (Class IIb, Level of Evidence B) followed by a recent approval of the Penumbra clot suction system. But, clinical trials are being conducted to define its role in the management of an acute embolic stroke. As recommended by American Heart Association (AHA) other currently available endovascular devices or techniques should be used within a clinical trial (Class IIb, Level of Evidence C) (2). With the rapid advancement in technology and the introduction of user-friendly systems, more effective and safer endovascular treatments will be available for a routine clinical use. In this chapter, we describe various concepts of endovascular revascularization and discuss some frequently used devices and their limitations.

TABLE 1   Definition of Classes and Levels of Evidence Used in American Heart Association Recommendations

Classification	
Class I	Conditions for which there is evidence for and/or general agreement that the procedure or treatment is useful and effective
Class II	Conditions for which there is conflicting evidence and/or a divergence of opinion about the usefulness/efficacy of a procedure or treatment
Class IIa	The weight of evidence or opinion is in favor of the procedure or treatment
Class IIb	Usefulness/efficacy is less well established by evidence or opinion
Class III	Conditions for which there is evidence and/or general agreement that the procedure or treatment is not useful/effective and in some cases may be harmful
Level of evidence	
A	Data derived from multiple randomized clinical trials
B	Data derived from a single randomized trial or nonrandomized studies
C	Consensus opinion of experts
Level of evidence for diagnostic recommendation	
A	Data derived from multiple prospective cohort studies that used a reference standard applied by a masked evaluator
B	Data derived from a single grade A study or one or more case–control studies or studies that used a reference standard applied by an unmasked evaluator
C	Consensus opinion of experts

Source: Reproduced with permission from Ref. (2).

MECHANICAL REVASCULARIZATION

Endovascular mechanical revascularization techniques offer several distinct potential advantages over endovascular delivery of pharmacological fibrinolytics. There are several reasons why mechanical revascularization should be considered for treatment in a patient with an acute ischemic stroke. Mechanical devices could provide the following: (i) a potentially more rapid, efficacious, and safer method of clot removal compared to fibrinolytic agent treatment; (ii) an alternative treatment when thrombolytic agents are contraindicated; (iii) a combination therapy with fibrinolytic agents to accelerate the rate of chemical clot lysis; and (iv) a quick reduction of clot burden in large, easily accessed, proximal cerebral vessels, followed by clean-up pharmacologic thrombolysis of embolized fragments in smaller distal vessels. Another more recently introduced endovascular concept is the augmentation of the cerebral blood flow and brain perfusion by partial and transitory obstruction of the abdominal aorta using a double balloon system (5). The principle is based on increased peripheral resistance which probably results in enhancement and recruitment of collateral blood supply to the cerebral ischemic area. Also promising are results from an endovascular induced local and moderate hypothermia as an adjunct therapy to mechanical or chemical revascularization in acute ischemic stroke. We will discuss briefly both treatment options.

Mechanical therapies often work more rapidly, can achieve recanalization within few minutes, and potentially have lower intracerebral and systemic hemorrhage risk because of the avoidance of pharmacological lysis. A recanalization of the occluded site and near normal global perfusion (thrombolysis in myocardial

TABLE 2 Recanalization and Reperfusion Scoring System in Acute Ischemic Stroke

Grade	TIMI Reperfusion	Score	AOL Recanalization
0	No perfusion	0	No recanalization of the primary occlusive lesion
1	Perfusion past the initial occlusion, but no distal branch filling	I	Incomplete or partial recanalization of the primary occlusive lesion with no distal flow
2	Perfusion with incomplete or slow distal branch filling	II	Incomplete or partial recanalization of the primary occlusive lesion with any distal flow
3	Full perfusion with filling of all distal branches, including M3, 4	III	Complete recanalization of the primary occlusive lesion with any distal flow

Abbreviations: TIMI=thrombolysis in myocardial infarction; AOL=arterial occlusive lesion
Source: Adapted with permission from Ref. (6).

infarction, TIMI 2–3; Table 2) is associated with a better functional outcome (modified Rankin scale, 0–2) as compared with TIMI 0–1 perfusion score (6). However, as previously discussed, attention has to be paid to the use of terminology when assessing the benefits of revascularization devices. Although recanalization entails a flow restoration of the occluded vessel segment, reperfusion of distal arterial system including terminal branches and thus the brain tissue may be difficult to assess angiographically (7). The main potential disadvantage of mechanical revascularization is the possibility of occlusion or damage of perforating arteries, vessel dissection, or endothelial injury, which could lead to intracranial hemorrhage or endothelial flap stenosis and occlusion. Other problems include clot fragmentation because of microcatheter or device manipulation within the clot with distal embolic infarction and reduction in distal perfusion. However, embolic event may also occur during IV and/or IA thrombolysis. New anterior cerebral artery stroke during T-occlusion thrombolysis of the internal carotid artery (ICA) has been described (8).

IA mechanical interventions in acute stroke may be classified into three categories: endovascular thrombectomy, mechanical clot disruption or fragmentation, and augmented fibrinolysis devices (9).

Thrombectomy
Endovascular thrombectomy devices are designed to extract occlusive thrombi from target vessels through a transcatheter approach and can be classified into two general categories: (i) clot retrieval devices that physically grasp cerebral thrombi and pull them out of the cerebral circulation and (ii) suction thrombectomy devices that aspirate occlusive thrombus material from the vessel.

1. *Clot retrieval devices* were first developed to capture errant coils and other foreign bodies that had embolized within the cerebral circulation during endovascular procedures. These devices can ensnare a thrombus and then withdraw it out of the body, through the guide catheter, or release it into a safer extracranial territory. Some specific examples of clot retrieval devices available today are the MERCI retrieval device, the Microsnare, Neuronet, In-Time, Ensnare, Retriever, the Alligator, and the Penumbra retrieval devices.

    (a) *MERCI Retriever X5/X6/LX (10)* (*Concentric Medical*, Fig. 1). This was the first device approved by the FDA specifically for a mechanical thrombectomy in

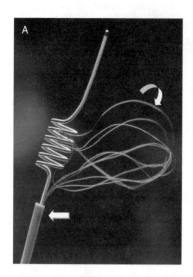
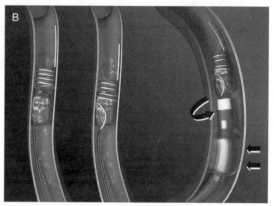

FIGURE 1 (*A*) MERCI Retriever. First FDA-approved device in the United States for mechanical thrombectomy. The attached nylon fibers (*bent arrow*) prevent stretching and fracture of the device during clot and foreign body retrieval and are supposed to enable an improved capture of clots. The corkscrew-like wire tip, which is available in different diameters, has been pushed through the delivery microcatheter (*arrow*). *Source*: © 2008 Concentric Medical, Mountain View, CA, All rights reserved. (*B*) Illustration of a partly deployed MERCI Retriever within the occlusive clot, which is removed by pulling back the device together with the microcatheter. Blood flow reversal is achieved by proximal inflation of a temporary balloon (*double arrow*) in the internal carotid or vertebral artery. During clot retrieval blood is aspirated through the large guide catheter (*curved arrow*). This is supposed to prevent distal emboli. *Source*: © 2008 Concentric Medical, Mountain View, CA, All rights reserved. (See for clinical studies and illustrative cases Part 2, Chapter 9.)

acute ischemic stroke. The X5 and X6 devices consist of a platinum-tipped nitinol wire with a moderately stiff, gradually enlarging helix that is deployed through a microcatheter. In addition, a 9-F balloon-tipped guide catheter is used for flow arrest or reversal within the ICA or the vertebral artery during retrieval. The basic approach is to navigate the microcatheter distal to the embolus and deploy the first two to three loops of the device. Then, the device is withdrawn to engage the embolus and deploy the remaining loops. To help incorporate the embolus, the device is torqued three to five times clockwise. The balloon in the internal or common carotid artery is inflated and suction applied as the distal device is withdrawn through the carotid artery and into the guide catheter. The MERCI Retriever X5 and X6 devices were tested in the MERCI trial. The trial evaluated the safety and efficacy of these devices to restore patency of occluded intracranial vessels within the first 8 h of acute ischemic stroke. The MERCI trial was conducted in two parts (10). Part I enrolled 55 patients and part II enrolled an additional 96 patients, for a total of 151 patients. Recanalization was achieved in 46% of patients with markedly improved clinical outcomes (90-day mRS, 0–2 in 46% of recanalizers vs. 10% of nonrecanalizers; $p < 0.0001$). Symptomatic intracranial hemorrhages occurred in 7.8% of the patients treated with the device alone (10) (see also Part 2, Chapter 9).

The encouraging results of the MERCI trial led the FDA in 2004 to designate the MERCI Retriever as the first revascularization device labelled specifically for use in acute ischemic stroke. The FDA approved this technology only for patients who are ineligible for treatment with IV t-PA or who fail IV t-PA therapy.

A recent advancement of the family of MERCI Retrievers is the LX type. This device has concentric helical loops with polymer filaments attached, increasing clot traction, and it has achieved higher recanalization rates than the X5/X6 Retrievers in preclinical studies. More recent data from the Multi-MERCI Trial (11)using the modified clot retriever L5 were more promising. Overall recanalization rate in 164 patients enrolled was 54.9% with the device alone and 68.3% with use of adjuvant therapy (prior use of IV t-PA and adjuvant IA t-PA was allowed). Patients joining the study were admitted with a severe ischemic stroke and a baseline NIHSS of 19.3±6.4. The site of occlusion were ICA/ICA-T in $n=52$ patients, MCA in $n=60$ patients, and vertebro-basilar artery in $n=14$ patients. Favorable outcome at 90 days was seen in 36% (mRS≤2); mortality at 90 days was 34%.

(b) *The Amplatz Goose Neck Microsnare (12) (ev3, Inc. (Microvena) Plymouth, MN,* Fig. 2). The Amplatz Goose Neck Microsnare device is a wire loop snare that exits the microcatheter at a 90° angle, which was designed to improve its ability to retrieve foreign bodies. This device, and many others, involves the use of a 6F introducer in the femoral artery through which a 6F guiding catheter is inserted into the extracranial segment of the ICA (12). A microcatheter is positioned with its tip just proximal to the occlusion. A retrieval snare having the same diameter of the occluded vessel is then introduced. The loop of the snare is pushed out of the microcatheter just enough for it to open fully and take its built-in shape perpendicular to the catheter and the vessel. The microcatheter is then pushed together with the snare into the embolus. After this, the snare is pulled back slightly into the microcatheter, so that only a small eye can be seen outside the catheter tip on fluoroscopy. Then, the microcatheter and snare are pulled out a few centimeters. If the embolus is caught in the snare, the whole assembly of the snare, the

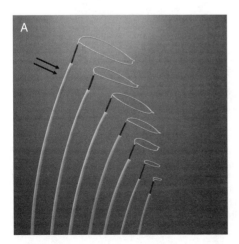

FIGURE 2 (*A*) The Amplatz Goose Neck Microsnare. View of the distal tip of several different sizes of snares. The 90° angle of the snare, which is delivered through the microcatheter (*double arrow*) to the target site, was designed to improve its retrieval abilities. *Source*: Permission from ev3 Inc., Plymouth, MN.

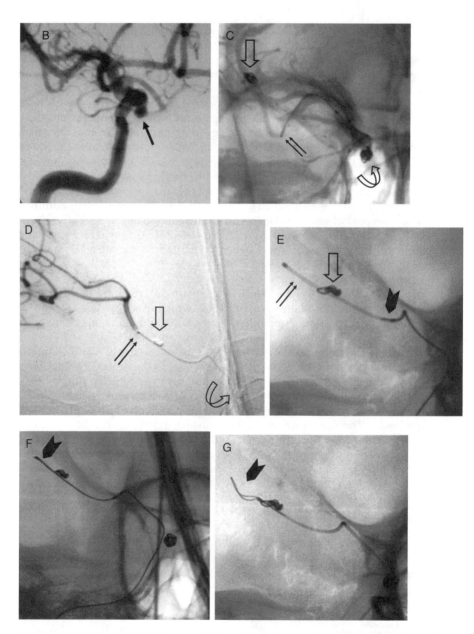

FIGURE 2 (*Continued*) (*B*) Right superior hypophyseal artery aneurysm (*arrow*). (*C*) Retrieval of a coil (*open arrow*) with a Microsnare from the right middle cerebral artery that was dislodged during embolization of the aneurysm (*bent arrow*). Images show different steps of coil retrieval using a microcatheter (*double arrow*) and the snare. (*D*) The microcatheter (*double arrow*) is placed distal to the coil mass (*open arrow*). (*E*) and (*F*) The snare (*arrow head*) is placed through the microcatheter. (*F*) The snare is placed inside the artery and distal to the coil mass. (*G*) The snare is gently pulled back with some rotation to allow to catch the coil mass and is then pulled back toward the microcatheter.

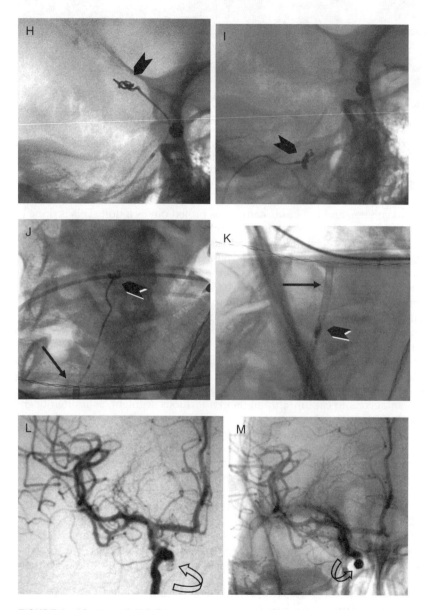

FIGURE 2 (*Continued*) (*H*) The coil mass is locked between the microcatheter and the snare. (*I*) The entire system (snare and microcatheter) is pulled back through the larger lumen guide catheter (*arrow*). (*J,K*) The coil mass is retrieved through the guide catheter (*arrow*). (*L*) Subtracted and (*M*) nonsubtracted right internal carotid artery follow-up angiograms show a restored blood flow within the intracranial circulation and an obliterated aneurysm using coils (*bent arrow*).

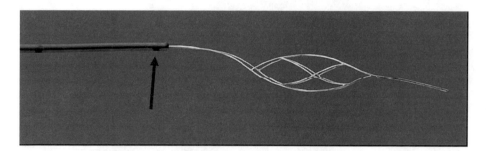

FIGURE 3   The Neuronet retrieval device (Guidant Endovascular, Santa Clara, CA). The device has an FDA approval in the United States for foreign body retrieval. View of the distal tip of the self-expanding nitinol basket, which is released by retraction of the microcatheter (*arrow*). *Source*: Reproduced with permission from Ref. (13).

microcatheter, and the guide catheter is pulled out as a unit. This is done to minimize the risk of dislodging the embolus from the snare.

(c) *Neuronet (13) (self-expanding nitinol basket; Guidant,* Fig. 3). This microgu-idewire-based device consists of a self-expanding nitinol basket that can be pushed through a standard microcatheter (13). The device should be advanced distally to the thrombus. The basket has more struts distally than proximally and is attached to the microwire excentrically to load the thrombus. After the microcatheter, which acts as a sheath, is removed, the embolus is retracted with the expanded basket. This device is most effective in straighter vessel segments, such as the M1 segment (9).

(d) *In-Time Retriever Device (Boston Scientific Neurovascular, Fremont, CA,* Fig. 4). This device has four to six wire loops and tends to bow when opened but has no specific opening to capture the embolus. Theoretically, this device may be advantageous to capture thrombus in a tortuous segment, as it often opens eccentrically.

(e) *EnSnare (Medical Device Technologies/InterV/Angiotech, Gainesville, FL).* The EnSnare has a tulip-shaped three-loop design but requires a 0.027-inch lumen. It opens distally, which may reduce the chance to capture emboli.

(f) *The Retriever (Boston Scientific, Neurovascular, Fremont, CA).* This device is another microsnare similar to the Amplatz Goose Neck Microsnare, described above. The major difference between these two microsnares is that The Retriever does not exit the microcatheter at a 90° angle, but rather it exits parallel to the microcatheter. It is also a slightly smaller profile, and therefore possibly less likely to injure distal small intracranial arteries, but it is also more difficult to navigate to these distal arteries compared to the Amplatz Goose Neck snare device.

(g) *The Alligator Retrieval Device (14) (Chestnut Medical Technologies, Menlo Park, CA,* Fig. 5). This device has three microprongs on the end of a microwire that can be pushed through the tip of a microcatheter to open the jaws; then it can be pulled back inside the microcatheter to close the jaws. This device is easier to navigate compared to the other thrombectomy devices, and it seems to grasp the foreign body more securely than most other retrieval devices and is successfully been used to retrieve foreign bodies from distal cerebrovascular segments.

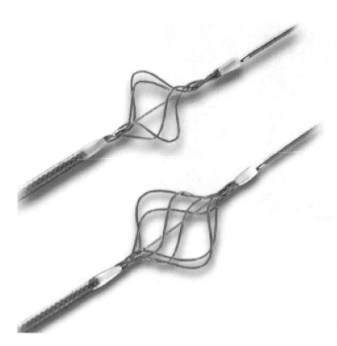

FIGURE 4 In-time foreign body retrieval device for neurovascular and peripheral application. View of the distal tip of the in-time device in two different configurations. *Source*: Courtesy of Boston Scientific, Fremont, CA.

(h) Other mechanical thrombectomy device include the *Penumbra System*, a clot retriever from Penumbra Inc. with a structure similar to a stent (Penumbra Inc., San Leandro, CA) that is not yet FDA approved for ischemic stroke (Fig. 6). The device is navigated through a microcatheter into the clot, which then can be grabbed by the device and removed through the guide catheter.

(i) *The Phenox Clot Retriever (15)* (Fig. 7) consists of a dense palisade of perpendicularly oriented stiff polyamid microfilaments attached to core wire (Phenox GmbH, Bochum, Germany). The device is introduced into the target vessel through a 0.021- or 0.027-inch microcatheter, deployed distally to the thrombus, and slowly pulled back under continuous aspiration of blood through the guiding catheter. So far, only a few patients have been treated with this system (15).

2. *Suction thrombectomy devices*

Suction thrombectomy devices use vacuum aspiration to remove occlusive clot in acute ischemic stroke. Compared with mechanical disruption devices, suction thrombectomy has reduced risk of causing uncontrolled thrombus fragmentation and distal embolization. Simple syringe suction applied to an endovascular catheter was successful in treating large, ICA thrombi in small case series (9). More sophisticated, vortex aspiration devices have been developed for the extracerebral circulation, using high-pressure streams to generate Venturi forces that physically fragment, draw in, and aspirate thrombi.

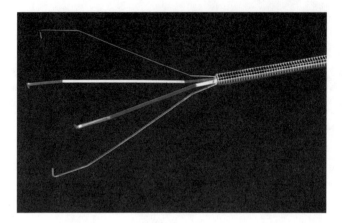

FIGURE 5 Alligator Retrieval Device (ARD) for neurovascular and peripheral application (Chestnut Medical Technologies, Inc., Menlo Park, CA). View of the distal end of the device. The device is made of a 0.016-inch stainless steel wire with micro-fabricated precision grasping arms attached to the tip and is placed through a microcatheter. The device is available in 2–5 mm maximal diameter with the jaws fully open. The jaws are closed on re-sheathing the microcatheter. *Source*: Reproduced with permission from Ref. (14).

(a) *AngioJet (Possis Medical, Minneapolis, MN) and Oasis (16) (Boston Scientific, Natick, MA, Fig. 8A).* These are endovascular thrombectomy devices that combine local vortex suction with mechanical disruption for what has been coined rheolytic thrombectomy (16). These 4- or 5-F catheters use either a single (Oasis) retrograde high-pressure saline jet (16) or multiple (Angio-Jet) retrograde high pressure fluid jets directed into the primary evacuation

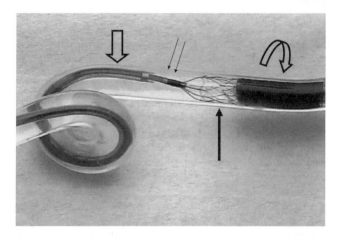

FIGURE 6 Penumbra clot retriever system is not FDA approved in the United States for clot removal (Penumbra Inc.). The distal nitinol basket, designed like a retrievable stent (*arrow*), is pushed through a microcatheter (*double arrow*) and grabs the clot (*bent arrow*, in vitro illustration). The entire system is navigated through a flexible 6 Fr guide catheter (Neuron Intracranial Access System) which tapers distally to a 5 Fr size and can easily be positioned into the intracranial circulation. *Source*: Permission from Penumbra Inc.

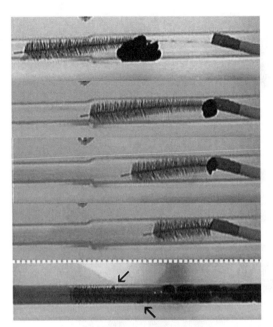

FIGURE 7 Phenox Clot Retriever consists of a dense palisade of perpendicular-oriented stiff polyamid microfilaments attached to core wire (Phenox GmbH). The device is introduced into the target vessel through a 0.021- or 0.027-inch microcatheter, deployed distally to the thrombus, and slowly pulled back under continuous aspiration of blood through the guiding catheter. *Source*: Reproduced with permission from Ref. (18).

lumen to create a hydrodynamic vortex that draws in, traps, and fragments adjacent thrombus (Fig. 8B). The debris is then simultaneously removed through the recovery lumen. The technology is based on the Bernoulli Principle. The initial generation AngioJet successfully treated some internal carotid and vertebrobasilar thromboses in case reports (16,17), although lack of flexibility made navigation in the intracranial circulation difficult. The AngioJet or Oasis may have some advantages over other mechanical devices for their ability to remove more solid organized embolic material. However, because of stiffness their major limitation is the inability to safely navigate distal to the petrous carotid segment and the carotid siphon, thus requiring an alternative technique when occlusion is located distally (16). Presently, there are no clinical trials for acute stroke in progress.

(b) *The NeuroJet (Possis Medical)*. This suction thrombectomy device is a single-channel device that uses the same physics as the AngioJet, but it is designed specifically for intracranial navigation. The device has the same size as a standard microguidewire, and it is placed through a 3-F catheter. Nesbit et al. (9) reported dramatic successes using this technique in some cases. However, failure of the technique is still related mainly to its ability to navigate through the small, tortuous, and fragile intracranial circulation. Between April 2000 and July 2003, the device underwent safety and efficacy trial for thromboembolic occlusions of MCA, vertebral and basilar arteries and terminal ICA. As two perforations occurred with subarachnoid hemorrhage in 22 patients treated, the Thrombectomy in Middle Cerebral Artery Embolism (TIME) trial was prematurely terminated. Thus, the NeuroJet has been redesigned and is now available as the AngioJet® Rheolytic Thrombectomy system (Fig. 8), but not approved for the treatment of acute ischemic stroke.

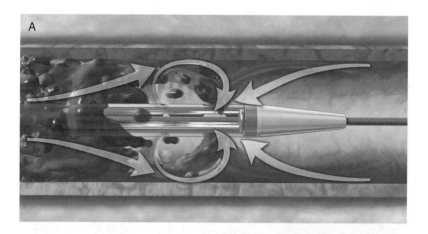

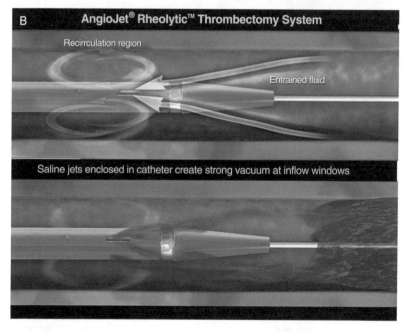

FIGURE 8   (*A*) Illustrative view of the distal tip of the AngioJet Rheolytic Thrombectomy device (Possis Medical, Inc., Minneapolis, MN) as it is advanced using the over-the-wire technique in to the clot, prior to activation of the device. (*B*) Illustration of the Bernoulli Principle involved that drives the Angio-Jet suction-thrombectomy device. The saline jets within the tip of the catheter and forces high pressure saline retrograde back into the catheter lumen, which then creates a low pressure recirculation region. This draws the entrained fluid, with blood clot, from the arterial lumen into the device lumen. *Source*: Permission from Possis Medical, Inc., Minneapolis, MN. (See also color plate section.)

Clot Disruption/Fragmentation

Mechanical clot disruption includes any technique by which the interventionalist mechanically fragments or completely destroys the thrombus within the artery. This may be accomplished simply by using guide wire manipulation or in a more complex fashion such as with laser shock-wave devices. As the thrombus is disrupted and flow reestablished, small emboli are created and carried into distal branches. A recently published in vitro study compared several embolectomy systems (18). All the tested devices generated clot fragments during passage through the clot and retrieval. But differences were significant between the devices, which were evaluated in a plastic tube (slip boundary condition) filled with human clot and attached to a mock flow loop. If fragmented emboli are small enough, they will pass through the increasingly small distal circulation. In case of larger clot fragments, a further reperfusion may require endogenous or exogenous enzymatic thrombolysis. Because smaller emboli may facilitate exogenous thrombolysis, mechanical clot disruption may also be applied as an augmented fibrinolysis technique.

(a) *Simple microguidewire.* This is the most basic of these devices and the easiest to apply. In IA thrombolysis, a microcatheter is navigated over a microguidewire up to the proximal portion of the thrombus. The microguidewire with a soft and flexible tip can usually be easily advanced through the thrombus into the distal vessel. Different shapes can be given to the microcatheter tip to avoid vessel perforation. Multiple passes through the clot with the wire and microcatheter is one form of mechanical disruption that may fragment the thrombus if it is not organized. As an individual technique, it is only marginally effective; however, in combination with fibrinolytic agents, this disruption aids in the process by increasing the surface area of the thrombus exposed to the thrombolytic. Mechanical manipulation incrementally improves the recanalization rate up to 75% (19–21).

(b) *Penumbra System (Penumbra Inc., Fig. 9).* Penumbra has developed besides its clot grabber, a second system for clot retrieval. A wire with an olive-shaped tip is navigated into the clot through a larger braided microcatheter. Simultaneously, suction is applied to the microcatheter allowing aspiration of the fragmented clot. Penumbra has received a FDA approval for clot removal based on results from single-arm, multicenter trial conducted in the United States and Europe. Enrolled were 125 patients at 24 international centers (22). The average time from symptom onset to arterial puncture was 4.1 h. The baseline NIHSS was 17.6 with angiographically confirmed TIMI 0 flow in 96% of patients. ICA and vertebrobasilar occlusion was observed in 18% and 9%, respectively. In 81.6% of the cases a revascularization (TIMI 2 or 3) was achieved using the Penumbra system. Procedural but not device-related serious adverse events were encountered in 4 (3.2%) of the treated cases. Although mRS≤2 was achieved only by 25% of the patients, it needs to be noted that 46% of the patients had at least a 4-point improvement in NIHSS at discharge. In addition, 27% of patients had either a ≥10-point NIHSS improvement or NIHSS 0-1 at discharge. Good clinical outcome after 30 days, defined as ≥4-point NIHSS improvement or mRS≤2, was recorded in 46% of patients in whom recanalization was achieved versus only 22% of cases where the occluded vessel was not recanalized ($p < 0.05$).

(c) *Microsnares or net devices.* The various microsnares and nets described earlier can also be used to more aggressively fragment thrombus (Fig. 2). One must be careful to avoid dissections and perforations when using these devices as a mechanical disruption device. These devices will result in variable-sized fragments and, as an isolated technique, may result in multiple distal branch occlusions. As an adjunctive technique, the use of snares should result in more fragmentation and, theoretically, more rapid recanalization than does the use of microguidewires (23).

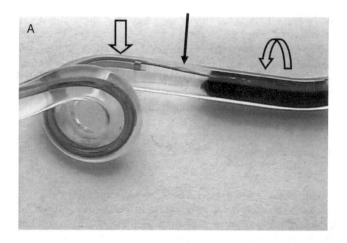

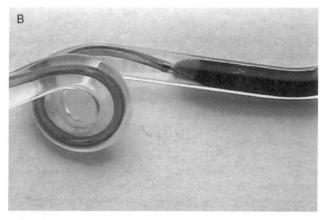

FIGURE 9   (A) In vitro illustration of the Penumbra clot fragmentation and (B) suction system, FDA approved in the United States for clot removal (Penumbra Inc.). The Separator (*arrow*) has an olive-shaped plastic structure attached proximal to the wire tip (*arrow*). The system is pushed back and forth through the clot (*bent arrow*) under simultaneous suction through the guide catheter (*open arrow*). The principle is based on thrombus debulking approach in thromboembolic ischemic stroke. The entire system is navigated through a flexible 6 Fr guide catheter (Neuron Intracranial Access System) which tapers distally to a 5 Fr size and can easily be positioned into the intracranial circulation. *Source*: Courtesy of Penumbra Inc.

(d) *Laser thrombolysis.* At least two devices have been tested at this time that use laser energy to assist clot fragmentation for cerebrovascular occlusion in an acute ischemic stroke. The laser is designed to effectively disrupt or dissolve the clot without damaging the endothelium. Some technical challenges remain and only further improvements will allow their safe use in the clinical setting.
  (i) *Endovascular Photo Acoustic Recanalization (EPAR, EndoVasix Inc., Belmont, CA,* Fig. 10). This technology was used for the first and most extensive trial on laser-based thrombolysis for stroke. A laser power source generates energy for the system. The energy is delivered by fiber optics to the tip of the catheter,

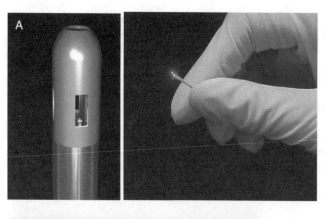

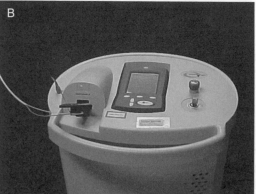

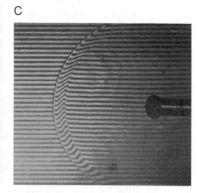

FIGURE 10 (*A*) View of the distal flexible tip of the 3 Fr EPAR (Endovascular PhotoAcoustic Recanalization) device based on laser technology. The hydrophilic coated catheter is placed over a standard 0.014-inch microwire into the clot (EndoVasix, Inc.). (*B*) Catheter attached to the EPAR laser energy source. The energy is delivered through fiberoptics to the tip of the catheter. (*C*) Absorption of laser light by darkly pigmented material (i.e., clot) converts the photo energy to acoustic energy, which emulsifies clot inside the catheter tip (EndoVasix, Inc.). (See also color plate section.)

at the treatment site. Absorption of laser light by darkly pigmented materials, that is, the clot, occurs inside the 1-mm catheter tip, and the system is designed to minimize scattering of laser light. Absorption converts photo energy into acoustic energy, which then causes the clot to emulsify inside the catheter tip. The study involved 34 patients in the United States and Germany who all presented to the health center with severe ischemic stroke, measured by a median NIHSS score of 19 (24). If the anterior circulation was involved, the patients were treated within 6-h time window of symptom onset. In case of a posterior circulation stroke, the patients were treated up to 24 h after symptom onset. Of the 34 vessel segments treated, 14 (41.1%) improved by at least one point on the TIMI flow after the treatment. Additional treatment with IA infusion of t-PA was carried out in 13 patients. A fatal adverse event associated with use of the device occurred in one patient. Symptomatic hemorrhage occurred in two patients (5.9%).Two vessel perforations were encountered during the procedure. The mortality rate was 38.2%. This was not unexpected given the severity of stroke at the time of hospital admission center (24).

(ii) *LaTIS laser device (LaTIS, Inc., Coon Rapids, MN)*. This device uses laser energy to ablate clots. The device was evaluated in a safety and feasibility trial at two centers in the United States. Arteries 2–5 mm in diameter could be treated, including the ICA, M1 or M2 branch of the MCA, A1 branch of the ACA, basilar artery, PCA, and vertebral artery. Patients could receive treatment as late as 8 h after symptom onset in the anterior circulation and within 24 h in the posterior circulation. A preliminary report of safety and feasibility results noted difficulty in delivery of the laser device to the site of the clot in two of the initial five patients treated. After catheter revision, the Phase I trial has resumed at two centers in the United States (25).

Augmented Fibrinolysis

Several mechanical techniques may enhance pharmacological fibrinolysis. The use of mechanical devices such as microcatheters, guidewires, snares, nets, and balloons, when used in addition to fibrinolytics, may help to accomplish this goal. Qureshi et al. (22) described an increase in recanalization rates after combined aggressive mechanical clot disruption and thrombolytic agents.

Ultrasonification

Ultrasonification is used in conjunction with thrombolytic therapy (25). Nonthermal effects of low-frequency ultrasound energy have been found to accentuate enzymatic fibrinolysis in vitro (27,28). In vitro flow model studies of externally applied, low-frequency, pulse wave ultrasonography suggest that direct and transcranial ultrasound combined with t-PA significantly shortens the time to vessel recanalization as compared with t-PA alone (29,30).

The mechanism of action is debated, but there is a scientific evidence for at least four contributing effects: (i) rectified diffusion, which provides a pumping effect and enables drug transport into the thrombus; (ii) reformation and opening of the fibrin matrix of clot exposed to ultrasound resulting in enhanced drug diffusion; (iii) cleavage of fibrin polymers and surface expansion for thrombolytic effect; and (iv) improved binding of alteplase to fibrin.

Local direct ultrasound thrombolysis with miniaturized transducers attached to catheters have already reached clinical investigation (25,31). Tachibana et al. (32) showed an improved in vitro clot lysis with a microtransducer operating at 225 kHz, and similar in vitro results were found for a combined application of ultrasound (170 kHz, 0.5 W/cm^2) and urokinase.

Currently, there is only one ultrasound thrombolytic infusion catheter available in the United States (EKOS Corporation, Bothell, WA), which combines the use of an ultrasound transducer at the microcatheter tip with simultaneous infusion of a thrombolytic agent through the microcatheter (Fig. 11).

In a preclinical study investigating the efficacy of the device in peripheral vascular occlusion, thrombi were induced bilaterally in the superficial femoral arteries of nine dogs (33). Although urokinase (5000 IU/kg) was delivered to vessels on both sides, the ultrasound transducer of the catheter was activated on only one side. Follow-up angiography after treatment showed a good flow (i.e., TIMI grade 2 or 3;

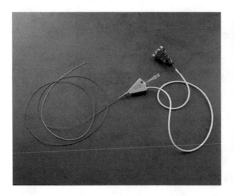 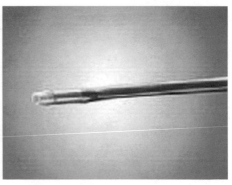

FIGURE 11 View of the EKOS microcatheter and distal tip. The microcatheter attached to the external energy source has the ability to generate ultrasonic waves while embedded in the clot and simultaneously allows a local intra-arterial infusion of thrombolytic agents. *Source*: Courtesy of EKOS Corporation.

Table 2) in 9 (100%) of the ultrasound-treated vascular segments and in 6 (67%) of the controls that were not treated with ultrasound ($p=0.058$). Angioscopy and histopathology revealed more thrombi in the vessels that did not receive ultrasound treatment. Mahon et al. (34) published the North American clinical experience with the EKOS MicroLysUS infusion catheter for the treatment of embolic stroke. Fourteen patients with anterior ($n=10$) and posterior ($n=4$) circulation embolic occlusion were treated (NIHSS score, 9–23 [mean, 18.2] and 11–27 [mean, 18.75], respectively) using the EKOS catheter combined with a simultaneous IA thrombolysis 3–6 and 4–13 h after symptom onset, respectively. Three deaths occurred at 24 h: two from intracranial hemorrhage and one from cerebral swelling. One patient died at 1 week and another at 1 month following the treatment. Average time to recanalization was 46 min. No catheter related adverse events were encountered. TIMI grade 2–3 flow was achieved in eight patients in the first hour. Mean NIHSS scores in eight of nine survivors at 90 days were 5 in the anterior-circulation group and 3 in the posterior-circulation group; mean mRS scores at 90 days were 2 and 3, respectively (33). In this safety and feasibility study, ultrasound was used in conjunction with IA t-PA or Reteplase infusion. The EKOS catheter was placed in the proximal portion of the clot. After a bolus of thrombolytic agent was injected through the catheter, the patient received a continuous IA infusion and simultaneous ultrasound transmission for up to 60 min. The EKOS device was used in a study, which evaluated the feasibility and safety of a combined IV and IA treatment for acute ischemic stroke (Interventional Management of Stroke (IMS) II Study) and is currently being used in the IMS III trial (see for more details on clinical trials Part 2, Chapter 9).

Stenting and Angioplasty

(a) *Intracranial Angioplasty.* Intracranial percutaneous transluminal angioplasty (PTA) in acute stroke can be used as a primary technique to mechanically fragment the thromboembolus or combined with IV or IA thrombolysis (Fig. 12). It can also be useful for treatment of an acute ischemic stroke associated with an occlusion of a hemodynamic significant intracranial atherosclerotic lesion when

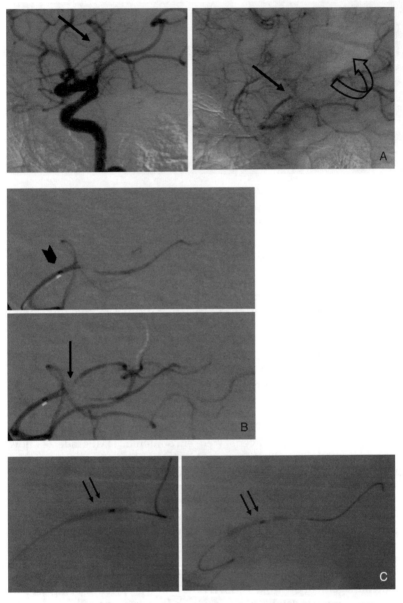

FIGURE 12 Sixty-year-old male presenting with a left-hemispheric stroke (NIHSS = 12) 4 hrs after initial ictus. (*A*) Initial left internal carotid artery angiogram in lateral view shows a thromboembolic occlusion of the left angular artery (*arrow*) with a large area of hypoperfusion in the capillary phase (*bent arrow*). (*B*) Follow-up angiogram after local intra-arterial infusion of 20 mg of t-PA (5 mg as bolus and 15 mg infused over 1 h)through the microcatheter (*arrow head*) shows partial recanalization with remnant clot at the angular artery bifurcation (*arrow*). (*C*) Percutaneous angioplasty (PTA) of the upper and lower branches (*double arrows*) with a low-profile noncompliant balloon at 6 atm (Maverick 1.5 × 9 mm, BSC, Natick, MA).

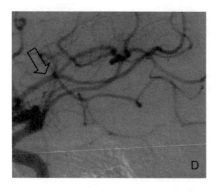

FIGURE 12 (*Continued*) (*D*) Post-PTA follow-up angiogram shows a complete recanalization of the angular artery and excellent distal blood flow (TIMI 3). Three days after the procedure the patients presented with a left facial palsy and a left arm weakness 4/5 (NIHSS < 5).

chemical thrombolysis is ineffective or only partially successful. Ringer et al. (35) performed angioplasty in selected patients if thrombolysis resulted in inadequate or failed recanalization. Five of nine patients had successful recanalization and none presented with a reocclusion. Nakano et al. (36) primarily used PTA rather than thrombolytics when early ischemic findings were present on initial CT and/ or when lenticulostriate arteries were involved. The authors also used PTA when a superselective microcatheter angiography distal to the occlusion site confirmed

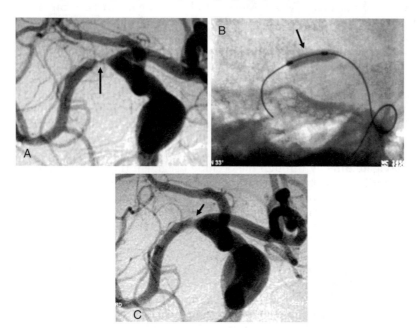

FIGURE 13 Fifty-nine-year-old male with recurrent episodes of transitory ischemic attacks on antiplatelet therapy and a previous history of left hemiparesis associated with a right hemispheric hemorrhagic infarction. (*A*) Right internal carotid artery angiogram shows a short and concentric atherosclerotic lesion at the origin of the right middle cerebral artery (*arrow*). (*B*) Percutaneous transluminal angioplasty with a noncompliant 3 × 9 mm balloon at 6 atm (*arrow*; Maverick, BSC, Natick, MA). (*C*) Post-angioplasty angiography shows an excellent revascularization with a visible shelf corresponding to the remaining compressed plaque and probably a small plaque dissection (*arrow*).

the presence of a large embolus or a high-grade stenosis suggestive of a thrombosis. Initial recanalization rate in a small case series ($n=10$) was 100% and a reocclusion occurred in two patients. There were no hemorrhagic or technical complication reported (35). Ueda et al. (38) experienced no reocclusion when PTA was combined with thrombolysis for acute thrombotic stroke. Our experience shows that angioplasty appears particularly useful in patients with underlying intracranial atherosclerotic lesions, which may progress to an acute thrombotic occlusion most likely to plaque rupture (Fig. 13).

(b) *Stenting for Acute Stroke.* Stenting of an occluded ICA or an occluded intracranial artery in selected cases presenting with an acute stroke has gained attention in recent years. We will discuss the rational for the use of stents.

(i) *Stenting of acute occlusion of the internal carotid artery*

The prognosis for patients presenting with acute stroke caused by an acute ICA occlusion and poor collateral blood supply is generally considered poor. This often results in a "T" occlusion with a massive clot burden for the patient. It is estimated that 16%–55% of these patients will die of complications from infarction, 40%–69% will be left with great disability, and only 2%–12% of patients will make a good recovery (37). The optimal treatment for these patients has not been established and represents a challenging and complex problem. Results of urgent surgical recanalization are not ideal (39,40). Meyer et al. (38) identified two important prognostic factors correlating with poor surgical outcome, that is, the presence of an associated MCA occlusion and lack of collateral flow. Unfortunately, concurrent intracranial occlusion of the ipsilateral MCA territory is commonly observed in patients with an acute symptomatic occlusion of the ICA and usually correlates with a decreased flow in MCA and poor or absent collateral blood flow. Several studies strongly suggest that an early revascularization with local IA thrombolytics or mechanical devices is vital for a clinical improvement in patients with an ICA occlusion (40–45). To gain access to the intracranial circulation through the ipsilateral occluded ICA, it is necessary to either recanalize the ICA or navigate directly through the occluded segment (Fig. 14). Several recent studies have shown that neither IV nor IA thrombolysis is effective for recanalization of an occluded cervical ICA (40,46). Higher doses of thrombolytic agents do not seem to correlate with the success rate (40,46). Mechanical thrombectomy has been described as technically feasible, with only small expenditures of time. This may serve as an alternative to chemical thrombolysis for ICA recanalization. Endarterectomy and angioplasty in severe ICA stenosis, however, are usually postponed for days or weeks after the initial ictus. However, during the first hours and days after a stroke, the risk of reocclusion or recurrent arterio-arterial embolism remains. To reduce this risk, some investigators have developed protocols for endovascular treatment that include stent implantation in the proximal ICA segment with or without IA thrombolysis (IAT). The patient, however, has to be placed on (dual) antiplatelet therapy following stenting. Previously, Wang et al. (47) reported data on six patients who underwent urgent catheter navigation through the occluded ICA, thrombolysis, and PTA. Stent implantation was performed in three patients who subsequently had a favorable outcome at a mean follow-up

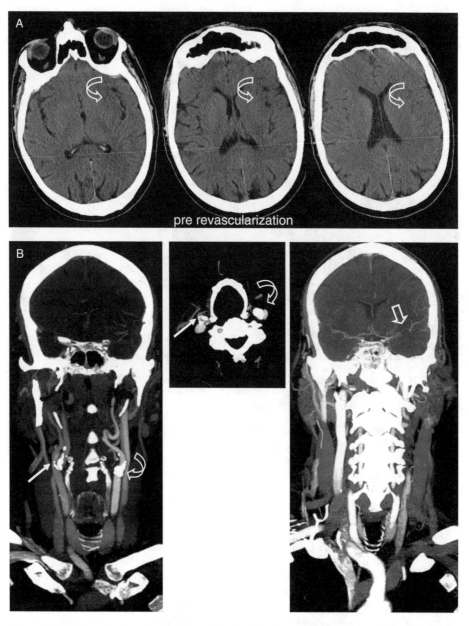

Figure 14   A 62-year-old male presents with a right hemiparesis and aphasia; time of symptom onset is unclear. Patient is admitted for an endovascular treatment. (*A*) Brain CT without contrast shows effacement of the left sylvian fissure due to swelling of the insula and operculum, some loss of gray–white-matter differentiation, and mild hypodensity (*bent arrow*). (*B*) CT angiograms in coronal (*left*) and axial (*center*) planes show a severe calcification of both internal carotid arteries at the carotid bulb/bifurcation level (*arrow*) and a high-grade stenosis of the left internal carotid artery origin (*bent arrow*). A study of the intracranial circulation (*right*) shows a possible thromboembolic occlusion of the left middle cerebral artery M1 segment/bifurcation.

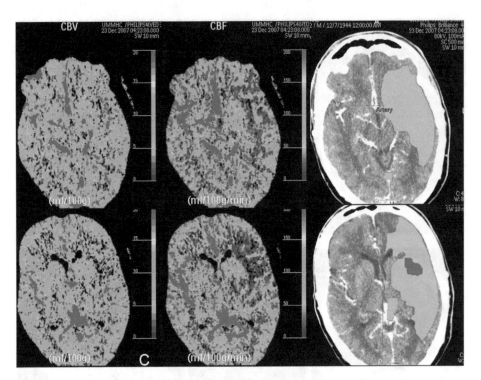

FIGURE 14 (*Continued*) (*C*) CT perfusion studies show a mismatch (*right*) between cerebral blood volume (*left*) and cerebral blood flow (*center*) indicating the penumbra (*green*). Note red represents the dead tissue. (See also color plate section.)

of 8 months. Nedeltchev et al. (48) combined IAT and stent implantation of the proximal ICA segment in 25 patients within the therapeutic time window of 6 h. ICA recanalization was successful in 21 patients. Good recanalization of the MCA was achieved in 11 patients. In nine of these patients, recanalization of the MCA was achieved by using mechanical revascularization only. Symptomatic intracerebral hemorrhage occurred in two patients. When the investigators compared their endovascular group to the medical group (*n* = 31), at 3 months, 56% of the endovascular group and 26% of the medical group had a favorable outcome. Mortality rate was 20% in the endovascular and 16% in the medical group (48). Jovin et al. (49) and Imai et al. (50) have also confirmed the benefit of emergent stenting of extracranial ICA occlusion in acute stroke. Jovin et al. (49) achieved a revascularization in 92% of 25 patients treated. At 30-day follow-up, 40% and 88% of patients who presented with an acute stroke and a subacute stroke, respectively, had an mRS ≤ 2. Imai et al. (50) had a 100% technical success rate in 17 high-grade stenotic or completely occluded ICA treated. Fifty-nine percent of these patients recovered or were considered to have a nondisabling stroke at 90 days after the procedure (50). The major risks include thrombus fragmentation and distal emboli, vessel perforation, and dissection. Microemboli, however, may remain both clinically and angiographically silent.

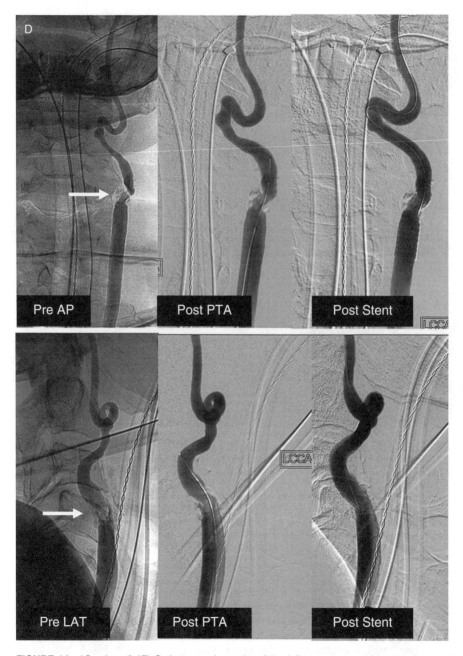

FIGURE 14 (*Continued*) (*D*) Catheter angiography of the left common carotid artery in anterior–posterior (AP) and lateral views shows a high-grade stenosis of the internal carotid artery origin (*arrow*) due to a calcified atherosclerotic lesion with occlusion of the external carotid artery. Angioplasty of the stenosis with a low-profile PTA balloon (Gateway 4 × 20 mm, BSC, Natick, MA) followed by a 5 × 20 mm PTA balloon dilatation (Aviator Plus, Cordis, Miami Lakes, FL), and placement of a Precise 8 × 30 mm carotid stent (Cordis, Miami Lakes, FL).

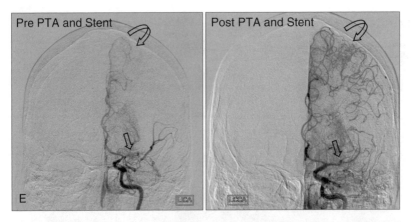

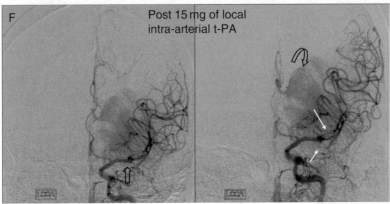

FIGURE 14 (*Continued*) (*E*) Intracranial studies show an improved collateral blood supply through the left anterior cerebral artery after angioplasty and stenting. Noted is a filling of the watershed area and of the distal middle cerebral artery territory in a retrograde fashion. The left middle cerebral artery bifurcation occlusion remains unchanged (*open arrow*) with hypoperfusion of the insula and temporal lobe. (*F*) Follow-up angiograms after local intraarterial thrombolysis (5 mg of t-PA as bolus, followed by infusion of further 10 mg) show recanalization of the occluded middle cerebral artery (*open arrow*) and improved distal flow; some clots are recognized within proximal M2 branches (*arrow*). Hyperperfusion of basal ganglia and the insula is seen with early transmedullary venous drainage (*bent arrow*) into the deep internal venous system.

Our own experience and reported literature (47–50) do not support the notion that catheter navigation through an acute occluded cervical ICA may result in any of the aforementioned complications.

(ii) *Stenting for symptomatic middle cerebral artery stenosis*

The most recognized stroke syndromes occur in the MCA region, in large part related to the extensive MCA blood supply to the lateral two-third hemisphere and deep basal ganglia. Although thromboembolism is the predominant mechanism affecting the MCA territory, primary atherosclerosis at this site occurs in a subset of patients. There appears to be a higher prevalence of MCA atherosclerotic disease in African

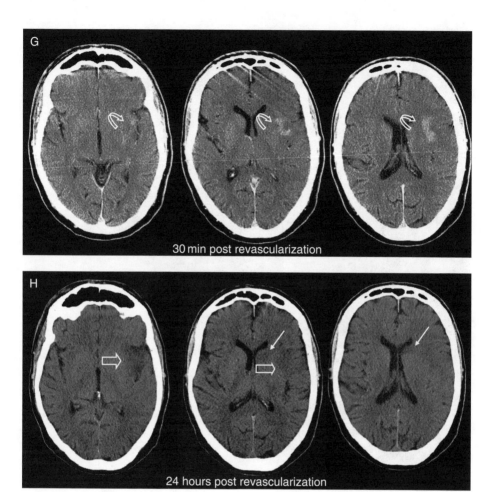

FIGURE 14 (*Continued*) (*G*) Follow-up CT 30 min after the recanalization procedure shows some contrast extravasations in the insula area and along the cella media of the left lateral ventricle (*bent arrow*). This study could also represent hemorrhagic transformation of the ischemic area. (*H*) On a 24-h follow-up study, the contrast material has disappeared and the nonsalvageable ischemic area is clearly demarcated as hypodensity of the insula (*open arrow*) and the left caudate (*arrow*).

Americans and Asians as compared with Caucasians (51,52). Many patients with intracranial atherosclerosis have recurrent cerebral ischemic events despite standard medical therapy with antiplatelet agents or oral anticoagulants (Fig. 15). In the Extracranial/Intracranial Bypass Trial, patients with symptomatic MCA stenosis randomized to medical therapy had an annual ipsilateral stroke rate of 7.8% and a total stroke rate of 9.5% (53,54). Only about one third of patients had a warning transient ischaemic attack (TIA) prior to stroke (54). The most common presentation was a cerebral infarction without a warning TIA. In these patients, the stenosis progresses as a result of atherosclerotic disease rather than a thromboembolic process. Anticoagulants would therefore appear to

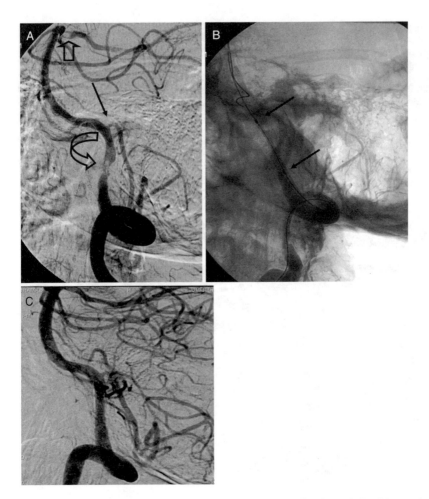

FIGURE 15 A 74-year-male with a posterior circulation infarction admitted for an intraarterial thrombolysis. (*A*) Angiogram of the left vertebral artery (VA) in oblique projection after completion of an local intraarterial infusion of t-PA shows remnant clot in the left distal VA riding on an atherosclerotic plaque (*curved arrow*). Some clot may be present in the origin of the left posterior inferior cerebellar artery (PICA, *arrow*) and the left P1 segment of the posterior cerebral artery (PCA, *open arrow*). (*B*) Placement of a balloon-expandable coronary stent (heparin-coated BX Sonic 3×13 mm at 10 atm, Cordis J&J, Miami Lakes, FL) over a 0.014-inch wire. Note the proximal and distal markers of the stent and contrast stagnation during stent placement. (*C*) Follow-up angiography in lateral view after stent implantation shows a smooth vessel boundary and an excellent flow to the posterior circulation.

aid only in prevention of an acute final occlusion caused by a thrombus and not in preventing progression of the disease to an inevitable occlusion (55). The high recurrent stroke rates in these patients indicate the need for more aggressive treatment methods for patients with symptomatic MCA athero-occlusive disease. PTA has recently been proposed as a promising treatment for patients with ongoing cerebral ischemic events despite standard medical therapy (56–58). However, PTA is associated with an acute vessel occlusion because of intimal damage, elastic recoil, and thrombosis (55,57). Patient frequently do not tolerate an acute occlusion of the MCA and develop a massive stroke or die. PTA has also been complicated by symptomatic recurrent stenosis, which may require multiple retreatments. Stents have improved these complications in coronary and peripheral vascular beds (59), and advantages of stent-assisted angioplasty include coverage of the plaque and reduced risk of dissection and prevention of vessel recoil and rupture (60). Therefore, the availability of recently introduced flexible stents, the development of potent antiplatelet inhibitors, and increasing evidence from experimental and clinical studies of intracranial stents have encouraged the use of stents in the management of ischemic intracranial cerebrovascular disease (61–65). Recently, Levy et al. (66) published the first case of stent-assisted angioplasty for M2 bifurcation in the setting of an acute stroke, which led to vessel recanalization after failed thrombolytic therapy. The rationale for using the balloon-expandable coronary stent was that it allowed the occlusive material, which becomes morselized by the angioplasty balloon, to be held in place against the vessel wall by the stent struts (67). By using extremely slow inflation techniques, the vessel is able to accommodate slight dilatation, which may be caused by the stent pressing thrombus against the intima and decrease the likelihood of rupture. Additionally, the stents are

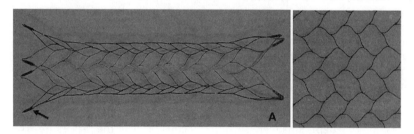

Enterprise – Closed cell design

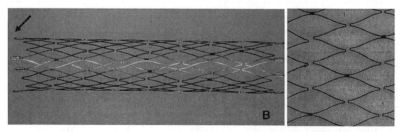

Neuroform – Open cell design

FIGURE 16 Low-profile, highly flexible self-expanding nitinol (nickel–titanium alloy) cerebrovascular stents, which are deployed through a microcatheter. Arrows indicate radio-opaque platinum markers at the end of the stent. (*A*) Retrievable closed cell design stent (Enterprise, Cordis Neurovascular J&J, Miami Lakes, FL). (*B*) Nonretrievable semi-open cell design (Neuroform, BSC, Natick, MA).

deployed at pressures well below nominal pressure (4.5 atm, as opposed to 8 or 10 atm), resulting in deployment of the stent at two-thirds of the intended diameter (deployment is estimated to be 2.5–2.8 mm, rather than 3 mm). This, in turn, leads to a reduction in the relative porosity of the stent, by decreasing the distance of the interstices between each stent strut. This phenomenon helps to jail pieces of thrombus or fragmented atherosclerotic material against the arterial lumen and prevent acute reocclusion.

(iii) *Retrievable stents*:
Stiffer balloon-expandable coronary stents, initially used for acute revascularization in stroke, are gradually being replaced by intracranial self-expanding stents navigated into the intracranial system through tiny microcatheters. Stenting of clot in acute stroke has been previously reported with successful recanalization in up to 80% of cases with both balloon expandable and self-expanding (66–69). A low-profile closed-cell self-expanding stent is an excellent platform for further development of a retrievable stent for an acute stroke (Fig. 16). A retrievable stent can partially be deployed into the clot with or without adjunctive antiplatelet or fibrinolytic therapy (70). If TIMI II or III flow is obtained, the stent can be retrieved. However, the benefit of using this system could be a final deployment of the stent in the event that sufficient flow is not achieved.

MISCELLANEOUS
Augmented Cerebral Blood Perfusion
Another more recently introduced endovascular concept is the augmentation of the cerebral blood flow and brain perfusion by partial and transitory obstruction of the abdominal aorta using a double balloon system. The principle is based on increased peripheral resistance and recruitment of collateral blood supply to the ischemic area (Fig. 17). A previous report showed some beneficial effect of aorta-obstruction in patients presenting with cerebral vasospasm associated with a subarachnoid hemorrhage resulting from an aneurysm rupture (5). Twenty-four patients were treated and a mean flow velocity increase in both the middle cerebral arteries over 15% was noted. Aneurysms were secured by coils prior to the procedure. The NIHSS decreased ≥2 points in 20 patients (83%). Currently, the Safety and Efficacy of NeuroFlo Treatment for Ischemic Stroke (SENTIS) trial is ongoing to investigate the beneficial value in acute ischemic stroke.

Induced Hypothermia
Induced hypothermia is considered to be one of the most potent methods of neuroprotection. Moderate surface and endovascular cooling of core body temperature to 32–33°C over 24–48 h has shown to improve survival and short-term neurological recovery in survivors of cardiac arrest compared with standard treatment (71–73). Multiple mechanisms for hypothermia-induced neuroprotective effect have been discussed, such as reduced metabolic rate and energy depletion. In the range of 22°C–37°C, brain oxygen consumption is reduced by approximately 5%/°C body temperature drop (74). Other neuroprotective mechanisms involve reduction of glutamate release under hypothermia (75), decreased generation of free radicals, reduced vascular permeability and blood–brain barrier disruption, and edema (76–79). In animal studies a moderate hypothermia has shown a better outcome

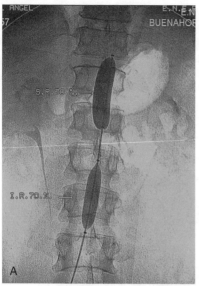

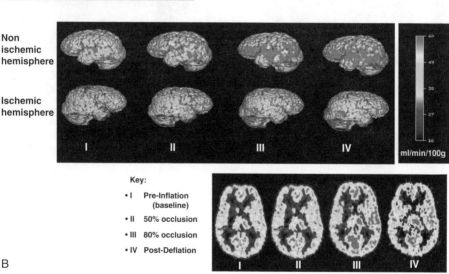

FIGURE 17 (*A*) Cerebral perfusion augmentation with a partial aortic occlusion. NeuroFlo System (Coaxia, Maple Grove, MN) has been inflated in the abdominal aorta of a patient. (*B*) A 38-year-old male (NIHSS = 11) presenting with a hemiplegia associated with a thromboembolic middle cerebral artery occlusion as shown on an MRA study. The patient was treated 10 h after the acute ischemic stroke with a NeuroFlo system. Images represent a sequence of PET images on the patient. The scale indicates the level of perfusion (ml/min/100 g) (*upper right*). The individual panels are as follows: I (baseline, before treatment), II (approximately 30%–50% balloon occlusion), III (70%–80% balloon occlusion), and IV Deflation (after both balloons are deflated, 60 min of inflation time). A progressive and significant increased perfusion (30%) is seen with a maximum in the cortical rim; reduction of the penumbra. Follow-up MRA showed no recanalization (not shown). Final MRI showed a small basal ganglia infarct. At 30 days the patient presented with a NIHSS of 5 and mRs = 2. *Source*: Permission from Dr. WD Heiss, Max-Planck-Institute, Germany. (See also color plate section.)

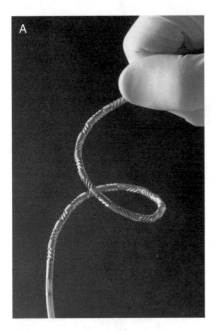

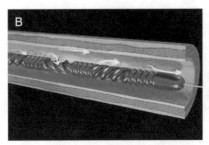

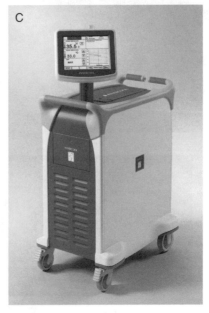

Figure 18 The catheter (*A*) which serves as an endovascular heat exchanger (*B*) is positioned in the inferior vena cava. The Celsius Control System consists of a disposable and flexible heat-transfer catheter, the administration cassette, and a console. (*C*) The catheter holds metallic temperature control element (TCE) that can be cooled or warmed by sterile saline circulating within the console. This system does not require intravenous infusion of cold fluid or extra-corporal heat exchange of patient's blood. To avoid embolic complications, the TCE and the catheter are heparin coated. *Source*: Permission from INNERCOOL therapies.

than sever hypothermia (80). Lyden et al. (81) consider a severe hypothermia as core body temperature <28°C while moderate hypothermia is defined as 28°C–34°C.

Two trials using surface cooling (82) and endovascular cooling (83) were designed to study effects of hypothermia in acute ischemic stroke. Albeit both trials showed feasibility, numbers of patient were small to be conclusive on safety and clinical efficacy. In both the hypothermia and the control, the clinical outcomes were similar. Mean diffusion-weighted imaging (DWI) lesion growth in the hypothermia group ($n=12$) was 90.0±83.5% compared with 108.4±142.4% in the control group ($n=11$) (NS). Mean DWI lesion growth in patients who cooled well ($n=8$) was 72.9±95.2% (NS) (83).

In animal models of focal ischemic stroke, effect of hypothermia on infarct size and improvement in behavioral outcome varies depend on ischemia duration and timing of hypothermia. The greatest benefits are achieved when hypothermia precedes the ischemic insult or is initiated immediately following the ischemia (84–86). Other animal studies show that moderate hypothermia of 32°C induced 1 h after MCA infarction for the period of 5 h did delay the infarct evolution but did not reduce the final infarct size on follow-up (87). However, the author found a significant infarct size reduction and improved animal behavioral outcome if hypothermia was combined with decompressive craniectomy.

Unlike surface cooling, which requires a tremendous effort from the nursing staff to maintain the hypothermia in some trial up to 72 h and includes the use of cooling blankets, ice water and frequent whole body rubs (82), endovascular cooling with newer generation of devices is fully controlled, and the target core temperature of 32–33°C can be reached within 3 h (vs. 6 h with surface cooling) (83,88). An 8.5 F (ICEY, Alsius Corportion, Irvine, CA), a 10.7 F or a 14 F catheter (Celsius Control System, INNERCOOL therapies, San Diego, CA) is placed simply through a femoral venous access into the inferior vena cava. The Celsius Control System consists of a disposable heat-transfer catheter, administration cassette, and a console (Fig. 18). The distal segment of the catheter has a flexible, metallic temperature control element (TCE) that can be cooled or warmed by sterile saline circulating within the console. The administration cassette connects the catheter to the console. This system does not require IV infusion of cold fluid or extra-corporal heat exchange of patient's blood. To avoid embolic complications, the TCE and the catheter are heparin coated. INNERCOOL received FDA clearance in January 2003 for the Celsius Control System to induce, maintain, and reverse mild hypothermia in neurosurgical patients in surgery and recovery.

Hypothermia-related and most commonly documented complications are singultus, shivering, pulmonary infection, arterial hypotension, bradycardia, arrhythmia, and thrombocytopenia (82,83). But, a coagulopathy was not encountered. Shivering may be excessive requiring combination therapy of meperidine busprione (89) or even intubation, sedation, and application of muscle relaxant (82). Although important, at present there is not enough clinical experience on beneficial or detrimental effects of hypothermia in hemorrhagic transformation of ischemic stroke. Undoubtedly, direct or indirect cooling of the brain in ischemic stroke is a potent neuroprotective solution which could be combined with a chemical or mechanical revascularization.

CONCLUSION

Emerging endovascular treatment strategies which include the use of microsnares, angioplasty balloons, thrombectomy, devices, ultrasonography, lasers, stents and other devices appear promising. Safety trials for several novel mechanical devices are currently under investigation, and many more are being planned for the near future. There is room for extensive improvements in our endovascular armamentarium and techniques. The next several years will undoubtedly witness rapid technologic advance in clot retrieval devices as mechanical endovascular instruments proliferate, which improve on or complement the existing devices. Combined with flow augmentation and local hypothermia, adjunctive treatments may be useful to expand the therapeutic window for mechanical and/or chemical revascularization. As the market is being flooded with various systems, the devices have to be demonstrated as user-friendly, safe, and effective with improved clinical results prior to their widespread use for acute ischemic stroke.

REFERENCES

1. Zeumer H, Hacke W, Ringelstein EB. Local intraarterial thrombolysis in vertebrobasilar thromboembolic disease. AJNR Am J Neuroradiol 1983; 4(3):401–404.
2. Adams HP, Jr,. del Zoppo G, Alberts MJ, et al. Guidelines for the early management of adults with ischemic stroke: a guideline from the American Heart Association/American Stroke Association Stroke Council, Clinical Cardiology Council, Cardiovascular Radiology and Intervention Council, and the Atherosclerotic Peripheral Vascular Disease and Quality of Care Outcomes in Research Interdisciplinary Working Groups: The American Academy of Neurology affirms the value of this guideline as an educational tool for neurologists. Stroke 2007; 38(5):1655–1711.
3. Siepmann G, Müllner-Jensen M, Goossens-Merkt H, Lachenmayer L, Zeumer H. Local intraarterial fibrinolysis in acute middle cerebral artery occlusion. In: Hacke W, del Zoppo GJ, Hirschberg M, eds. Thrombolytic Theropy in Acute Ischemic Stroke. Heidelberg, Germany: Spinger; 1991:68–71.
4. Zeumer H, Freitag HJ, Grzyska U, et al. Local intraarterial fibrinolysis in acute vertebrobasilar occlusion. Technical developments and recent results. Neuroradiology 1989; 31(4):336–340.
5. Lylyk P, Vila JF, Miranda C, et al. Partial aortic obstruction improves cerebral perfusion and clinical symptoms in patients with symptomatic vasospasm. Neurol Res 2005; 27(Suppl 1):S129–S135.
6. Khatri P, Neff J, Broderick JP, et al. Revascularization end points in stroke interventional trials: Recanalization versus reperfusion in IMS-I. Stroke 2005; 36(11):2400–2403.
7. Tomsick T. TIMI, TIBI, TICI: I came, I saw, I got confused. AJNR Am J Neuroradiol 2007; 28(2):382–384.
8. King S, Khatri P, Carrozella J, et al. Anterior cerebral artery emboli in combined intravenous and intra-arterial t-PA treatment of acute ischemic stroke in the IMS I and II trials 2007;(28)10:1890–1894.
9. Nesbit GM, Luh G, Tien R, et al. New and future endovascular treatment strategies for acute ischemic stroke. J Vasc Interv Radiol 2004; 15(1 Pt 2):S103–S110.
10. Smith WS, Sung G, Starkman S, et al. Safety and efficacy of mechanical embolectomy in acute ischemic stroke: results of the MERCI trial. Stroke 2005; 36(7):1432–1438.
11. Smith WS, Sung G, Saver J, et al. Mechanical thrombectomy for acute ischemic stroke. Final results of the multi MERCI trial. Stroke 2008; 39:1205–1212.
12. Wikholm G. Transarterial embolectomy in acute stroke. AJNR Am J Neuroradiol 2003; 24(5):892–894.
13. Mayer TE, Hamann GF, Brueckmann HJ. Treatment of basilar artery embolism with a mechanical extraction device: necessity of flow reversal. Stroke 2002; 33(9):2232–2235.
14. Henkes H, Lowens S, Preiss H, et al. A new device for endovascular coil retrieval from intracranial vessels: alligator retrieval device. AJNR Am J Neuroradiol 2006; 27(2): 327–329.
15. Henkes H, Reinartz J, Lowens S, et al. A device for fast mechanical clot retrieval from intracranial arteries (phenox clot retriever). Neurocrit Care 2006; 5(2):134–140.
16. Bellon RJ, Putman CM, Budzik RF, et al. Rheolytic thrombectomy of the occluded internal carotid artery in the setting of acute ischemic stroke. AJNR Am J Neuroradiol 2001; 22(3):526–530.
17. Kawamura A, Tilem M, Gossman DE, et al. Rheolytic thrombectomy for thromboembolic occlusion of the internal carotid artery complicating coronary intervention. J Invasive Cardiol 2006; 18(3):E108–E110.
18. Liebig T, Reinartz J, Hannes R, et al. Comparative in vitro study of five mechanical embolectomy systems: effectiveness of clot removal and risk of distal embolization. Neuroradiology 2008; 50(1):43–52.
19. Barnwell SL, Clark WM, Nguyen TT, et al. Safety and efficacy of delayed intraarterial urokinase therapy with mechanical clot disruption for thromboembolic stroke. AJNR Am J Neuroradiol 1994; 15(10):1817–1822.
20. Mericle RA, Luft AR, Lopes DK, et al. Mechanical revascularization of cerebral arterial occlusions for acute thromboembolic stroke. Neurosurgery 1998; 43(3):700.

21. Nesbit GM, Clark WM, O'Neill OR, et al. Intracranial intraarterial thrombolysis facilitated by microcatheter navigation through an occluded cervical internal carotid artery. J Neurosurg 1996; 84(3):387–392.
22. McDougall CG, Clark W, Mayer T, et al. The Penumbra stroke trial: Safety and effectiveness of a new generation of mechanical devices for clot removal in acute ischemic stroke. The 2008 International Stroke Conference, New Orleans, LA,February 20–22, 2008.
23. Qureshi AI, Siddiqui AM, Suri MF, et al. Aggressive mechanical clot disruption and low-dose intra-arterial third-generation thrombolytic agent for ischemic stroke: a prospective study. Neurosurgery 2002; 51(5):1319–1327.
24. Berlis A, Lutsep H, Barnwell S, et al. Mechanical thrombolysis in acute ischemic stroke with endovascular photoacoustic recanalization. Stroke 2004; 35(5):1112–1116.
25. http://www.emedicine.com/neuro/topic702.htm (accessed December 2007).
26. Daffertshofer M, Hennerici M, Daffertshofer M, et al. Ultrasound in the treatment of ischaemic stroke. Lancet Neurol 2003; 2(5):283–290.
27. Sehgal CM, Leveen RF, Shlansky-Goldberg RD. Ultrasound-assisted thrombolysis. Invest Radiol 1993; 28(10):939–943.
28. Spengos K, Behrens S, Daffertshofer M, et al. Acceleration of thrombolysis with ultrasound through the cranium in a flow model. Ultrasound Med Biol 2000; 26(5):889–895.
29. Behrens S, Daffertshofer M, Spiegel D, et al. Low-frequency, low-intensity ultrasound accelerates thrombolysis through the skull. Ultrasound Med Biol 1999; 25(2):269–273.
30. Behrens S, Spengos K, Daffertshofer M, et al. Potential use of therapeutic ultrasound in ischemic stroke treatment. Echocardiography 2001; 18(3):259–263.
31. Goyen M, Kroger K, Buss C, et al. Intravascular ultrasound angioplasty in peripheral arterial occlusion. Preliminary experience. Acta Radiol 2000; 41(2):122–124.
32. Tachibana K. Enhancement of fibrinolysis with ultrasound energy. J Vasc Interv Radiol 1992; 3(2):299–303.
33. Atar S, Luo H, Nagai T, et al. Arterial thrombus dissolution in vivo using a transducer-tipped, high-frequency ultrasound catheter and local low-dose urokinase delivery. J Endovasc Ther 2001; 8(3):282–290.
34. Mahon BR, Nesbit GM, Barnwell SL, et al. North American clinical experience with the EKOS microlysus infusion catheter for the treatment of embolic stroke. AJNR Am J Neuroradiol 2003; 24(3):534–538.
35. Ringer AJ, Qureshi AI, Fessler RD, et al. Angioplasty of intracranial occlusion resistant to thrombolysis in acute ischemic stroke. Neurosurgery 2001; 48(6):1282–1288.
36. Nakano S, Yokogami K, Ohta H, et al. Direct percutaneous transluminal angioplasty for acute middle cerebral artery occlusion. AJNR Am J Neuroradiol 1998; 19(4):767–772.
37. Ueda T, Hatakeyama T, Kohno K, et al. Endovascular treatment for acute thrombotic occlusion of the middle cerebral artery: local intra-arterial thrombolysis combined with percutaneous transluminal angioplasty. Neuroradiology 1997; 39(2):99–104.
38. Meyer FB, Sundt TM Jr., Piepgras DG, et al. Emergency carotid endarterectomy for patients with acute carotid occlusion and profound neurological deficits. Ann Surg 1986; 203(1):82–89.
39. Walters BB, Ojemann RG, Heros RC. Emergency carotid endarterectomy. J Neurosurg 1987; 66(6):817–823.
40. Christou I, Felberg RA, Demchuk AM, et al. Intravenous tissue plasminogen activator and flow improvement in acute ischemic stroke patients with internal carotid artery occlusion. J Neuroimaging 2002; 12(2):119–123.
41. Spearman MP, Jungreis CA, Wechsler LR. Angioplasty of the occluded internal carotid artery. AJNR Am J Neuroradiol 1995; 16(9):1791–1796.
42. Jansen O, von Kummer R, Forsting M, et al. Thrombolytic therapy in acute occlusion of the intracranial internal carotid artery bifurcation. AJNR Am J Neuroradiol 1995; 16(10):1977–1986.
43. Rudolf J, Neveling M, Grond M, et al. Stroke following internal carotid artery occlusion—a contra-indication for intravenous thrombolysis?. Eur J Neurol 1999; 6(1):51–55.
44. Trouillas P, Nighoghossian N, Derex L, et al. Thrombolysis with intravenous t-PA in a series of 100 cases of acute carotid territory stroke: determination of etiological, topographic, and radiological outcome factors. Stroke 1998; 29(12):2529–2540.

45. von Kummer R, Holle R, Rosin L, et al. Does arterial recanalization improve outcome in carotid territory stroke? Stroke 1995; 26(4):581–587.
46. Endo S, Kuwayama N, Hirashima Y, et al. Results of urgent thrombolysis in patients with major stroke and atherothrombotic occlusion of the cervical internal carotid artery. AJNR Am J Neuroradiol 1998; 19(6):1169–1175.
47. Wang H, Lanzino G, Fraser K, et al. Urgent endovascular treatment of acute symptomatic occlusion of the cervical internal carotid artery. J Neurosurg 2003; 99(6):972–977.
48. Nedeltchev K, Brekenfeld C, Remonda L, et al. Internal carotid artery stent implantation in 25 patients with acute stroke: preliminary results. Radiology 2005; 237(3):1029–1037.
49. Jovin TG, Gupta R, Uchino K, et al. Emergent stenting of extracranial internal carotid artery occlusion in acute stroke has a high revascularization rate. Stroke 2005; 36(11):2426–2430.
50. Imai K, Mori T, Izumoto H, et al. Emergency carotid artery stent placement in patients with acute ischemic stroke. AJNR Am J Neuroradiol 2005; 26(5):1249–1258.
51. Caplan LR, Gorelick PB, Hier DB. Race, sex and occlusive cerebrovascular disease: a review. Stroke 1986; 17(4):648–655.
52. Li H, Wong KS, Li H, et al. Racial distribution of intracranial and extracranial atherosclerosis. J Clin Neurosci 2003; 10(1):30–34.
53. The EC/IC Bypass Study Group Failure of extracranial-intracranial arterial bypass to reduce the risk of ischemic stroke. Results of an international randomized trial. N Engl J Med 1985; 313(19):1191–1200.
54. Bogousslavsky J, Barnett HJ, Fox AJ, et al. Atherosclerotic disease of the middle cerebral artery. Stroke 1986; 17(6):1112–1120.
55. Connors JJ, III. Intracranial angioplasty. In: Connors JJ III, Wojak JC, eds. Interventional Neuroradiology. Philadelphia:Saunders Co., 1999:500–505.
56. Lee JH, Kwon SU, Suh DC, et al. Percutaneous transluminal angioplasty for symptomatic middle cerebral artery stenosis: long-term follow-up. Cerebrovasc Dis 2003; 15 (1–2):90–97.
57. Marks MP, Marcellus M, Norbash AM, et al. Outcome of angioplasty for atherosclerotic intracranial stenosis. Stroke 1999; 30(5):1065–1069.
58. Mori T, Fukuoka M, Kazita K, et al. Follow-up study after intracranial percutaneous transluminal cerebral balloon angioplasty. AJNR Am J Neuroradiol 1998; 19(8):1525–1533.
59. Kimura T, Yokoi H, Nakagawa Y, et al. Three-year follow-up after implantation of metallic coronary-artery stents. N Engl J Med 1996; 334(9):561–566.
60. Lylyk P, Cohen JE, Ceratto R, et al. Angioplasty and stent placement in intracranial atherosclerotic stenoses and dissections. AJNR Am J Neuroradiol 2002; 23(3):430–436.
61. Al-Mubarak N, Gomez CR, Vitek JJ, et al. Stenting of symptomatic stenosis of the intracranial internal carotid artery. AJNR Am J Neuroradiol 1998; 19(10):1949–1951.
62. Gress DR, Smith WS, Dowd CF, et al. Angioplasty for intracranial symptomatic vertebrobasilar ischemia. Neurosurgery 2002; 51(1):23–27.
63. Kim JK, Ahn JY, Lee BH, et al. Elective stenting for symptomatic middle cerebral artery stenosis presenting as transient ischaemic deficits or stroke attacks: short term arteriographical and clinical outcome. J Neurol Neurosurg Psychiatry 2004; 75(6):847–851.
64. Levy EI, Hanel RA, Bendok BR, et al. Staged stent-assisted angioplasty for symptomatic intracranial vertebrobasilar artery stenosis. J Neurosurg 2002; 97(6):1294–1301.
65. Mori T, Kazita K, Mori K. Cerebral angioplasty and stenting for intracranial vertebral atherosclerotic stenosis. AJNR Am J Neuroradiol 1999; 20(5):787–789.
66. Levy EI, Ecker RD, Horowitz MB, et al. Stent-assisted intracranial recanalization for acute stroke: early results. Neurosurgery 2006; 58(3):458–463.
67. Levy EI, Rinaldi MJ, Howington JU, et al. Should interventional cardiologists treat ischemic strokes? A global perspective. J Invasive Cardiol 2002; 14(11):646–651.
68. Fitzsimmons BF, Becske T, Nelson PK, et al. Rapid stent-supported revascularization in acute ischemic stroke. AJNR Am J Neuroradiol 2006; 27(5):1132–1134.
69. Levy EI, Mehta R, Gupta R, et al. Self-expanding stents for recanalization of acute cerebrovascular occlusions. AJNR Am J Neuroradiol 2007; 28(5):816–822.
70. Wakhloo AK, Gounis MJ. Retrievable closed-cell intracranial stent for foreign body and clot removal. Neurosurgery 2008; 62(4)(in press).

71. Bernard SA, Gray TW, Buist MD, et al. Treatment of comatose survivors of out-of-hospital cardiac arrest with induced hypothermia. N Engl J Med 2002; 346(8):557–563.
72. Holzer M, Müllner M, Sterz F, et al. Efficacy and safety of endovascular cooling after cardiac arrest: cohort study and bayesian approach. Stroke 2006; 37(7):1792–1797.
73. Hypothermia after Cardiac Arrest Study Group. Mild therapeutic hypothermia to improve the neurologic outcome after cardiac arrest. N Engl J Med 2002; 346(8):549–556.
74. Hagerdal M, Harp J, Nilsson L, et al. The effect of induced hypothermia upon oxygen consumption in the rat brain. J Neurochem 1975; 24(2):311–316.
75. Nakashima K, Todd MM. Effects of hypothermia on the rate of excitatory amino acid release after ischemic depolarization. Stroke 1996; 27(5):913–918.
76. Baker CJ, Fiore AJ, Frazzini VI, et al. Intraischemic hypothermia decreases the release of glutamate in the cores of permanent focal cerebral infarcts. Neurosurgery 1995; 36(5): 994–1001.
77. Colbourne F, Sutherland G, Corbett D. Postischemic hypothermia. A critical appraisal with implications for clinical treatment. Mol Neurobiol 1997; 14(3):171–201.
78. Dietrich WD, Busto R, Globus MY, et al. Brain damage and temperature: cellular and molecular mechanisms. Adv Neurol 1996; 71:177–194.
79. Schwab S, Schwarz S, Spranger M, et al. Moderate hypothermia in the treatment of patients with severe middle cerebral artery infarction. Stroke 1998; 29(12):2461–2466.
80. Maier CM, Ahern K, Cheng ML, et al. Optimal depth and duration of mild hypothermia in a focal model of transient cerebral ischemia: effects on neurologic outcome, infarct size, apoptosis, and inflammation. Stroke 1998; 29(10):2171–2180.
81. Lyden PD, Krieger D, Yenari M, et al. Therapeutic hypothermia for acute stroke. Int J Stroke 2006; 1(1):9–19.
82. Krieger DW, De Georgia MA, Abou-Chebl A, et al. Cooling for acute ischemic brain damage (COOL AID): an open pilot study of induced hypothermia in acute ischemic stroke. Stroke 2001; 32(8):1847–1854.
83. De Georgia MA, Krieger DW, Abou-Chebl A, et al. Cooling for acute ischemic brain damage (COOL AID): a feasibility trial of endovascular cooling. Neurology 2004; 63(2):312–317.
84. Welsh FA, Sims RE, Harris VA. Mild hypothermia prevents ischemic injury in gerbil hippocampus. J Cereb Blood Flow Metab 1990; 10(4):557–563.
85. Dietrich WD, Busto R, Alonso O, et al. Intraischemic but not postischemic brain hypothermia protects chronically following global forebrain ischemia in rats. J Cereb Blood Flow Metab 1993; 13(4):541–549.
86. Yanamoto H, Nagata I, Niitsu Y, et al. Prolonged mild hypothermia therapy protects the brain against permanent focal ischemia. Stroke 2001; 32(1):232–239.
87. Doerfler A, Schwab S, Hoffmann TT, et al. Combination of decompressive craniectomy and mild hypothermia ameliorates infarction volume after permanent focal ischemia in rats. Stroke 2001; 32(11):2675–2681.
88. Georgiadis D, Schwarz S, Kollmar R, et al. Endovascular cooling for moderate hypothermia in patients with acute stroke: first results of a novel approach. Stroke 2001; 32(11):2550–2553.
89. Mokhtarani M, Mahgoub AN, Morioka N, et al. Buspirone and meperidine synergistically reduce the shivering threshold. Anesth Analg 2001; 93(5):1233–1239.

8

The Future of Neuroprotection

Kenneth M. Sicard[1] and Marc Fisher[1]

[1]Department of Neurology, University of Massachusetts Medical School, Worcester, Massachusetts, U.S.A.

RATIONALE FOR NEUROPROTECTIVE STRATEGIES

Embolic or in situ thrombotic occlusion of an artery supplying the brain causes focal brain ischemia, which can ultimately lead to irreversible tissue injury and infarction via a complex array of pathogenic mechanisms, termed the "ischemic cascade" (1). Thrombolytic drugs or mechanical devices can reperfuse occluded vessels, improving outcome following acute ischemic stroke (AIS). Intravenous tissue plasminogen activator (t-PA) has regulatory approval for AIS treatment within 3 h of symptom onset and, more recently, the MERCI clot retriever has been approved for removal of intracranial thrombi in AIS treatment (see Part 2, Chapter 7) (2,3). However, only 3% of AIS patients receive specific therapy (4). This percentage can be increased by extending the 3-h time window for thrombolysis and/or administering neuroprotective pharmacological agents. Neuroprotection, another therapeutic approach for acute ischemic stroke, attempts to impede the cellular mechanisms that lead to irreversible ischemic tissue injury. However, this approach has not been successful in clinical trials for several reasons (5).

The neuroprotection hypothesis posits that ischemic brain tissue can be prevented from evolving into infarction by the delivery of drugs that intervene on key aspects of the ischemic cascade (1). Neuroprotective drugs can be delivered into the target ischemic but not the irreversibly injured tissue because such tissue has residual blood flow and a reasonably prolonged time window for potential tissue salvage, which is likely directly linked to the severity of reduction in blood flow (2). In experimental stroke models and stroke patients, it has been observed that residual cerebral blood flow levels vary in the ischemic zone and that progression to irreversible injury is slowest in that part of the ischemic zone with the least severe reduction in blood flow. These observations support the potential utility of neuroprotective drugs as monotherapy for acute ischemic stroke. The combination of neuroprotection and reperfusion therapy may synergistically maximize ischemic tissue salvage (3). The concept of neuroprotection monotherapy is supported by numerous animal studies of a wide variety of neuroprotective drugs that have shown significant amounts of ischemic tissue salvage in permanent occlusion stroke models with delayed initiation of therapy (6). What types of neuroprotective drugs are likely to be most effective and when will they be maximally effective during the evolution of focal ischemic brain injury remain largely unknown. The ischemic cascade has multiple pathways and different facets are likely to be activated depending on factors such as the duration of ischemia, location of ischemia, severity of blood flow reduction, the general metabolic environment, and brain temperature (6). Drugs with multiple mechanisms of action and/or which target a final common pathway of tissue injury are most likely to be efficacious.

THE HISTORY OF NEUROPROTECTION: A LACK OF POSITIVE RESULTS
Inadequate Preclinical Testing
A large number of neuroprotective drugs have demonstrated effectiveness in preclinical models but failed to achieve positive results when brought forward into clinical development (7). Despite encouraging preclinical data, none of these neuroprotective agents improved outcome on the prespecified primary endpoint measures in clinical trials. Most of these drugs were tested because they interfere with one or more of the pathogenic pathways of the ischemic cascade (e.g., glutamate excitotoxicity, calcium overload, oxidative stress, and inflammation) while other agents enhance pro-survival pathways or recovery pathways such as those mediated by growth factors. The major problems accounting for the failure of prior clinical trials can be attributed to (a) inadequate preclinical testing, (b) inadequate clinical testing, and (c) narrow therapeutic index.

One important reason for the widespread failure of some neuroprotective drugs in acute ischemic stroke trials was the inadequacy of preclinical evaluation, related to the lack of widely accepted standards for neuroprotective studies in acute stroke. For example, there is only one published report on the anti-inflammatory agent, LeukArrest (Hu23F2G), in a transient middle cerebral artery occlusion (MCAO) stroke model in the rabbit. LeukArrest was administered to rabbits 20 min after ischemia and the animals were observed for 8 h post-ischemia before infarct volumes were determined (3). It was unknown whether this agent provided benefit over a longer period, whether it reduces the severity of neurological deficits, what its effects are in a permanent ischemia model, in other animal species, or in older animals. Similarly, the glutamate receptor antagonist, Gavestinel, was shown to reduce infarct volumes at 24 h post-ischemia in a permanent MCAO stroke model in the rat when administered up to 6 h after onset of MCAO. However, no data were reported on long-term neurological outcome in older animals, or in a second species (7). In addition to incomplete study designs, it is likely that some animal studies with negative results were not published, producing a publication bias, which may explain why some clinical neuroprotection trials were negative.

Inadequate Clinical Testing
In animal studies, neuroprotective agents have typically been administered before or shortly after ischemia. Likewise, preclinical studies suggest a narrow therapeutic time window for most pharmacologic neuroprotective interventions to prevent infarction (8). However, the typical upper time limit for enrollment in prior phase III clinical trials was 6–8 h or longer after the onset of stroke. For example, almost 30 clinical studies of the calcium antagonist, nimodipine, enrolled patients with time windows ranging 6–48 h after stroke, despite the fact that data from preclinical studies suggested that intracellular calcium overload likely plays a maximum pathophysiological role within minutes of ischemia. It is not surprising then that preclinical studies, which administered nimodipine before or immediately after ischemia, showed this agent to be neuroprotective whereas clinical trials did not. The same argument can be made for the antiglutaminergic agents that are likely to intervene at early sites in the ischemic

cascade. In essence, the time window for most prior clinical studies on neuroprotective agents does not reflect those used in animal studies and, in fact, some clinical studies included extended time windows from 12 to 48 h (9–11).

In addition to time window considerations, insufficient preclinical data were collected on drug pharmacokinetics. Some drug development programs failed to demonstrate that their drugs crossed the blood–brain barrier at therapeutic concentrations in animals or humans. Other trials did not establish dose–response curves, with most drugs advancing to phase III trials with minimal data on effective plasma levels and the minimal dose needed to achieve a 95% maximal effect. In several instances, there was a marked difference between the doses used in clinical trials versus the doses used in animals. Consequently, the chosen doses in trials may not have been sufficient to achieve the plasma and central nervous system levels needed to adequately salvage ischemic tissue.

Several other clinical study design issues may have contributed to a lack of positive results. First, prior phase III trials studied a heterogenous population of stroke patients (9,12,13). For example, some enrolled patients with mild and severe deficits, patients with mild deficits, are more likely to recover spontaneously and those with severe deficits are unlikely to achieve good recovery with or without treatment, making it difficult to access the effects of drug treatment. Second, most prior investigations included patients with different stroke subtypes, including lacunar and subcortical white matter infarcts which may not respond to neuroprotective agents that target gray matter injury (5). In fact, no prior neuroprotection clinical trials studied a homogenous population of stroke patients as was done in the Prolyse in Acute Cerebral Thromboembolism II (PROACT-II) trial of intra-arterial ProUrokinase (14), which included patients with angiographically determined MCAOs.

Narrow Therapeutic Index

Certain neuroprotective agents caused side effects in humans, which limited achieving drug concentrations shown as therapeutic in preclinical animal studies. For example, the N-methyl D-aspartate (NMDA) antagonist, Selfotel, was protective in animals at a plasma level of 40 µg/ml but the highest tolerated level in stroke patients was only half of this target level (21 µg/ml), which caused significant neurological and psychiatric side effects (15,16).

FORMATION OF STAIR CRITERIA

The variability of preclinical and clinical evaluation paradigms and lack of clinical success of neuroprotective drugs led to the organization of the first Stroke Therapy Academic Industry Roundtable (STAIR) meeting in 1999 and the subsequent publication of recommendations for the preclinical evaluation of purported neuroprotective drugs (6,17–20).

The primary recommendations for preclinical development of neuroprotective drugs for acute ischemic stroke are overviewed in Table 1. The most important aspects of the STAIR recommendations are using appropriate animal stroke models that allow for assessment of drug treatment effects with an extended time window of efficacy in relationship to the period of penumbral survival; adequate quality control of preclinical experiments, evaluating both histological (infarct volume) and behavioral outcome measures over an extended time period; and robustness

TABLE 1 STAIR Recommendations Ecommendations for Preclinical Reclinical Stroke Drug Development

1. Evaluate the candidate drug in permanent and temporary occlusion models and in both rodent and gyrencephalic species.
2. Evaluate an adequate dose–response effect over a reasonable time window.
3. Appropriate physiological monitoring and blinding should be performed.
4. Histological and functional outcome measures should be assessed with prolonged survival to ensure that early treatment effects are not lost.
5. If feasible, treatment effects should be confirmed in both sexes and aged animals.
6. Treatment effects should be replicated in several laboratories, including both industry and academic locations.
7. Data, both positive and negative, should be published.

of treatment effects in multiple stroke models and laboratories. Dose–response and toxicology evaluations are also critical. These STAIR preclinical recommendations were widely heeded and now are accepted as a reasonable template for evaluation prior to initiation of clinical development.

THE HOPE PROVIDED BY THE SAINT-I TRIAL AND THE DISAPPOINTMENT OF SAINT-II

Although not optimal, the preclinical studies of NXY-059 (Cerovive) were comprehensive and attempted to follow the STAIR recommendations. NXY-059 was shown to reduce infarct volume in rats subjected to 2 h of MCAO when given within 3 h of reperfusion but not at 6 h (21). In a study of the dose–response and time window in a permanent model of MCAO in the rat, treatment initiated within 4 h significantly reduced infarct volume (22). Later studies using a permanent occlusion model in primates showed improved neurological deficits when the drug was started within 4 h of the onset of ischemia (23). At neuroprotective doses in animals, NXY-059 was found to be safe and tolerable in stroke patients (24).

The clinical trials of NXY-059 also followed many STAIR recommendations for clinical drug development programs for stroke therapy, including treatment duration, dose range and route of administration, time from onset of stroke to initiation of treatment, pharmacokinetic and side effect profiles, among others (17,25). Dose selection, dosing paradigm, and time windows for treatment were based on preclinical and early-phase human trials. Patients were enrolled up to 6 h after stroke onset but sites were mandated to maintain an average enrollment time of 4 h to avoid entering too many patients late in the enrollment window. A minimum National Institutes of Health Stroke Scale (NIHSS) score of 6 and limb weakness were required and the modified Rankin Scale (mRS) at 90 days was the primary outcome measure. However, instead of dichotomizing this scale, as was done in all prior clinical neuroprotection studies, effects of treatment across the entire range of the scale were evaluated (25). The result of shifting the mRS is to more likely capture the effect of treatment than a dichotomized "cure" approach previously used and seems a more appropriate approach for drugs that aim to *reduce* and not *reverse* the ischemic lesion volume. To date, the first Stroke-Acute-Ischemic NXY-Treatment (SAINT-I) trial is the first to achieve a statistically significant treatment effect on a prespecified primary outcome measure. Unfortunately, the SAINT-II trial did not reproduce these findings and NXY-059 was withdrawn from further development (25).

THE FUTURE OF NEUROPROTECTION: NEW RECOMMENDATIONS FOR CLINICAL TRIAL DESIGN

The failure of the SAINT-II trial to replicate the positive results of SAINT I raises a number of questions about the future of neuroprotection trials and casts doubt on the viability of the neuroprotection hypothesis (25). A gap remains between pre-clinical and clinical studies of neuroprotective drugs in acute stroke. To bridge this gap, new suggestions for the design of future animal and clinical neuroprotection development programs should be considered.

Change to a Biologically Relevant Endpoint

A reevaluation of the endpoint of acute stroke therapy is necessary. Preclinical studies focus on reduction of infarct volume, whereas phase III clinical studies use disability as the primary outcome measure and experts have raised concern over this disconnect (8). One approach to this problem would be to incorporate behavioral outcomes into animal modeling to evaluate the efficacy of neuroprotective drugs, but it is not known what relevance behavioral studies in rodents have to the commonly used outcome scales in clinical studies. A better translational approach would be to study whether these drugs salvage the ischemic penumbra in both preclinical and clinical studies. Diffusion-weighted (DWI) and perfusion-weighted (PWI) magnetic resonance imaging (MRI) provides an approximation of the penumbra, the target of acute neuroprotective therapy, with the "diffusion–perfusion mismatch" defined as the area of hypoperfusion on PWI that remains normal on DWI. Recent animal studies demonstrate that DWI/PWI imaging can be used to demonstrate that neuroprotective agents salvage ischemic penumbra and that protecting the penumbra reduces infarct volume (26,27). Several clinical studies support the usefulness of the MRI-based mismatch concept for patient selection and suggest that acute stroke therapies should target the penumbra to improve treatment effects, as a decrease in infarct volume is predictive of significant clinical improvement (12,27–30). We thus suggest that DWI and PWI MRI assume a greater role in the design of preclinical and clinical stroke neuroprotection studies.

Select Patients Who Match Animal Models

The SAINT trials, like most prior clinical neuroprotection studies, included a heterogeneous population of stroke patients and imaging was not performed either to confirm the presence of an ischemic penumbra or to determine the size and location of the infarct. Thus, it is unknown whether patients had small versus large vessel stroke, whether the stroke was in the anterior or posterior circulation, or whether patients had infarcts involving the cortex, white matter, or deep gray matter.

Conversely, all established animal models testing neuroprotective drugs are based on MCAO, which affects the cortex and striatum. Moreover, most neuroprotective drugs have little effect on white matter and are likely to maximally protect gray matter such as cortex (5). Future clinical trials should therefore focus on selecting patients with MCA infarcts and exclude small vessel and posterior circulation strokes. Diffusion-weighted MRI or perfusion computed tomography (CT) will be useful in future trials as they can identify the location of ischemia and characterize regions that represent the penumbra (31).

The above discussion notwithstanding, it is important to consider two important facts regarding lacunar (small vessel) stroke. First, they comprise a quarter of all strokes and are not benign (32). Second, the causes, mechanisms, and location of small vessel stroke differ substantially from large vessel ischemic stroke (32). In light of these facts, it is reasonable to enroll patients with acute lacunar stroke in separate clinical trials examining the effectiveness of agents proven to be therapeutic in relevant animal models of focal, acute white matter injury. Such experimental models already exist and include a rodent photoembolic stroke model that is directly analogous to human acute ischemic optic neuropathy caused by sudden loss of vascular supply to retinal ganglion axons of the optic nerve (33,34). Use of such animal models may represent a valuable source of information on the pathogenesis and pathophysiology of human vascular white matter disease and should be used for the preclinical development of neuroprotective agents that can then be tested clinically.

Evaluate Drugs That Work on Multiple Ischemic Pathways

Given the failure of many previously evaluated neuroprotective drugs that targeted a single aspect of the complex ischemic cascade, agents with multiple effects on the ischemic cascade should be considered as they are more likely to have positive effects. This multimodal approach can be achieved with combinations of drugs each acting on a single pathway, or with a single agent with multiple effects such as hypothermia, caffeinol, and hypoxia-inducible factor activators (35–37). The single agent approach is preferable to avoid drug interactions and to simplify regulatory approval.

Evaluate Neuroprotection Separately from Reperfusion

Initial clinical trials of neuroprotectants should not include patients who have received thrombolytic therapy, such as with intravenous t-PA. This is probably necessary to avoid difficulties with the interpretation of trial endpoints, be they imaging-based or a clinical endpoint such as change in deficit. The use of t-PA can have a ceiling effect on the outcome measure and make it difficult to observe any benefit from the neuroprotective drug. After a neuroprotective agent has demonstrated efficacy by itself, then further trials can be carried out to determine synergistic or harmful effects when it is combined with thrombolysis.

CONCLUSION

In the past, the concept of neuroprotection for acute ischemic stroke was widely explored but was without success for a variety of reasons. The mistakes of the past should not be repeated or success will remain elusive. Careful linking of preclinical and clinical trials is needed and trial participants must be properly selected. Improving trial design and outcome assessments as well as studying agents with multiple effects on the ischemic cascade will improve the probability of developing an efficacious neuroprotective agent for acute ischemic stroke.

REFERENCES

1. Fisher M. The ischemic penumbra: identification, evolution and treatment concepts. Cerebrovasc Dis 2004; 17(Suppl 1):1–6.
2. Fisher M, Ratan R. New perspectives on developing acute stroke therapy. Ann Neurol 2003; 53(1):10–20.

3. Cheng YD, Al-Khoury L, Zivin JA. Neuroprotection for ischemic stroke: two decades of success and failure. NeuroRx 2004; 1(1):36–45.
4. Heuschmann PU, Kolominsky-Rabas PL, Roether J, et al. Predictors of in-hospital mortality in patients with acute ischemic stroke treated with thrombolytic therapy. JAMA 2004; 292(15):1831–1838.
5. Gladstone DJ, Black SE, Hakim AM. Toward wisdom from failure: lessons from neuro-protective stroke trials and new therapeutic directions. Stroke 2002; 33(8):2123–2136.
6. Recommendations for standards regarding preclinical neuroprotective and restorative drug development. Stroke 1999; 30(12):2752–2758.
7. Bordi F, Pietra C, Ziviani L, et al. The glycine antagonist GV150526 protects somatosen-sory evoked potentials and reduces the infarct area in the MCAo model of focal ischemia in the rat. Exp Neurol 1997; 145(2 Pt 1):425–433.
8. Grotta JC. Acute stroke therapy at the millennium: consummating the marriage between the laboratory and bedside. The Feinberg lecture. Stroke 1999; 30(8):1722–1728.
9. Clark WM, Wechsler LR, Sabounjian LA, et al. A phase III randomized efficacy trial of 2000 mg citicoline in acute ischemic stroke patients. Neurology 2001; 57(9):1595–1602.
10. Wahlgren NG, Ranasinha KW, Rosolacci T, et al. Clomethiazole acute stroke study (CLASS): results of a randomized, controlled trial of clomethiazole versus placebo in 1360 acute stroke patients. Stroke 1999; 30(1):21–28.
11. Yamaguchi T, Sano K, Takakura K, et al. Ebselen in acute ischemic stroke: a placebo-controlled, double-blind clinical trial. Ebselen Study Group. Stroke 1998; 29(1):12–17.
12. Albers GW, Thijs VN, Wechsler L, et al. Magnetic resonance imaging profiles predict clinical response to early reperfusion: the diffusion and perfusion imaging evaluation for understanding stroke evolution (DEFUSE) study. Ann Neurol 2006; 60(5):508–517.
13. Lyden P, Shuaib A, Ng K, et al. Clomethiazole acute stroke study in ischemic stroke (CLASS-I): final results. Stroke 2002; 33(1):122–128.
14. Furlan A, Higashida R, Wechsler L, et al. Intra-arterial prourokinase for acute ischemic stroke. The PROACT II study: a randomized controlled trial. Prolyse in Acute Cerebral Thromboembolism. JAMA 1999; 282(21):2003–2011.
15. Labiche LA, Grotta JC. Clinical trials for cytoprotection in stroke. NeuroRx 2004; 1(1):46–70.
16. Davis SM, Lees KR, Albers GW, et al. Selfotel in acute ischemic stroke: possible neuro-toxic effects of an NMDA antagonist. Stroke 2000; 31(2):347–354.
17. Recommendations for clinical trial evaluation of acute stroke therapies. Stroke 2001; 32(7):1598–1606.
18. Fisher M. Stroke Therapy Academic Industry Roundtable. Recommendations for advancing development of acute stroke therapies: Stroke Therapy Academic Industry Roundtable 3. Stroke 2003; 34(6):1539–1546.
19. Fisher M, Albers GW, Donnan GA, et al. Stroke Therapy Academic Industry Roundtable. Enhancing the Development and Approval of Acute Stroke Therapies: Stroke Therapy Academic Industry Roundtable IV.. Stroke 2005; 36(8):1808–1813.
20. Fisher M, Hanley DF, Howard G, et al. Recommendations from the STAIR V meeting on acute stroke trials, technology and outcomes. Stroke 2007; 38(2):245–248.
21. Kuroda S, Tsuchidate R, Smith ML, et al. Neuroprotective effects of a novel nitrone, NXY-059, after transient focal cerebral ischemia in the rat. J Cereb Blood Flow Metab 1999; 19(7):778–787.
22. Sydserff SG, Borelli AR, Green AR, et al. Effect of NXY-059 on infarct volume after transient or permanent middle cerebral artery occlusion in the rat; studies done on dose, plasma concentration and therapeutic time window. Br J Pharmacol 2002; 135(1):103–112.
23. Marshall JW, Cummings RM, Bowes LJ, et al. Functional and histological evidence for the protective effect of NXY-059 in a primate model of stroke when given 4 hours after occlusion. Stroke 2003; 34(9):2228–2233.
24. Lees KR, Sharma AK, Barer D, et al. Tolerability and pharmacokinetics of the nitrone NXY-059 in patients with acute stroke. Stroke 2001; 32(3):675–680.
25. Lees KR, Zivin JA, Ashwood T, et al. NXY-059 for acute ischemic stroke. N Engl J Med 2006; 354(6):588–600.

26. Ebisu T, Mori Y, Katsuta K, et al. Neuroprotective effects of an immunosuppressant agent on diffusion/perfusion mismatch in transient focal ischemia. Magn Reson Med 2004; 51(6):1173–1180.

27. Warach S, Pettigrew LC, Dashe JF, et al. Effect of citicoline on ischemic lesions as measured by diffusion-weighted magnetic resonance imaging. Citicoline 010 investigators. Ann Neurol 2000; 48(5):713–722.

28. Hacke W, Albers G, Al-Rawi Y, et al. The Desmoteplase in Acute Ischemic Stroke Trial (DIAS): a phase II MRI-based 9-hour window acute stroke thrombolysis trial with intravenous desmoteplase. Stroke 2005; 36(1):66–73.

29. Furlan AJ, Eyding D, Albers GW, et al. Dose Escalation of Desmoteplase for Acute Ischemic Stroke (DEDAS): evidence of safety and efficacy 3 to 9 hours after stroke onset. Stroke 2006; 37(5):1227–1231.

30. Warach S, Kaufman D, Chiu D, et al. Effect of the Glycine Antagonist Gavestinel on cerebral infarcts in acute stroke patients, a randomized placebo-controlled trial: the GAIN MRI substudy. Cerebrovasc Dis 2006; 21(1–2):106–111.

31. Wintermark M, Reichhart M, Thiren JP, et al. Prognostic accuracy of cerebral blood flow measurement by perfusion computerized tomography, at the time of emergency room admission, in acute stroke patients. Ann Neurol 2002; 51(4):417–432.

32. Wardlaw JM. What causes lacunar stroke? J Neurol Neurosurg Psychiatry 2005; 76(5):617–619.

33. Danylkova NO, Alcala SR, Pomeranz HD, et al. Neuroprotective effects of brimodidine treatment in a rodent model of ischemic optic neuropathy. Exp Eye Res 2007; 84(2):293–301.

34. Bernstein SL, Guo Y, Kelman SE, et al. Functional and cellular responses in a novel rodent model of anterior ischemic optic neuropathy. Invest Opthalmol Vis Sci 2003; 44(10):4153–4162.

35. De Georgia MA, Krieger DW, Abou-Chebl A, et al. Cooling for acute ischemic brain damage (COOL AID): a feasibility trial of endovascular cooling. Neurology 2004; 63(2):312–317.

36. Aronowski J, Strong R, Shirzadi A, et al. Ethanol plus caffeine (caffeinol) for treatment of ischemic stroke: preclinical experience. Stroke 2003; 34(5):1246–1251.

37. Ratan RR, Siddiq A, Aminova L, et al. Translation of ischemic preconditioning to the patient: prolyl hydroxylase inhibition and hypoxia inducible factor-1 as novel targets for stroke therapy. Stroke 2004; 35(11 Suppl 1):2687–2689.

9

Acute Ischemic Stroke: Paradigm for Treatment

Italo Linfante[1] and Ajay K. Wakhloo[2]

[1]Division of Neuroimaging and Intervention, Department of Radiology,
University of Massachusetts Medical School, Worcester, Massachusetts, U.S.A.

[2]Department of Radiology, Neurology and Neurosurgery,
University of Massachusetts Medical School, Worcester, Massachusetts, U.S.A.

INTRODUCTION

Stroke is the third cause of death and leading cause of disability in the United States and Europe. According to data from the American Stroke Association, each year about 700,000 individuals experience a new or recurrent stroke; 160,000 of these events are fatal. In terms of care and disability, it is estimated that the annual cost of stroke totals approximately $56.8 billion (1)[1].

The development of several treatment options for acute stroke has changed the historical perception that stroke was untreatable into the realization that stroke is a medical emergency with potential treatments. The time-sensitive window of opportunity for the treatment of stroke is due to the characteristics of the ischemic penumbra. Neuronal electrical function is lost in the ischemic penumbra when cerebral blood flow (CBF) falls below a critical threshold of approximately 20 ml of blood per 100 g of brain tissue per minute (normal = 50 ml blood per 100 g of brain tissue per minute). At this level, the penumbra is thought to be capable of rescue. Irreversible damage occurs when blood flow falls below 10 ml of blood per 100 g brain tissue per minute.

The goals for the treatment of acute thromboembolic stroke are to diagnose early, initiate rapid thrombolysis, restore normal CBF, prevent iatrogenic hemorrhagic events, and preserve function. Neurointerventional procedures for acute stroke treatment consist of IA administration of thrombolytics, mechanical thrombectomy, and hypothermic devices.

Over the past decade, multicenter clinical trials performed in acute ischemic stroke patients showed that thrombolytic therapy can improve their clinical outcome. As a result of these trials, the use of intravenous (IV) tissue plasminogen activator (t-PA) for the treatment of acute ischemic stroke within 3 h after symptom onset has been approved in the United States, Canada, Australia, and the European Union. However, IV fibrinolytic therapy is used in less than 2% of patients being admitted for stroke. As in myocardial ischemia, a more aggressive education of the community in recognizing stroke is mandatory to accelerate an early detection, commence a fast treatment, and improve outcome. Nilasena and coworkers (2) from the National Stroke Project of the US Centers for Medicare and Medicaid Service analyzed 14,295 inpatient Medicare medical records from a national sample of patients with acute stroke who were treated between April 1998 and March 1999. Fibrinolytic therapy was employed in only 1.7% of patients. In a study of Cleveland hospitals, only 1.8% of patients received IV t-PA (3). Furthermore, the 5-year recurrence rate

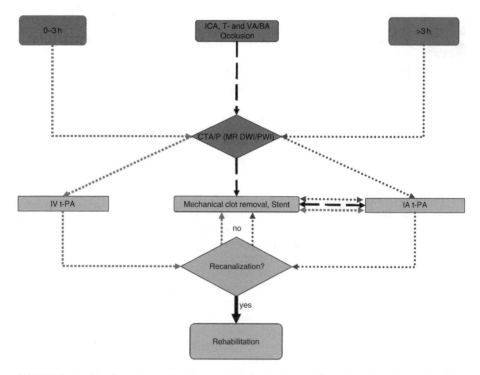

FIGURE 1   Imaging-based paradigm for acute stroke treatment. (See also color plate section.)

for stroke has been reported anywhere from 24% to 42% (4–7). The etiology of the stroke must be addressed to minimize the risk of an additional stroke.

Research in the treatment of acute ischemic stroke is focusing mainly on three aspects: (i) imaging, to improve the selection of patients for treatment and outcome; (ii) revascularization treatment, both IV and intra-arterial (IA); and (iii) neuroprotection. As a result, several multicentric controlled trials in these three fronts are either completed or being performed.

In this chapter, we summarize data on the advancement of imaging and treatment of acute ischemic stroke and on pharmacological and mechanical IA thrombolysis. Both a concise and treatment-focused imaging and fast and early revascularization are the main pillars for a successful outcome. Fig. 1 summarizes the rationale for an IV and/or IA treatment based on imaging.

IMAGING

Several authors have reported that computerized tomography (CT) and magnetic resonance imaging (MRI) can provide important data on the pathophysiology of cerebral ischemia as well as structural and functional information on potentially salvageable tissue (8–14) (see also Part 2, Chapter 5 for details).

Computerized Tomography

In recent years, the use of dynamic CT perfusion (CTP) imaging and CT angiography (CTA) to acquire information on acute stroke has shown remarkable progress (15–17).

For dynamic CTP imaging, 50–100 ml of iodinated contrast material is intravenously injected while continuous scanning is performed over one anatomic location of 5–10 mm thickness, generally the opercular area for approximately 45 s (17). Data are reconstructed at 0.5- to 1.0-s intervals using CTP analysis software commercially available (17). Perfusion maps of CBV and CBF are reconstructed using integration of tissue–time curves (17) (Fig. 2). Dynamic CTP imaging has shown a good correlation with MRI for CBF and mean transit time (MTT) abnormalities in acute stroke (17). CTA has demonstrated to be accurate in the evaluation of cervical and large-vessel intracranial occlusion and may be valuable to help triage acute stroke patients for IA fibrinolysis (15). Lastly, transcranial Doppler (TCD) has shown to be a useful diagnostic tool and may be a therapeutic adjuvant in fibrinolysis (18). CT unlike MRI is readily accessible for imaging of both extracranial and intracranial arteries and is gradually replacing catheter angiography in most centers. Multidetector CT angiography (MDCTA) with its high contrast-resolution allows the differentiation of normal, stenotic or occlusive disease and a characterization of atherosclerotic plaques and can provide sufficient information for the appropriate treatment. CTA can be performed in an emergency setting even in severely ill patients or in patients not suitable for MRI, provided no contraindication for iodinated contrast material exists. Images can be displayed with 3D reformatting software. CTA may allow differentiation between dissection and atherosclerotic occlusive disease by visualizing the intimal flap or atherosclerotic plaque. Although spatial resolution of digital subtraction angiography (DSA) remains superior to CTA, it is an excellent imaging tool in the acute ischemic setting. Due to the adjacent bone density, petrous portion of the carotid artery remains a challenge, albeit development of newer algorithms will overcome this obstacle.

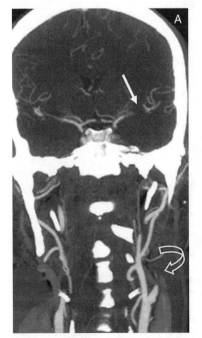

FIGURE 2 A 54-year-old man who develops a sudden onset of right face > arm > leg weakness, dysarthria and mild expressive aphasia. He arrives in the emergency department 2 h and 45 min after symptom onset presenting with fluctuating symptoms. Computer tomography (CT) is negative for intracranial hemorrhage. (*A*) Three-dimensional reformatted CT angiography (CTA) in coronal projection shows an occluded left internal carotid artery (LICA) distal to the ostium (*curved arrow*) and an occluded left middle cerebral artery at the bifurcation (*arrow*). Owing to a recent history of surgery, an IV t-PA treatment is contraindicated.

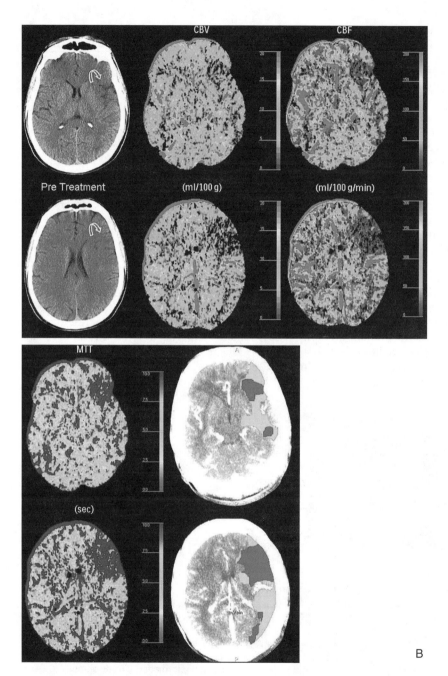

FIGURE 2 (*Continued*) (*B*) CT perfusion maps of cerebral blood flow (CBF), cerebral blood volume (CBV), mean transit time (MTT), and time-to-peak (TTP) after injection of 40 ml of Isovue-370. There is evidence of changes in the CBV images in the left frontal lobe and slightly larger area of increased MTT and TTP in the left frontal lobe as well as parieto-temporal areas. A "mismatch" between CBF and CBV is seen (*right image*). (See also color plate section.)

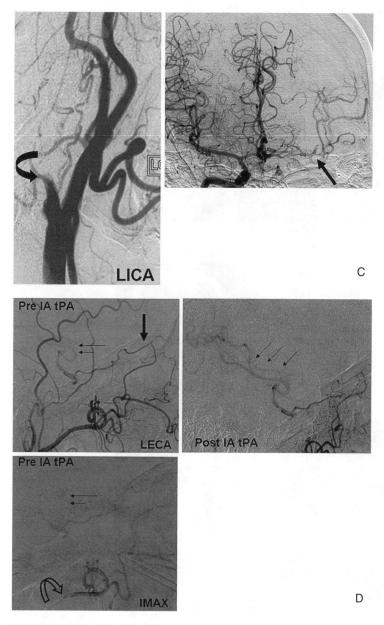

FIGURE 2 (*Continued*) (*C*) Catheter angiography confirms the finding of an occluded LICA (*curved arrow*) and a poor collateralization of the left hemisphere through the right ICA. Because of a clot within the M1/M2 bifurcation, an incomplete filling of the left MCA territory (*arrow*) is seen. (*D*) Injection of left external carotid artery (ECA) in lateral view shows poor filling of left MCA branches (double arrow) through ophthalmic artery anastomosis (arrow). Superselective micro-catheter injection (curved arrow) of the left internal maxillary artery (IMAX) prior to local intra-arterial t-PA infusion. Follow-up IMAX angiogram after 30 mg t-PA infusion shows partial recanalization and improved MCA perfusion.

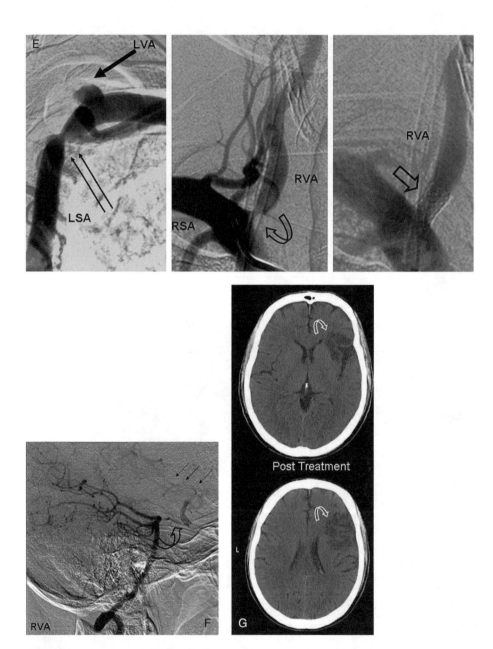

FIGURE 2 (*Continued*) (*E*) The patient has also a poor collateral blood supply through the posterior circulation because of a stenosis of the left subclavian artery (LSA, *double arrow*), an occluded left vertebral artery (LVA), and a high-grade stenosis of the right vertebral artery origin (RVA, *curved arrow*). Acute stenting and improvement of the collateral blood supply (*block arrow*). (*F*) Follow-up angiogram and contrast material injection into the right subclavian artery shows blood supply to the left MCA territory (*small arrows*) through the posterior communicating artery (*curved arrow*). (*G*) Follow-up CT 24 h after admission shows an ischemic area within the insula and operculum (*curved arrow*) corresponding to changes seen on the initial CBF map. (See also color plate section.)

Magnetic Resonance Imaging

Diffusion (DWI)-, perfusion (PWI)-, and T2*-weighted imaging play a major role in the evaluation of acute stroke patients (9–12). In DWI, the addition of two magnetic field gradients positioned before and after the 180° radio frequency pulse makes a T2-weighted sequence sensitive to the Brownian motion of the molecules of water (19). An Echo Planar readout sequence allows the acquisition of the entire DWI data set in a matter of seconds (10,20). The b-factor permits the transformation of the DW images into a map where each pixel represents a measurement of the Apparent Diffusion Coefficient (ADC) of water (19). In acute stroke imaging, DWI and the ADC map are the most sensitive, the earliest detectors of ischemia, and can differentiate between various degrees of cerebral ischemia (9,11,12). In PWI, a bolus of Gadolinium is administered IV during the acquisition of a T2*-weighted sequence. Changes in signal intensity over time can provide data on tissue perfusion. Indices of CBF and cerebral blood volume (CBV) can be derived. The combination of DWI and PWI sequences (Fig. 3) has demonstrated that tissue viability can be assessed on acute stroke patients in the time window for thrombolysis (9,11,12). Therefore, treatment decisions can be made on the actual state of ischemic tissue rather than on rigid time intervals.

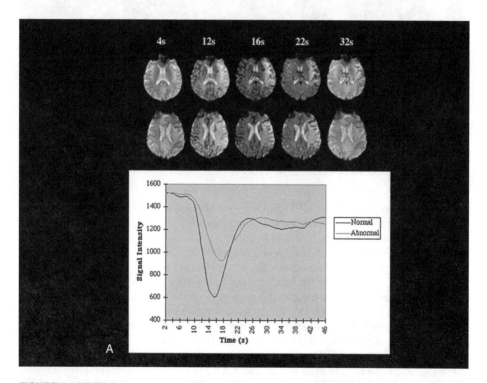

FIGURE 3 (*A*) Perfusion-weighted MR imaging (PWI) in a patient with left middle cerebral artery (MCA) occlusion. Gadolinium (Gd)-based contrast agent has been injected intravenously and causes signal loss in an echo-planar MR sequence. Areas that are well perfused appear dark while ischemic territory does not change signal characteristics. Changes in signal intensity over time can be quantified to derive indices of blood volume and blood flow (Courtesy of Dr. G. Schlaug, Beth Israel Deaconess Medical Center and Harvard Medical School, Boston, MA).

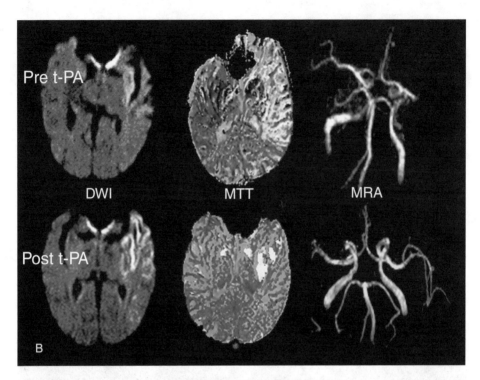

FIGURE 3 (*Continued*) (*B*) Diffusion-weighted MR imaging (DWI), mean transit time (MTT) and 3D time-of-flight (TOF) MR angiography (MRA) before (*upper row*) and after intravenous (IV) infusion of t-PA (*lower row*) with successful recanalization of the left occluded MCA. The final infarcted area corresponds to territory presenting initially with DWI changes but is smaller than the territory presenting with MTT changes prior to treatment. The difference between DWI and MTT changes indicate the brain tissue, which is salvageable if reperfusion is achieved. Reproduced with permission from Ref. (33).

It has been argued that MRI cannot detect acute intracranial hemorrhage (ICH); therefore, MRI cannot be used as the sole imaging modality before thrombolysis. However, MRI is intrinsically able to detect hyperacute ICH. Such capability is based on the magnetic susceptibility effect of deoxyhemoglobin. In ICH, hemoglobin leaks into an environment with a low O_2 concentration, low pH, and high CO_2. Because of the Bohr Effect, such changes promote the formation of deoxyhemoglobin that extends from the periphery of the hematoma toward the center. Deoxyhemoglobin has four unpaired electrons and is paramagnetic ($x > 0$). As such, it produces magnetic inhomogeneities that result in local T2* relaxation enhancement (21). The MR contrast of deoxyhemoglobin is highly dependent on the mode of imaging acquisition. For instance, deoxyhemoglobin-induced signal loss (darkening) is most pronounced in sequences that are T2*-weighted, such as conventional gradient echo (GE) as well as both spin-echo and GE echo-planar sequences. Two well-controlled clinical trials recently proved that MRI is as sensitive as or perhaps more sensitive than CT to detect acute ICH (22,23).

Magnetic Resonance Angiography (MRA) allows examination of the intracranial and extracranial vasculature noninvasively and without the need for iodinated contrast agents or ionizing radiation. Information can be acquired on blood flow and flow velocity, as well as on blood volume if phase-contrast (PC) angiography

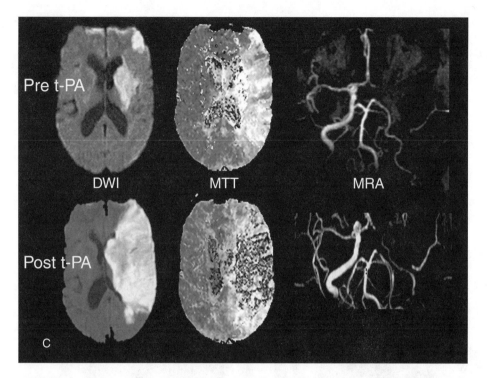

FIGURE 3 (*Continued*) (*C*) Unsuccessful IV t-PA treatment in another patient with a left MCA occlusion. Initial DWI changes are small while the tissue at risk for infarction, but potentially salvageable, is demarcated by the more extensive MTT changes. Follow-up studies show DWI and MTT changes of the entire left MCA territory corresponding to a massive infarction of the dominant hemisphere. Reproduced with permission from Ref. (33).

techniques are used. The most commonly used techniques are time-of-flight (TOF) and contrast-enhanced (CE)-MRA. MRA, however, is sensitivity to motion, susceptibility and pulsatility artifacts, signal loss to slow, oscillating flow, disturbed and turbulent flow. CE-MRA uses gadolinium as a contrast agent which is injected intravenously to further shorten the T1 relaxation in flowing blood. In some centers, this method has replaced all existing imaging modalities for carotid artery examination. However, the technique is limited due to a venous contamination which reduces the signal clarity. In addition, more recent reports have described in more than 200 patients, who were exposed to gadolinium containing contrast agents, a nephrogenic systemic fibrosis (NSF) with renal insufficiency (24). A combination of impaired renal function or concurrent inflammatory condition and exposure to gadolinium-based contrast agent may be involved in triggering a nephrogenic systemic fibrosis (25). Thus, a CTA may be considered in selected patients. Furthermore, anatomical details on MRA are poorer when compared with images obtained from a catheter angiography, especially, when the information on collateral blood circulation is of importance.

Catheter Angiography
DSA still offers the highest sensitivity for investigating cerebrovascular disease in the chronic and acute setting. Angiography also helps the planning of an endovascular

approach and device selection. The femoral artery is the most common site of arterial access for cerebral diagnostic angiography and intervention, but other alternatives are radial, brachial, or direct carotid approaches. One of the most important advantages of the angiography is the ability to evaluate the entire cerebrovascular arterial and venous systems. Capillary blush gives information on brain perfusion prior to and following an intervention. Flat panel detectors have replaced image intensifiers and provide high-resolution angiograms including soft tissue images of the surrounding structures and the brain (cone beam reconstruction). Improvement of angiography equipment, catheter technology, and introduction of iso-osmolar nonionic contrast materials have all helped minimize complications of diagnostic neuroangiography that should not exceed 0.5% (26). But, as recently demonstrated on DWI/MRI, silent ischemic changes resulting from microemboli are seen in 1.7%

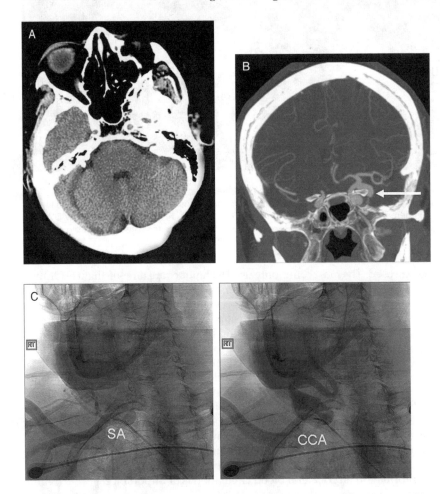

FIGURE 4 (A) Axial CT scan of the posterior fossa without contrast in a 79-year-old female presenting with left-sided throbbing headaches. (B) CT angiography shows a large left posterior communicating artery aneurysm (*arrow*). (C) Catheter angiography of the right subclavian and common carotid artery shows an extreme tortuous and diseased vascular system. The entire aortic arch is extensively calcified (not shown).

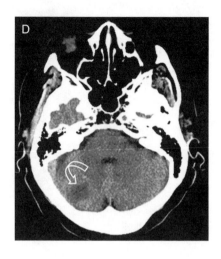

FIGURE 4 (*Continued*) (*D*) Follow-up CT in preparation for the aneurysm treatment and several days after the angiogram shows a small asymptomatic right superior cerebellar artery stroke (*curved arrow*) most likely due to a clinically silent thromboembolic event during catheter angiography.

of cases and in almost 22.9% of patients with risk factors such as atherosclerotic disease, vasculitis and hypercoagulable states (Fig. 4) (27).

TREATMENT

Several controlled and noncontrolled clinical trials showed that the early reperfusion of acute cerebral ischemia leads to better neurological outcomes (Table 1). Historically, the background data to support this concept arose from the National Institute of Neurological Disorders and Stroke (NINDS) t-PA stroke trial (28).

NINDS (National Institute of Neurological Disorders and Stroke) t-PA Stroke Trial

The NINDS t-PA trial was a randomized, multicenter, placebo-control study in which a dose of 0.9 mg/kg of t-PA was tested versus placebo in acute stroke patients presenting within 3 h after symptom onset. The study was composed of two parts. In part 2 (333 patients enrolled), clinical outcome was assessed at 3 months by using four clinical scales (Table 2): Barthel Index, modified Rankin Scale (mRS), the

TABLE 1 Clinical Acute Stroke Trials

	NINDS		PROACT II		IMS	IMS II	MERCI
		Controls		Controls			
Patients	168	165	121	59	80	81	141
Time window (h)	0–3	0–3	0–6		0–3	0–3	0–8
Base NIHSS	14	15	17	17	18	19	20
TIMI 2–3(%)			66	18	56	60	46
Sympt ICH (%)	7	1	10	2	6	10	8
mRS 0–1%	39	26	26	7	30	33	
mRS 0–2%			40	25	43	46	23
Death at 3 months %	21	24	25	27	16	16	43

Abbreviations: NINDS=National Institute of Neurological Disorders and Stroke; PROACT=prolyse in acute cerebral thromboembolism; IMS=interventional management of stroke, MERCI=mechanical embolus removal in cerebral ischemia; NIHSS=National Institutes of Health Stroke Scale; TIMI=thrombolysis in myocardial infarction; ICH=intracerebral hemorrhage; mRS=modified Rankin Scale.
Source: Adapted from Refs. (28, 40, 42–44).

TABLE 2 Frequently Used Scales to Assess Neurological Status and Clinical Outcome in Patients with Stroke

A. The National Institute Health Stroke Scale (NIHSS)

Instructions	Scale Definition	Score
1a. Level of Consciousness: The investigator must choose a response if a full evaluation is prevented by such obstacles as an endotracheal tube, language barrier, orotracheal trauma/bandages. A 3 is scored only if the patient makes no movement (other than reflexive posturing) in response to noxious stimulation.	0 = **Alert**; keenly responsive. 1 = **Not alert**; but arousable by minor stimulation to obey, answer, or respond. 2 = **Not alert**; requires repeated stimulation to attend, or is obtunded and requires strong or painful stimulation to make movements (not stereotyped). 3 = Responds only with reflex motor or autonomic effects or totally unresponsive, flaccid, and areflexic.	
1b. LOC Questions: The patient is asked the month and his/her age. The answer must be correct—there is no partial credit for being close. Aphasic and stuporous patients who do not comprehend the questions will score 2. Patients unable to speak because of endotracheal intubation, orotracheal trauma, severe dysarthria from any cause, language barrier, or any other problem not secondary to aphasia are given a 1. It is important that only the initial answer be graded and that the examiner not "help" the patient with verbal or nonverbal cues.	0 = **Answers** both questions correctly. 1 = **Answers** one question correctly. 2 = **Answers** neither question correctly.	
1c. LOC Commands: The patient is asked to open and close the eyes and then to grip and release the nonparetic hand. Substitute another one step command if the hands cannot be used. Credit is given if an unequivocal attempt is made but not completed due to weakness. If the patient does not respond to command, the task should be demonstrated to him or her (pantomime), and the result scored (i.e., follows none, one or two commands). Patients with trauma, amputation, or other physical impediments should be given suitable one-step commands. Only the first attempt is scored.	0 = **Performs** both tasks correctly. 1 = **Performs** one task correctly. 2 = **Performs** neither task correctly.	

TABLE 2 *(Continued)*

Instructions	Scale Definition	Score
2. Best Gaze: Only horizontal eye movements will be tested. Voluntary or reflexive (oculocephalic) eye movements will be scored, but caloric testing is not done. If the patient has a conjugate deviation of the eyes that can be overcome by voluntary or reflexive activity, the score will be 1. If a patient has an isolated peripheral nerve paresis (CN III, IV, or VI), score a 1. Gaze is testable in all aphasic patients. Patients with ocular trauma, bandages, pre-existing blindness, or other disorder of visual acuity or fields should be tested with reflexive movements, and a choice made by the investigator. Establishing eye contact and then moving about the patient from side to side will occasionally clarify the presence of a partial gaze palsy.	0 = **Normal.** 1 = **Partial gaze palsy:** gaze is abnormal in one or both eyes, but forced deviation or total gaze paresis is not present. 2 = **Forced deviation,** or total gaze paresis not overcome by the oculocephalic maneuver.	
3. Visual: Visual fields (upper and lower quadrants) are tested by confrontation, using finger counting or visual threat, as appropriate. Patients may be encouraged, but if they look at the side of the moving fingers appropriately, this can be scored as normal. If there is unilateral blindness or enucleation, visual fields in the remaining eye are scored. Score 1 only if a clear-cut asymmetry, including quadrantanopia, is found. If patient is blind from any cause, score 3. Double simultaneous stimulation is performed at this point. If there is extinction, patient receives a 1, and the results are used to respond to item 11.	0 = **No visual loss.** 1 = **Partial hemianopia.** 2 = **Complete hemianopia.** 3 = **Bilateral hemianopia** (blind including cortical blindness).	
4. Facial Palsy: Ask—or use pantomime to encourage—the patient to show teeth or raise eyebrows and close eyes. Score symmetry of grimace in response to noxious stimuli in the poorly responsive or non-comprehending patient. If facial trauma/bandages, orotracheal tube, tape or other physical barriers obscure the face, these should be removed to the extent possible.	0 = **Normal** symmetrical movements. 1 = **Minor paralysis** (flattened nasolabial fold, asymmetry on smiling). 2 = **Partial paralysis** (total or near-total paralysis of lower face). 3 = **Complete paralysis** of one or both sides (absence of facial movement in the upper and lower face).	

(Continued)

TABLE 2 Frequently Used Scales to Assess Neurological Status and Clinical Outcome in Patients with Stroke (*Continued*)

Instructions	Scale Definition	Score
5. Motor Arm: The limb is placed in the appropriate position: extend the arms (palms down) 90° (if sitting) or 45° (if supine). Drift is scored if the arm falls before 10 s. The aphasic patient is encouraged using urgency in the voice and pantomime, but not noxious stimulation. Each limb is tested in turn, beginning with the nonparetic arm. Only in the case of amputation or joint fusion at the shoulder, the examiner should record the score as untestable (UN), and clearly write the explanation for this choice.	0 = **No drift**; limb holds 90° (or 45°) for full 10 s. 1 = **Drift**; limb holds 90° (or 45°), but drifts down before full 10 s; does not hit bed or other support. 2 = **Some effort against gravity**; limb cannot get to or maintain (if cued) 90° (or 45°), drifts down to bed, but has some effort against gravity. 3 = **No effort against gravity**; limb falls. 4 = **No movement.** UN = **Amputation** or joint fusion, explain: **5a. Left Arm** **5b. Right Arm**	
6. Motor Leg: The limb is placed in the appropriate position: hold the leg at 30° (always tested supine). Drift is scored if the leg falls before 5 s. The aphasic patient is encouraged using urgency in the voice and pantomime, but not noxious stimulation. Each limb is tested in turn, beginning with the nonparetic leg. Only in the case of amputation or joint fusion at the hip, the examiner should record the score as untestable (UN), and clearly write the explanation for this choice.	0 = **No drift**; leg holds 30° position for full 5 s. 1 = **Drift**; leg falls by the end of the 5-s period but does not hit bed. 2 = **Some effort against gravity**; leg falls to bed by 5 s, but has some effort against gravity. 3 = **No effort against gravity**; leg falls to bed immediately. 4 = **No movement.** UN = **Amputation** or joint fusion, explain: **6a. Left Leg** **6b. Right Leg**	
7. Limb Ataxia: This item is aimed at finding evidence of a unilateral cerebellar lesion. Test with eyes open. In case of visual defect, ensure testing is done in intact visual field. The finger-nose-finger and heel-shin tests are performed on both sides, and ataxia is scored only if present out of proportion to weakness. Ataxia is absent in the patient who cannot understand or is paralyzed. Only in the case of amputation or joint fusion, the examiner should record the score as untestable (UN), and clearly write the explanation for this choice. In case of blindness, test by having the patient touch nose from extended arm position.	0 = **Absent.** 1 = **Present in one limb.** 2 = **Present in two limbs.** UN = **Amputation** or joint fusion, explain:	

TABLE 2 (*Continued*)

Instructions	Scale Definition	Score
8. Sensory: Sensation or grimace to pinprick when tested, or withdrawal from noxious stimulus in the obtunded or aphasic patient. Only sensory loss attributed to stroke is scored as abnormal and the examiner should test as many body areas [arms (not hands), legs, trunk, face] as needed to accurately check for hemisensory loss. A score of 2, "severe or total sensory loss," should only be given when a severe or total loss of sensation can be clearly demonstrated. Stuporous and aphasic patients will, therefore, probably score 1 or 0. The patient with brainstem stroke who has bilateral loss of sensation is scored 2. If the patient does not respond and is quadriplegic, score 2. Patients in coma (item 1a=3) are automatically given a 2 on this item.	0 = **Normal;** no sensory loss. 1 = **Mild-to-moderate sensory loss;** patient feels pinprick is less sharp or is dull on the affected side; or there is a loss of superficial pain with pinprick, but patient is aware of being touched. 2 = **Severe to total sensory loss;** patient is not aware of being touched in the face, arm, and leg.	
9. Best Language: A great deal of information about comprehension will be obtained during the preceding sections of the examination. For this scale item, the patient is asked to describe what is happening in the attached picture, to name the items on the attached naming sheet and to read from the attached list of sentences. Comprehension is judged from responses here, as well as to all of the commands in the preceding general neurological exam. If visual loss interferes with the tests, ask the patient to identify objects placed in the hand, repeat, and produce speech. The intubated patient should be asked to write. The patient in a coma (item 1a=3) will automatically score 3 on this item. The examiner must choose a score for the patient with stupor or limited cooperation, but a score of 3 should be used only if the patient is mute and follows no one-step commands.	0 = **No aphasia;** normal. 1 = **Mild-to-moderate aphasia;** some obvious loss of fluency or facility of comprehension, without significant limitation on ideas expressed or form of expression. Reduction of speech and/or comprehension, however, makes conversation about provided materials difficult or impossible. For example, in conversation about provided materials, examiner can identify picture or naming card content from patient's response. 2 = **Severe aphasia;** all communication is through fragmentary expression; great need for inference, questioning, and guessing by the listener. Range of information that can be exchanged is limited; listener carries burden of communication. Examiner cannot identify materials provided from patient response. 3 = **Mute, global aphasia;** no usable speech or auditory comprehension.	

(*Continued*)

TABLE 2 Frequently Used Scales to Assess Neurological Status and Clinical Outcome in Patients with Stroke (*Continued*)

Instructions	Scale Definition	Score
10. Dysarthria: If patient is thought to be normal, an adequate sample of speech must be obtained by asking patient to read or repeat words from the attached list. If the patient has severe aphasia, the clarity of articulation of spontaneous speech can be rated. Only if the patient is intubated or has other physical barriers to producing speech, the examiner should record the score as untestable (UN) and clearly write an explanation for this choice. Do not tell the patient why he or she is being tested.	0 = **Normal.** 1 = **Mild-to-moderate dysarthria;** patient slurs at least some words and, at worst, can be understood with some difficulty. 2 = **Severe dysarthria;** patient's speech is so slurred as to be unintelligible in the absence of or out of proportion to any dysphasia, or is mute/anarthric. UN = **Intubated** or other physical barrier, explain:	
11. Extinction and Inattention (formerly Neglect): Sufficient information to identify neglect may be obtained during the prior testing. If the patient has a severe visual loss preventing visual double simultaneous stimulation, and the cutaneous stimuli are normal, the score is normal. If the patient has aphasia but does appear to attend to both sides, the score is normal. The presence of visual spatial neglect or anosagnosia may also be taken as evidence of abnormality. Since the abnormality is scored only if present, the item is never untestable.	0 = **No abnormality.** 1 = **Visual, tactile, auditory, spatial, or personal inattention** or extinction to bilateral simultaneous stimulation in one of the sensory modalities. 2 = **Profound hemi-inattention or extinction to more than one modality;** does not recognize own hand or orients to only one side of space.	

Source: Adapted from www.strokecenter.org.

TABLE 2 (*Continued*)

B. The Glasgow Coma Scale

Activity	Score
EYE OPENING	
None	1 = Even to supra-orbital pressure
To pain	2 = Pain from sternum/limb/supra-orbital pressure
To speech	3 = Non-specific response, not necessarily to command
Spontaneous	4 = Eyes open, not necessarily aware ____
MOTOR RESPONSE	
None	1 = To any pain; limbs remain flaccid
Extension	2 = Shoulder adducted and shoulder and forearm internally rotated
Flexor response	3 = Withdrawal response or assumption of hemiplegic posture
Withdrawal	4 = Arm withdraws to pain, shoulder abducts
Localizes pain	5 = Arm attempts to remove supra-orbital/chest pressure
Obeys commands	6 = Follows simple commands ____
VERBAL RESPONSE	
None	1 = No verbalization of any type
Incomprehensible	2 = Moans/groans, no speech
Inappropriate	3 = Intelligible, no sustained sentences
Confused	4 = Converses but confused, disoriented
Oriented	5 = Converses and oriented ____
	TOTAL (3–15): ____

Source: Adapted from Ref. (48).

(*Continued*)

TABLE 2 Frequently Used Scales to Assess Neurological Status and Clinical Outcome in Patients with Stroke (*Continued*)

C. Modified Rankin Scale (mRs)

Score

0	**No symptoms** at all
1	**No significant disability** despite symptoms; able to carry out all usual duties and activities
2	**Slight disability**: unable to carry out all previous activities, but able to look after own affairs without assistance
3	**Moderate disability**; requiring some help, but able to walk without assistance
4	**Moderately severe disability**; unable to walk without assistance and unable to attend to own bodily needs without assistance
5	**Severe disability**; bedridden, incontinent and requiring constant nursing care and attention
6	**Dead**

Source: Adapted from Refs. 49–51.

D. Barthel Index

Activity	Score
FEEDING	
0 = unable	
5 = needs help cutting, spreading butter, etc., or requires modified diet	
10 = independent	_____
BATHING	
0 = dependent	
5 = independent (or in shower)	_____
GROOMING	
0 = needs to help with personal care	
5 = independent face/hair/teeth/shaving (implements provided)	_____
DRESSING	
0 = dependent	
5 = needs help but can do about half unaided	
10 = independent (including buttons, zips, laces, etc.)	_____

TABLE 2 (*Continued*)

Activity	Score
BOWELS	
0 = incontinent (or needs to be given enemas)	
5 = occasional accident	
10 = continent	___
BLADDER	
0 = incontinent, or catheterized and unable to manage alone	
5 = occasional accident	
10 = continent	___
TOILET USE	
0 = dependent	
5 = needs some help, but can do something alone	
10 = independent (on and off, dressing, wiping)	___
TRANSFERS (BED TO CHAIR AND BACK)	
0 = unable, no sitting balance	
5 = major help (one or two people, physical), can sit	
10 = minor help (verbal or physical)	
15 = independent	___
MOBILITY (ON LEVEL SURFACES)	
0 = immobile or < 50 yards	
5 = wheelchair independent, including corners, > 50 yards	
10 = walks with help of one person (verbal or physical) > 50 yards	
15 = independent (but may use any aid; for example, stick) > 50 yards	___
STAIRS	
0 = unable	
5 = needs help (verbal, physical, carrying aid)	
10 = independent	
TOTAL (0–100):	___

Source: Adapted from Refs. (52–55).

Glasgow Coma Scale, and the National Institutes of Health Stroke Scale (NIHHS). Median NIHSS was 14 in the group given t-PA and 15 in the one given placebo. There was a significant difference in outcome in all four scales at 3 months in the t-PA group compared with the placebo group. In the t-PA group 39% of patients were left with minimal or no disability compared with 26% of the placebo group. There was no significant difference in mortality; however, there was a significant difference in the rate of ICH: 6.4% in the t-PA group (Fig. 5) versus 0.6% in the placebo group (Table 2). Data taken from the 275 patients of the placebo arm showed that 79% had moderate to severe disability or death. The authors found that an NIHSS ≥ 17 at stroke onset leads to a positive predictive value of 85% for poor outcome (100% confidence interval) and an NIHSS ≥ 22 at 24 h leads to a positive predictive value of

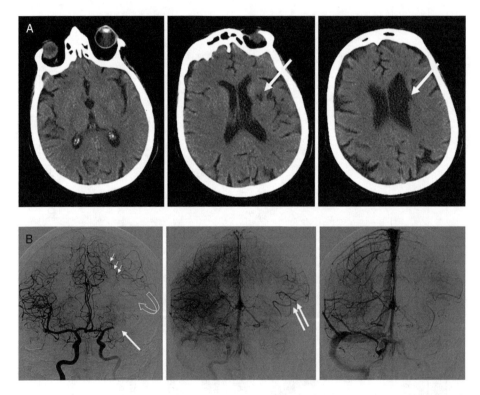

FIGURE 5 Seventy-three-year-old male with previous history of ischemic stroke suddenly develops a right-sided weakness and a global aphasia and is admitted to the emergency department 1 h after symptom onset. The NIH-Stroke Scale (NIHSS) at admission is 21. (*A*) Axial CT scans show no hemorrhage or larger areas of hypodensity or brain swelling. An old infarction within the left pyramidal tract is seen (*arrows*). As no contraindications are present, intravenous t-PA is given 2 h after symptom onset. No improvement of patient's neurological status is documented. Thus, 4 h after symptom onset a catheter angiography is acquired with potential endovascular thrombectomy. (*B*) Angiogram of the right internal carotid artery (ICA) shows a left middle cerebral artery (MCA) occlusion (*arrow*) involving a part of thalamo-perforators and a large hypoperfused MCA territory (*curved arrow*). Poor and slow collateral circulation through pial-pial anastomoses at the watershed area (*small arrows*) supplied through left anterior cerebral artery. Delayed contrast transit time and venous return in the left hemisphere.

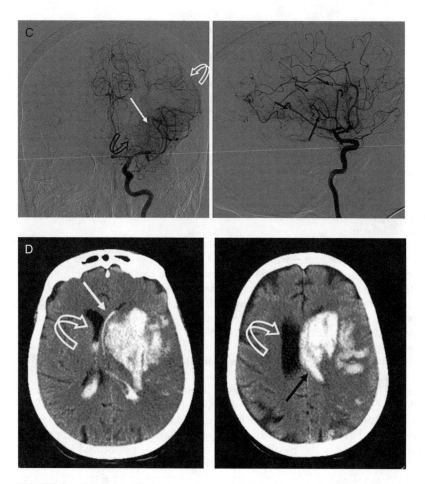

FIGURE 5 (*Continued*) (*C*) Angiogram of the left ICA a few minutes later shows recanalization of proximal left MCA with hyperperfusion of the deep basal ganglia and the insular-opercular area. Arteriovenous shunts with early cortical and deep venous drainage are seen (*curved arrows, left figure*). Truncation of distal MCA branches due to clot fracture and embolism (*small arrow, right plate*). (*D*) Follow-up axial CT scans 24 h after admission show a large intracerebral hematoma within the left pyramidal tract and the insular-opercular area. Compression and tamponade of the left lateral ventricle (*arrow*) and occlusive hydrocephalus of the contralateral ventricle (*curved arrow*).

98% for poor outcome (29). The NINDS t-PA stroke trial also gave important information on the natural history of acute stroke.

Data from the NINDS t-PA stroke trial were replicated by other well-designed studies. As a result of these trials, the use of IV t-PA for the treatment of acute ischemic stroke within 3 h after symptom onset was approved in the United States, Canada, Australia, and the European Union. However, there are several disadvantages with the use of IV t-PA. Data from the NIH in the United States estimates that IV t-PA is only used in 1%–2% of acute stroke patients presenting to the Emergency Room (30), although in specialized stroke centers the number can increase to 4.1% (31). Time and strict inclusion criteria seem to play primary roles in excluding patients for IV fibrinolytic treatment. Other important exclusion criteria are recent surgery and trauma. In addition to the NINDS exclusion criteria, some patients do not respond to treatment, and 12% will have reocclusion after initial reperfusion (32).

With regard to nonresponders, it has been noted that an internal carotid artery (ICA) occlusion may not reperfuse after 0.9 mg/kg of IV t-PA (33). In a retrospective analysis, the authors identified 36 consecutive patients who were treated with a standard IV t-PA protocol within 3 h after symptom onset of a stroke in the distribution of a documented ICA or middle cerebral artery (MCA) occlusion (33). Outcomes were assessed using the NIHSS and mRS. MRA or CTA was obtained before and after IV t-PA to evaluate recanalization. Although there was no difference in age and baseline NIHSS between the two groups, the MCA group had a lower day 3 NIHSS score compared with the ICA group. Similarly, the day 3 NIHSS was significantly lower in patients who had recanalization, regardless of the arterial occlusion.

Because of these limitations, IA thrombolysis has been considered as a possible treatment option for acute stroke patients (34,35). The endovascular approach presents several advantages, compared with standard IV treatment: (i) high intraclot concentration of the fibrinolytic agent; (ii) immediate assessment of arterial recanalization; (iii) treatment of severe strokes such as large artery occlusions and/or patients with contraindications for IV t-PA; and (iv) rapid evolution in design of new devices and fibrinolytic agents. Nevertheless, IA thrombolysis also has disadvantages, such as invasiveness, the time required to access the occluded vessel, and the need for a full-time interventional neuroradiology team, presently available mostly in secondary or tertiary medical centers.

Currently, several tools are available to achieve reperfusion; these include stents, balloons (Fig. 6), snares, and clot retrievers (see also Part 2, Chapter 7 for details). Pharmacological agents such as t-PA, urokinase, third-generation plasminogen activator, and glycoprotein IIb-IIIa antagonists have also been tested (35–39). We will summarize briefly the results of some clinical trials performed to address the safety and efficacy of the IA approach, such as the Prolyse in Acute Cerebral Thromboembolism (PROACT II), Emergency Management of Stroke (EMS), Interventional Management of Stroke (IMS), and Mechanical Embolus Removal in Cerebral Ischemia (MERCI) trials (Table 2).

PROACT II (Prolyse in Acute Cerebral Thromboembolism)

The safety and efficacy of using IA Prourokinase (Pro-UK) for the treatment of acute ischemic stroke was addressed by PROACT II (40), a randomized, placebo-controlled study with blinded follow-up. The trial enrolled 180 patients (121 treated and 59 controls) with MCA occlusions treated within 6 h after the symptom onset. The imaging study used to evaluate the patient was a noncontrast CT. The median baseline NIHSS was 17. Outcomes were neurological disability at 3 months; secondary outcomes were ICH and mortality. The authors reported that 40% of patients achieved favorable outcome (mRS ≤ 2) versus 25% in controls. The percentage of patients with reperfused occluded MCA was higher in treated patients (66% vs. 13%). With regard to safety, there was no difference in mortality (25%, treated group; 27%, placebo group). There was a statistically significant difference in symptomatic ICH: 10% in the Pro-UK arm versus 2% of patients treated with placebo. Based on these data, Pro-UK was not approved by the Federal and Drug

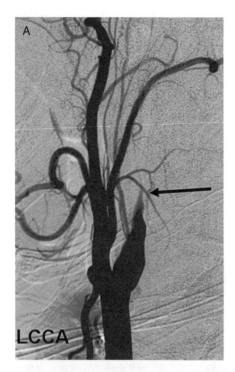

FIGURE 6 Thromboembolic occlusion of the left middle cerebral artery (MCA) bifurcation in a 40-year-old female presenting with aphasia and right-sided hemiparesis. She had an unremarkable CT at the time of admission; initial improvement on IV treatment was followed by worsening of symptoms. (*A*) Left common carotid angiogram shows a dissection with subsequent occlusion of the left internal carotid artery (*arrow*).

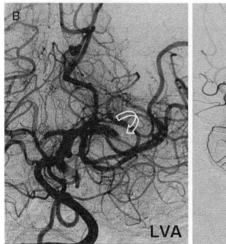
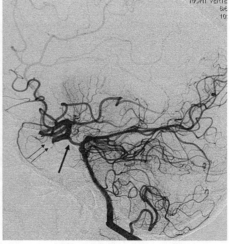

FIGURE 6 (*Continued*) (*B*) Angiogram of the left vertebral artery in frontal and lateral view shows filling of the anterior circulation through a large posterior communicating artery (*arrow*) and a thromboembolic occlusion of the MCA bifurcation (*curved arrow*) with poor filling of the left hemisphere. Retrograde and partial filling of the left ICA (*double arrow*).

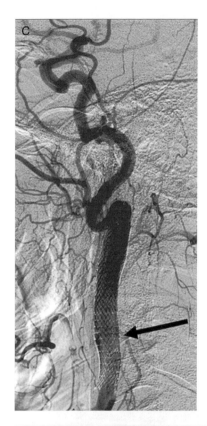

FIGURE 6 (*Continued*) (*C*) Stenting of the left internal carotid artery dissection with complete revascularization and reconstituted antegrade flow.

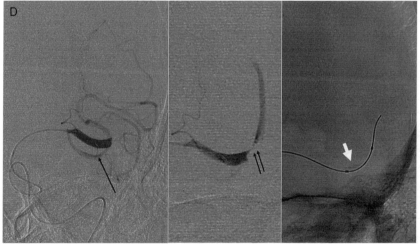

FIGURE 6 (*Continued*) (*D*) Selective catheterization of the left distal superior division of the MCA for intra-arterial delivery of t-PA (black arrow highlights the tip of the microcatheter, *left panel*). Continued clot formation in the turn of the superior division as it follows the Sylvian fissure (*double arrow*) and balloon angioplasty of the clot formation (*white arrow*).

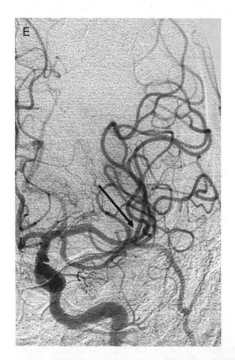

FIGURE 6 (*Continued*) (*E*) Immediate recanalization of the entire left distal middle cerebral artery with TIMI 3 flow. The patient improved neurologically within a few hours and had an NIH Stroke Scale score of less than 5. At 30 days office visit, the patient had no neurological deficit.

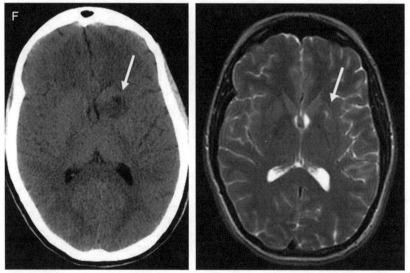

FIGURE 6 (*Continued*) (*F*) CT without contrast three days after stroke onset and treatment shows a small area of hypodensity in the anterior limb of the internal capsule with extension into the caudate, pallidum and putamen (*arrow, left panel*). Three-month follow-up T2W-MRI shows a residual hyperintensity in the anterior part of the putamen (*right panel*).

Administration (FDA) for use in the treatment of acute ischemic stroke. However, several large case series showed safety and efficacy data similar to that of currently used IA fibrinolytic agents such as UK and t-PA. Therefore, the American Stroke Association guidelines recognize IA fibrinolysis as a treatment option in selected patients.

EMS (Emergency Management of Stroke)

Because the NINDS t-PA stroke trial showed that early treatment is a predictor of good outcome, one of the criticisms of PROACT II was the time delay required to obtain angiography and to place the microcatheter in the occluded artery. Also, it has been observed that the administration of t-PA directly at the site of occlusion may increase the intraclot concentration of the agent, increasing the chance of successful thrombolysis. The safety and efficacy of combining IV and IA fibrinolysis was tested by the EMS bridging trial (41).

The EMS was a randomized, double-blind, placebo-controlled multicenter Phase I study of IV t-PA or placebo followed by immediate cerebral angiography and IA t-PA. Outcome was assessed by improvement on the NIHSS, Barthel Index, mRS, and the Glasgow Outcome Scale at 3 months post-stroke. Thirty-five patients were assigned randomly, 17 into the IV/IA group and 18 into the placebo/IA group. There was no difference in the 7- to 10-day or the 3-month outcomes, although there were more deaths in the IV/IA group. Recanalization was higher ($p < 0.03$) in the IV/IA group with thrombolysis in myocardial infarction (TIMI) 3 in 54% of the IV/IA patients versus 10% of the placebo/IA and correlated to the total dose of t-PA ($p < 0.05$) used. With regard to safety, there were eight ICH, but the number of symptomatic ICH was similar between the two groups.

IMS (Interventional Management of Stroke)

The IMS was a 17-center, open-label, single-arm, pilot study on the feasibility and safety of the combined use of IV and IA t-PA (42). Outcomes were compared with historical controls from the NINDS t-PA placebo group comparable for age and baseline NIHSS. Of 1477 patients screened, 80 acute stroke patients with a baseline NIHSS ≥ 10 were enrolled to receive IV t-PA (0.6 mg/kg) within 3 h after symptom onset. After IV t-PA, the patients had a cerebral angiogram. If the angiogram was suggestive of the presence of a stenosis secondary to a blood clot, a microcatheter was advanced to the site of occlusion. IA t-PA was then administered as 2-ml bolus until a total dose of 22 mg over 2 h of infusion or until thrombolysis was achieved. Sixty-two patients received combined IV/IA t-PA; the median baseline NIHSS score was 18. The median time to initiation of IV t-PA was 140 min, compared with 108 min for placebo and 90 min for the t-PA-treated arm of the NINDS t-PA trial. The 3-month mortality for the IMS study was not statistically different from that of the placebo group (24%) in the NINDS t-PA stroke trial. The rate of symptomatic ICH (6.3%) in the IMS subjects was similar to that in t-PA-treated patients (6.6%), but higher than the placebo group (1%) in the NINDS t-PA stroke trial. In the 62 subjects who received IA t-PA in addition to IV t-PA, complete recanalization (TIMI 3) occurred in 11% (7/62) and partial or complete recanalization (TIMI 2 or 3) in 56% (35/62) after a maximum of 2 h of infusion. Of the patients who achieved TIMI 2 or 3 flow, 34% had a favorable outcome (mRS of 0–1 at 3 months), as compared with 12% of those patients who achieved only TIMI 0 or 1 flow ($p < 0.013$). The observation that early treatment is a strong predictor of good outcome was also confirmed in the IMS study (42). Of those subjects who received IA t-PA within 3 h after symptom onset, 43% (7/16) had mRS of 0–1 at 3 months, as compared with 13% (3/24) of subjects who received IA t-PA within 3–4 h and 27% (6/22) of those who received IA t-PA after 4 h. Compared with the placebo-treated patients in the NINDS t-PA stroke trial, the patients in the IMS study had a significantly better outcome at 3 months for all outcome measures (odds ratios ≥ 2) when adjusted for age and NIHSS score ≥10 (42).

The primary goal of the IMS II study was to investigate the feasibility and safety of combining reduced-dose t-PA IV therapy with additional IA delivery of t-PA at the site of an arterial blockage in ischemic stroke patients within 3 h of onset (43). The IA t-PA was administered using the EKOS Micro-Infusion Catheter (see for details Part 2, Chapter 7). Patients ages 18 to 80 with a baseline NIHSS ≥ 10 (median baseline 19) were enrolled at one of 13 participating clinical centers from December 2003 through April 2005 (Table 2). IV t-PA was started at 0.6 mg/kg, infused over 30 min with 15% as bolus. Patients then underwent a diagnostic catheter angiography. If no thrombus or arterial occlusive lesions were identified, treatment was stopped. If a thrombus was identified, patients eligible for the EKOS catheter received a 2-mg hand bolus of drug administered into the proximal portion of the thrombus, and an infusion was begun at 10 mg/h for 2 h of treatment until the clot resolved. A maximal dose of 22 mg was administered. The mean age of the 81 patients enrolled in the trial was 64 years. Mean baseline NIHSS score was 19. Of the 81 patients, 26 received IV treatment only. Fifty-five patients received IV and IA treatment, 36 in conjunction with the EKOS microcatheter and 19 with a standard microcatheter. Three patients were treated with the EKOS system without ultrasound activation. The primary end point showed more complete recanalization at 60 min (60%; 33/55) with the EKOS ultrasound microcatheter (TIMI 2 and 3 grade reperfusion) as compared to subjects in the IMS I trial (56%; 35/62). Twelve patients (16.4%) died; symptomatic hemorrhages were greater in the IMS II trial (9.9%) as compared to IMS I (6.3%) and the NINDS t-PA trials (6.6%). Asymptomatic intracerebral hemorrhage less than 36 h from onset occurred in 32.1% of patients. Using the modified Rankin scale score of 0–2, 46% of patients in IMS II had good outcomes at 3 months, compared with 43% in IMS I, 39% in the NINDS t-PA stroke trial, and 28% in the NINDS placebo study. After adjustment for differences in baseline stroke severity, age, and time-to-treatment, the IMS II patients were 65% more likely to attain functional independence at 3 months, compared with patients treated with only IV t-PA in the NINDS t-PA stroke trial.

The currently in-progress IMS III trial is a randomized, open-label multicenter study that compares a combined IV and IA treatment approach to restoring blood flow to the brain to the current standard FDA-approved treatment approach of giving IV t-PA alteplase, alone. The treatment is initiated within 3 h of stroke onset. A projected 900 subjects with moderate to severe ischemic stroke (a baseline NIH Stroke Scale Score ≥ 10) and who are ages 18–80 are being enrolled at more than 40 centers in the United States and Canada. The IV t-PA group receives the full standard dose (0.9 mg/kg, 90 mg maximal (10% as bolus)) of t-PA intravenously over an hour. The combined IV/IA group receives a lower dose of t-PA (~0.6 mg/kg, 60 mg maximal) over 40 min followed by an immediate angiography. IA approach includes the use of the Concentric MERCI clot retriever, the EKOS catheter (see for details Part 2, Chapter 7), and the standard microcatheter combined with additional IA t-PA, depending on the lesion, experience, and training of the investigators.

A maximum dose of 22 mg of t-PA is administered intra-arterially, and IA treatment has to begin within 5 h and be completed within 7 h of stroke onset. A favorable clinical outcome is defined as a modified Rankin Score (mRS) of 0–2 at 3 months. Primary safety measures are mortality at 3 months and symptomatic ICH within the first 36 h after onset.

MERCI (Mechanical Embolus Removal in Cerebral Ischemia)

Several devices for mechanical thrombolysis—such as snares, laser devices positioned on a microcatheter, and angiojets—have been used in the attempt to recanalize an occluded vessel (36,44,45) (see also Part 2, Chapter 7). So far, only the MERCI retriever (Concentric Medical, Inc. Mountain View, CA) has been approved by the FDA for use in the treatment of ischemic stroke (44). The MERCI retriever was developed initially to capture foreign bodies (such as detachable coils or others) that accidentally embolize distally during endovascular procedures. The MERCI retriever X5 and X6 was approved by the FDA based on the results of the MERCI trial, a 25-center, noncontrolled, technical efficacy study (44). Acute stroke patients with exclusion criteria for IV t-PA up to 8 h after symptom onset were enrolled. During a period of 2.5 years 1800 patients were screened, 151 were enrolled, and 141 were treated with the device. The median age was 72 years, mean baseline NIHSS was 20, and median time from symptom onset to groin puncture was 4.3 h.

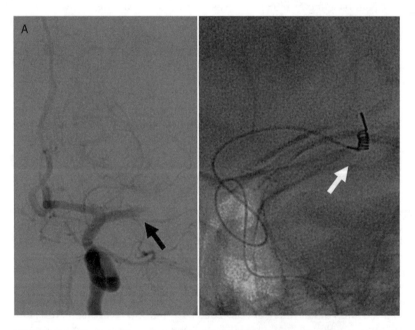

FIGURE 7 A 56-year-old woman with sudden onset of right hemiparesis and speech arrest arrived to the ER 2 h and 45 min after symptom onset. The patient was on aspirin 325 mg once a day for stroke prophylaxis. On examination, the patient had right hemiparesis (arm > leg > face), head and eyes deviation towards the left, and global aphasia. (*A*) Angiogram in the frontal projection showed occlusion of the distal segment of the left M1 (*black arrow*). The MERCI retriever is deployed in the M2 (superior division, white arrow).

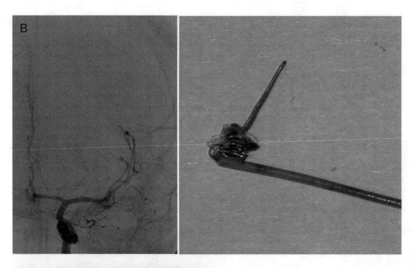

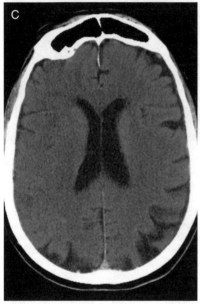

FIGURE 7 (*Continued*) (*B*) Successful recanalization of the occluded MCA is achieved (*left panel*). Multiple opercular MCA branches are occluded because of vasospasm and clot fragments. Photograph of the clot removed from the MCA with the retriever (*right panel*). (See also color plate section.) (*C*) CT post procedure shows a very small insular stroke. The patient recovered completely, without neurological deficit.

Primary outcome was recanalization, which was achieved in 48% of patients in whom the device was deployed (Fig. 7). Clinically significant procedural complications occurred in 10 of 141 patients (7.1%). Symptomatic ICH occurred in 7.8% (Fig. 8), most likely to arterial wall rupture. Disability-free outcome (i.e., mRS ≤ 2 at 90 days) was more frequent in patients who had recanalization, compared with those who did not (46% vs. 10%); however, only 22.6% of all patients had a mRS ≤ 2 at 90 days. Mortality was 43.5%, higher in patients who did not have recanalization (54.2%) versus patients who did (31.8%). More recent data from the Multi MERCI Trial presented at the International Stroke Conference (46) and using the modified

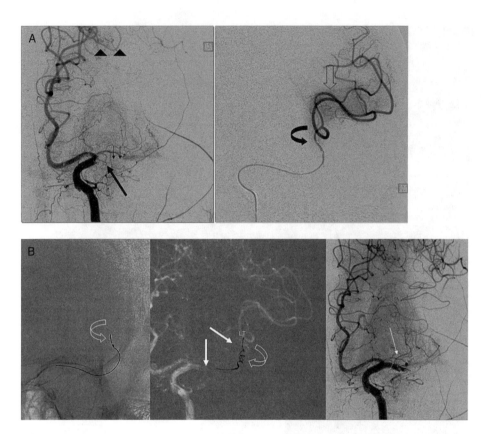

FIGURE 8 Eighty-four-year old female with recent history of a myocardial ischemia and arterial fibrillation. Three days after undergoing a coronary bypass surgery, the patient was found in the critical care unit nonresponsive, aphasic and hemiplegic. The initial CT of the brain was unremarkable; intravenous t-PA was contraindicated because of the recent history of surgery. (A) A catheter angiography of the left internal carotid artery 2 h after symptom onset shows an occluded left middle cerebral artery (MCA) (*arrow*) with involvement of lenticulostriate arteries supplying the basal ganglia (*small arrows*) and poor collateral blood supply to the left hemisphere through left anterior cerebral artery (*arrowheads*). A microcatheter is passed through the clot into the anterior division of MCA (*curved arrow*). Microcatheter angiogram shows patency of distal MCA branches and significant capillary blush of the operculum (*block arrow*). (B) The MERCI clot retriever is threaded through the microcatheter (*curved arrow*), and the clot is removed using dual-roadmap (simultaneous contrast injection through the guidecatheter and the microcatheter) to delineate the extension of vessel occlusion (*arrows*). Multiple passes are made, and partial revascularization of MCA-M1 segment and lenticulostriate arteries (*arrow*) is accomplished.

MERCI clot retriever L5 were more promising. Overall recanalization rate in 164 patients enrolled was 54.9% with the device alone and 68.3% with use of adjuvant therapy (prior use of IV t-PA and adjuvant IA t-PA was allowed). In the subgroup of 131 patients treated with the L5 device, the device recanalization was 57.3%, and the final recanalization with the use of adjuvant therapy was 69.5%. The baseline NIHSS was 19.3 ± 6.4. The site of occlusion was ICA/ICA-T in $n = 52$ patients, MCA in $n = 98$ patients, and vertebro-basilar artery in $n = 14$ patients. Favorable outcome

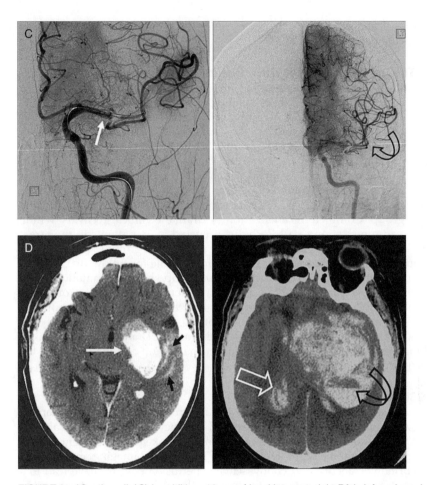

FIGURE 8 (*Continued*) (*C*) In addition, 10 mg of local intra-arterial t-PA is infused proximal to the occlusion site (*arrow*). Recanalization of entire M1 with some parts of clot left in both upper and lower MCA divisions. Slow and delayed antegrade filling of the left hemisphere (*curved arrow*). The patient deteriorates during the intervention and requires intubation. (*D*) CT following the procedure shows a large left basal ganglion bleed (*arrow*) and a subarachnoid hemorrhage (*small arrows*) mixed with contrast material most likely resulting from vessel rupture following clot retrieval. Follow-up CT 2 h later shows a massive left-hemispheric hematoma with separation of plasma and blood cellular components (*curved arrow*) due to inhibition of coagulation resulting from fibrinolysis. Note tamponade of ventricles (*block arrow*), midline shift, and brain herniation.

at 90 days was seen in 36% (mRS ≤ 2); mortality at 90 days was 34%. In the subgroup of 131 patients treated with L5 system, the favorable outcome was 37% while the mortality of 34% remained the same.

Early recanalization, with reperfusion and restoration of blood flow is the main goal of ischemic stroke treatment. However, recanalization is not yet a fully validated surrogate marker for good outcome. Therefore, even though the MERCI retriever can achieve high rates of recanalization, controlled trials on safety and efficacy are needed to assess whether the use of the device leads to better outcomes.

Several phase I and II trials using newer reperfusion devices and thrombolytic agents are being developed (36,45,47).

CLOTBUST (Combined Lysis of Thrombus in Brain Ischemia using Transcranial Ultrasound and systemic t-PA)

It has been hypothesized that TCD ultrasonography may help expose thrombi to t-PA as tested by the investigators in combined lysis of thrombus in brain ischemia using transcranial ultrasound and systemic t-PA (CLOTBUST) (18), a phase 2, multicenter, randomized clinical trial. Patients who had acute ischemic stroke due to occlusion of the MCA were treated with IV t-PA within 3 h after the onset of symptoms. The patients were assigned randomly to receive continuous 2-MHz TCD ultrasonography (63 patients) or placebo (63 patients). Symptomatic intracerebral hemorrhage occurred in three patients in the target group and in three in the control group. Complete recanalization or dramatic clinical recovery within 2 h after the administration of a t-PA bolus occurred in 31 patients in the target group (49%), as compared with 19 patients in the control group (30%; $p = 0.03$). Twenty-four hours after treatment of the patients eligible for follow-up, 24 (44%) in the target group and 21 (40%) in the control group showed dramatic clinical recovery ($p = 0.7$). At 3 months, 22 of 53 (42%) patients in the target group who were eligible for follow-up analysis and 14 of 49 (29%) in the control group had favorable outcomes (as indicated by a score of 0–1 on the mRS) ($p = 0.20$). The authors concluded that the association of continuous TCD and standard IV t-PA protocol may enhance t-PA-induced arterial recanalization and may increase the rate of recovery from acute MCA occlusions.

CONCLUSION

The historical perspective on the treatment of acute stroke has dramatically changed over the last decade and will continue to expand with new neuroendovascular technologies. After decades of conservative care for acute stroke patients, recent revolutions in stroke imaging, including DWI, PWI, CTA and CTP imaging, introduction of newer fibrinolytic agents, and endovascular reperfusion devices, have lead to a paradigm shift. Early recanalization is the main goal of ischemic stroke treatment to address the salvageable penumbra. However, recanalization per se is not yet a fully validated surrogate marker for good outcome. Neuroprotective agents will play a vital role to not only extend the time window for treatment but also stabilize impaired vascular wall integrity and prevent hemorrhagic transformation of the ischemic area.

REFERENCES

1. Heart Disease and Stroke Statistics—2005 Update. http://www.americanheart.org/presenter.jhtml?identifier=3000090 (accessed October 4, 2005).
2. Nilasena DS, Kresowik TF, Wiblin RT, et al. Assessing patterns of TPA use in acute stroke. Program and abstracts of the 27th International Stroke Conference; Feb 7–9, 2002; San Antonio, TX. Abstract 68.
3. Katzan IL, Furlan AJ, Lloyd LE, et al. Use of tissue-type plasminogen activator for acute ischemic stroke: the Cleveland area experience. JAMA 2000; 283(9):1151–1158.
4. Sacco RL, Wolf PA, Kannel WB, et al. Survival and recurrence following stroke. The Framingham Study. Stroke 1982; 13(3):290–295.
5. Sacco RL, Shi T, Zamanillo MC, et al. Predictors of mortality and recurrence after hospitalized cerebral infarction in an urban community: the Northern Manhattan Stroke Study. Neurology 1994; 44(4):626–634.

6. Petty GW, Brown RD Jr., Whisnant JP, et al. Survival and recurrence after first cerebral infarction: a population-based study in Rochester, Minnesota, 1975 through 1989. Neurology 1998; 50(1):208–211.
7. Stapf C, Mohr JP. Ischemic stroke therapy. Annu Rev Med 2002; 53:453–475.
8. Baird AE, Warach S. Magnetic resonance imaging of acute stroke. J Cereb Blood Flow Metab 1998; 18(6):583–609.
9. Kidwell CS, Alger JR, Saver JL. Beyond mismatch: evolving paradigms in imaging the ischemic penumbra with multimodal MRI. Stroke 2003; 34(11):2729–2735.
10. Sunshine JL, Tarr RW, Lanzieri CF, et al. Hyperacute stroke: ultrafast MR imaging to triage patients before therapy. Radiology 1999; 212(2):325–332.
11. Shih LC, Saver JL, Alger JR, et al. Perfusion-weighted magnetic resonance imaging thresholds identifying core, irreversibly infarcted tissue. Stroke 2003; 34(6):1425–1430.
12. Schellinger PD, Fiebach JB, Jansen O, et al. Stroke magnetic resonance imaging within 6 hours after onset of hyperacute cerebral ischemia. Ann Neurol 2001; 49(4):460–469.
13. Linfante I, Llinas RH, Caplan LR, et al. MRI features of intracerebral hemorrhage within 2 hours from symptom onset. Stroke 1999; 30(11):2263–2267.
14. Linfante I. Can MRI reliably detect hyperacute intracerebral hemorrhage? Ask the medical student. Stroke 2004; 35(2):506–507.
15. Sims JR, Rordorf G, Smith EE, et al. Arterial occlusion revealed by CT angiography predicts NIH stroke score and acute outcomes after IV t-PA treatment. AJNR Am J Neuroradiol 2005; 26(2):246–251.
16. Ezzeddine MA, Lev MH, McDonald CT, et al. CT angiography with whole brain perfused blood volume imaging: added clinical value in the assessment of acute stroke. Stroke 2002; 33(4):959–966.
17. Eastwood JD, Lev MH, Wintermark M, et al. Correlation of early dynamic CT perfusion imaging with whole-brain MR diffusion and perfusion imaging in acute hemispheric stroke. AJNR Am J Neuroradiol 2003; 24(9):1869–1875.
18. Alexandrov AV, Molina CA, Grotta JC, et al,. for the CLOTBUST Investigators. Ultrasound-enhanced systemic thrombolysis for acute ischemic stroke. N Engl J Med 2004; 351(21):2170–2178.
19. Le Bihan D, Breton E, Lallemand D, et al. MR imaging of intravoxel incoherent motions: application to diffusion and perfusion in neurologic disorders. Radiology 1986; 161(2):401–407.
20. Warach S, Chien D, Li W, et al. Fast magnetic resonance diffusion-weighted imaging of acute human stroke. Neurology 1992; 42(9):1717–1723.
21. Edelman RR, Johnson K, Buxton R, et al. MR of hemorrhage: a new approach. AJNR Am J Neuroradiol 1986; 7(5):751–756.
22. Fiebach JB, Schellinger PD, Gass A, et al. Stroke magnetic resonance imaging is accurate in hyperacute intracerebral hemorrhage: a multicenter study on the validity of stroke imaging. Stroke 2004; 35(2):502–506.
23. Kidwell CS, Chalela JA, Saver JL, et al. Comparison of MRI and CT for detection of acute intracerebral hemorrhage. JAMA 2004; 292(15):1823–1830.
24. Perazella MA. Nephrogenic systemic fibrosis, kidney disease, and gadolinium: is there a link? Clin J Am Soc Nephrol 2007; 2(2):200–202.
25. Sadowski EA, Bennett LK, Chan MR, et al. Nephrogenic systemic fibrosis: risk factors and incidence estimation. Radiology 2007; 243(1):148–157.
26. Johnston DC Chapman KM, Goldstein LB. Low rate of complications of cerebral angiography in routine clinical practice. Neurology 2001; 57(11):2012–2014.
27. Krings T, Willmes K, Becker R, et al. Silent microemboli related to diagnostic cerebral angiography: a matter of operator's experience and patient's disease. Neuroradiology 2006; 48(6):387–393.
28. The National Institute of Neurological Disorders and Stroke t-PA Stroke Study Group. Tissue plasminogen activator for acute ischemic stroke. N Engl J Med 1995; 333(24):1581–1587.
29. Frankel MR, Morgenstern LB, Kwiatkowski T, et al. Predicting prognosis after stroke: a placebo group analysis from the National Institute of Neurological Disorders and Stroke t-PA Stroke Trial. Neurology 2000; 55(7):952–959.

30. Reed SD, Cramer SC, Blough DK, et al. Treatment with tissue plasminogen activator and inpatient mortality rates for patients with ischemic stroke treated in community hospitals. Stroke 2001; 32(8):1832–1840.

31. Johnston SC, Fung LH, Gillum LA, et al. Utilization of intravenous tissue-type plasminogen activator for ischemic stroke at academic medical centers: the influence of ethnicity. Stroke 2001; 32(5):1061–1068.

32. Rubiera M, Alvarez-Sabin J, Ribo M, et al. Predictors of early arterial reocclusion after tissue plasminogen activator-induced recanalization in acute ischemic stroke. Stroke 2005; 36(7):1452–1456.

33. Linfante I, Llinas RH, Selim M, et al. Clinical and vascular outcome in ICA versus MCA occlusions after IV t-PA. Stroke 2002; 33(8):2066–2071.

34. Gonner F, Remonda L, Mattle H, et al. Local intra-arterial thrombolysis in acute ischemic stroke. Stroke 1998; 29(9):1894–1900.

35. Qureshi AI. Endovascular treatment of cerebrovascular diseases and intracranial neoplasms. Lancet 2004; 363(9411):804–813.

36. Molina CA, Saver JL. Extending reperfusion therapy for acute ischemic stroke: emerging pharmacological, mechanical, and imaging strategies. Stroke 2005; 36(10):2311–2320.

37. Qureshi AI, Siddiqui AM, Suri MF, et al. Aggressive mechanical clot disruption and low-dose intra-arterial third-generation thrombolytic agent for ischemic stroke: a prospective study. Neurosurgery 2002; 51(5):1319–1327.

38. Qureshi AI, Ali Z, Suri MF, et al. Intra-arterial third-generation recombinant tissue plasminogen activator (reteplase) for acute ischemic stroke. Neurosurgery 2001; 49(1):41–48.

39. Deshmukh VR, Fiorella DJ, Albuquerque FC, et al. Intra-arterial thrombolysis for acute ischemic stroke: preliminary experience with platelet glycoprotein IIb/IIIa inhibitors as adjunctive therapy. Neurosurgery 2005; 56(1):46–54.

40. Furlan AJ, Higashida RT, Wechsler L, et al. Intra-arterial prourokinase for acute ischemic stroke. The PROACT study: a randomized controlled trial. JAMA 1999; 282(21):2003–2011.

41. Lewandowski CA, Frankel M, Tomsick TA, et al. Combined intravenous and intra-arterial t-PA versus intra-arterial therapy of acute ischemic stroke: Emergency Management of Stroke (EMS) Bridging Trial. Stroke 1999; 30(12):2598–2605.

42. IMS Study Investigators. Combined intravenous and intra-arterial recanalization for acute ischemic stroke: the Interventional Management of Stroke Study. Stroke 2004; 35(4):904–911.

43. The IMS II Trial Investigators. The Interventional Management of Stroke (IMS) II Study. Stroke 2007; 38(7):2127–2135.

44. Smith WS, Sung G, Starkman S, et al. for the MERCI Trial Investigators. Safety and efficacy of mechanical embolectomy in acute ischemic stroke: results of the MERCI trial. Stroke 2005; 36(7):1432–1438.

45. Berlis A, Lutsep H, Barnwell S, et al. Mechanical thrombolysis in acute ischemic stroke with endovascular photoacoustic recanalization. Stroke 2004; 35(5):1112–1116.

46. Smith WS, Sung G, Saver J, et al. Mechanical thrombectomy for acute ischemic stroke. Final results of the Multi MERCI trial. Stroke 2008; 39(4):1205–1212.

47. Fisher M, for the Stroke Therapy Academic Industry Roundtable. Enhancing the development and approval of acute stroke therapies: Stroke Therapy Academic Industry Roundtable 4. Stroke 2005; 36(8):1808–1813.

48. Teasdale G, Jennett B. Assessment of coma and impaired consciousness. A practical scale. Lancet 1974; 13(7872):81–84.

49. Rankin J. Cerebral vascular accidents in patients over the age of 60. Scott Med J 1957; 2(2):200–215.

50. Bonita R, Beaglehole R. Recovery of motor function after stroke. Stroke 1988; 19(12):1497–1500.

51. Van Swieten JC, Koudstaal PJ, Visser MC, et al. Interobserver agreement for the assessment of handicap in stroke patients. Stroke 1988; 19(5):604–607.

52. Mahoney FI, Barthel D. Functional evaluation: the Barthel Index. Md State Med J 1965; 14:56–61.

53. Loewen SC, Anderson BA. Predictors of stroke outcome using objective measurement scales. Stroke 1990; 21(1):78–81.
54. Gresham GE, Phillips TF, Labi ML. ADL status in stroke: relative merits of three standard indexes. Arch Phys Med Rehabil 1980; 61(8):355–358.
55. Collin C, Wade DT, Davies S, Horne V. The Barthel ADL Index: a reliability study. Int Disability Study 1988; 10(2):61–63.

Index